The International Behavioural and Social Sciences Library

THE SUBCULTURE OF
VIOLENCE

TAVISTOCK

CRIME & DELINQUENCY
In 10 Volumes

THE SUBCULTURE OF VIOLENCE

Towards an Integrated Theory in Criminology

MARVIN E WOLFGANG AND
FRANCO FERRACUTI

First published in 1967 by
Tavistock Publications Limited

Reprinted in 2001 by
Routledge
2 Park Square, Milton Park, Abingdon, Oxon, OX14 4RN
or
270 Madison Avenue, New York, NY 10016

First issued in paperback 2010

Routledge is an imprint of the Taylor & Francis Group

British Library Cataloguing in Publication Data
A CIP catalogue record for this book
is available from the British Library

The Subculture of Violence
ISBN 978-0-415-26410-5 (hbk)
ISBN 978-0-415-60631-8 (pbk)
Crime & Delinquency: 10 Volumes
ISBN 978-0-415-26507-2
The International Behavioural and Social Sciences Library
112 Volumes
ISBN 978-0-415-25670-4

MARVIN E. WOLFGANG

FRANCO FERRACUTI

The Subculture of Violence

Towards an Integrated Theory in Criminology

TAVISTOCK PUBLICATIONS

London · New York · Sydney · Toronto · Wellington

First published in 1967
by Tavistock Publications Limited
2 Park Square, Milton Park, Abingdon,
Oxon, OX14 4RN
in 10 point Monotype Plantin, 2 point leaded
by Richard Clay (The Chaucer Press), Ltd., Bungay, Suffolk
© *Marvin E. Wolfgang and Franco Ferracuti 1967*
Foreword © *Hermann Mannheim 1967*
This work has been published in Italian under the title
Il Comportamento Violento: Moderni Aspetti Criminologici
by Dott. A. Giuffrè Editore, 1966

Distributed in the United States of America
by Barnes & Noble, Inc.

This book is dedicated to
Thorsten Sellin and Benigno Di Tullio

Contents

Foreword

Both on personal grounds and because of my special interest in its subject I am pleased to contribute the foreword to this important book. For several years I have been privileged to count the authors among my personal friends, and from the beginning I have been able to watch the progress of their joint efforts which have eventually led to the publication of the present volume.

As will be clear even to the most casual reader, this work is concerned with two focal problems, the methodological one of *integration* in criminological research and the substantive one of the *subculture of violence*. Which of the two has to be regarded as more important will largely depend on the individual tastes and scientific interests of the reader. Already in their preface the authors have provided a summary of the basic issues involved which could hardly be bettered, and very little has been left to me to add.

Let me first take up the methodological issue of integration. Already for a long time, ideas such as 'cross-cultural' and 'interdisciplinary' research and how to achieve closer cooperation between theory and practice in criminology have had a special attraction, not to say fascination, for me, and in 1957, in a lecture delivered at the First All-Canadian Congress of Corrections in Montreal, I took the opportunity offered to me to deal with some aspects of teamwork, mainly in a correctional setting. More recently, in my *Comparative Criminology* and in an address to the German Criminological Society, I briefly returned to the subject. By force of circumstances, all this had to remain at a rather superficial level. The work of Professors Wolfgang and Ferracuti, however, forces every criminologist to re-think the whole matter afresh. They have gone into it far more thoroughly and deeply than any of their predecessors and made the most determined and sophisticated onslaught on all those comparatively primitive and antiquated concepts with which we had to be content so far in criminological research.

First, what do we really mean by 'integration'? There are many fields in which the concept can be used. We speak of a well-integrated personality or marriage or society. What we have in mind is a person whose various faculties – intellectual, emotional, physical, and so forth – do not function in isolation, each of them regardless of the others or even in opposition to them as in the case of, say, a schizophrenic, but are well coordinated and balanced to form a real unit. And in the case of a marriage partnership we mean the union of two individuals who do not merely operate on more or less parallel lines, coming together only at certain points, notably for sexual and economic purposes, but achieve an ideal relationship in every sector of their lives. Complete integration of this kind can but rarely be found because personality differences and the centrifugal tendencies, the stresses and strains inherent in our surroundings, are too strong. *Mutatis mutandis* the same is true of the problem of integration in society at large. For the extreme case of a figure of world history fighting against almost overwhelming forces to achieve perfect integration and harmony the great Swiss poet Conrad Ferdinand Meyer has described the problem supremely well in a few lines referring to Martin Luther in his poem 'Hutten's Letzte Tage':

> *In seiner Seele kämpft was wird und war,*
> *Ein keuchend hart verschlungen Ringerpaar.*
> *Sein Geist ist zweier Zeiten Schlachtgebiet –*
> *Mich wundert's nicht, dass er Dämonen sieht!*

which might be freely and rather inadequately translated like this:

> *In his soul a war is raging between the past and the present –*
> *A pair of wrestlers closely embraced in deadly combat.*
> *His mind is the battlefield of two epochs –*
> *No wonder then that he should see demons!*

However, such extreme cases apart, even ordinary human beings are faced with the conflict between past and present which each succeeding generation has to face afresh and which causes maladjustment.

While our authors are, of course, not directly concerned with such world-historical perspectives, indirectly their own problems bear at least some affinity with them. Of what kind are the difficulties of scientific integration as seen in their investigation? The answer is provided, first of all, in a general way in the opening chapter, but quite naturally it has to be supplemented and made more specific subsequently in its application to criminological studies (Chapter II). As so often, it proves to be easier to say what integration is *not* than to give an exact and final positive definition of what it is or should be. Certainly, 'multidisciplinary cross-fertilization' is not enough. It is not enough to appoint a research team on which each of the relevant disciplines is represented if each member continues working along his usual lines, making no or inadequate concessions to the others. Even within one single discipline, be it sociology or biology, law, psychiatry, or psychology, members of different schools may sometimes fail to understand the minds of their co-workers and to achieve a really integrated approach. How much greater will be the corresponding difficulties where several disciplines are concerned which are so fundamentally apart in their historical development and in many essential characteristics and objectives as, for example, law, sociology, and psychiatry. The contrast between their past, their whole training and way of thinking, on the one hand, and what is now expected of them under the 'New Deal' in methodology and criminology on the other, may be too much for individual members of these professions. Integration, the authors stress, involves more than merely 'establishing a clearing-house of information to be shared' . . . 'dissemination is not integration'. It is certainly *more* than this, but where exactly is this plus to be found? There is a tentative answer already in the earlier part of Chapter I, but the authors are aware of its preliminary character and go on searching for something even more meaningful. Is it that 'related questions and hypotheses are tested in related ways'? Is it something connected with Max Weber's and Wilhelm Dilthey's concept of *Verstehen*, and what is the real meaning of that concept and is it capable at all of being defined in words? The example given in the book of how to carry out an analysis of the personality and work of a Leonardo da Vinci is helpful, but perhaps mainly to the converted, to those who already possess some insight, some comprehension of the objects for which the authors are fighting. The latter are indeed prepared for the movement towards integration to be slow and they realize that there can never be a perfectly integrated theory; there can never be complete fusion, a complete abandonment of disciplinary loyalties; the respect for the specific and traditional characteristics and idiosyncrasies of the individual disciplines would exclude

any such radicalism, nor can the effect of many years of strictly specialized – and all too often all too specialized – training be easily wiped out.
'The ultimate end of integration is grandiose and ambitious but worth
the candle.'

From this preliminary survey of the task to be performed, its difficulties and limitations, the authors move forward to attempts at classification and typology: integration should be achieved not only between
the different disciplines and between scientific theory and empirical
data, but also between theory and clinical practice. This tripartition still
looks rather general, but it is immediately supplemented by a list of
recommendations far more concrete and specific that might well become the ten commandments for any kind of team research. If it should
fail in its application to individual projects it will do so not because of its
own inner weakness but merely through the human frailty of those in
whose hands its application will be placed and for reasons similar to
those responsible for the failure so far of most attempts at federation in
the political sphere. In the latter, too, it has been our experience that
'Common Markets' and similar schemes, unless leading to complete
political union, are not quite enough and that such a union is still a
dream.

In Chapter II the discussion still continues on the level of general
criminological theory without being focused on any specific problem.
What is criminology and who is a criminologist? What are the major
trends in present-day criminology and the main arguments for and
against the 'positivist eclecticism' of a multi-factor theory? While the
preference of the authors clearly lies on the side of the critics of this
theory or pseudo-theory – and many of the criticisms here listed are no
doubt justified – they eventually reach a position to which adherents of
each of the opposing parties should be able to subscribe and which is in
fact not very dissimilar from the views I have expressed myself in previous writings. In any case, theirs is perhaps the most constructive
attempt so far made to end the wasteful struggle between the adherents
of Sutherland and those of the multi-factor theory. This is followed by
an evaluation of the 'cold' sociological versus the individualizing clinical
approach to criminology. As the authors recognize, the antagonism
between these two disciplines still tends to create a dangerous split
which makes truly integrated cooperation a very rare event. It should be
realized, by the way, that, on the one hand, the sociological way of
thinking – unless it is falsified by an abundance of irritating and unnecessary jargon – with the strong political, social, and economic

foundations on which it rests need not be 'cold' at all, and that, on the other hand, the clinical technique is sometimes highly impersonal and indifferent to the needs and the fate of the individual. In spite of certain tentative recommendations made by the authors, they admit that the outlook here is rather gloomy, although the younger generation of psychiatrists which is now growing up may well be less dogmatic and hidebound than some of their predecessors.

With Chapter III we enter what might be termed the special field of the investigation. While in no way taking final leave of their basic theme of integration, the authors realize that only by limiting research to a relatively narrow framework can they demonstrate to all comers how their ideas would work when applied to a specific topic. The subject chosen is the subculture of violence, and here our authors are in an exceptionally favourable position through their long and close association and their common interest in the subject. It is not just a case of an American sociologist and an Italian medically trained psychologist joining forces for this particular project; it is the collaboration of an American and an Italian scholar already deeply steeped in each other's language, culture, and ways of thinking, each of them having lived for considerable periods of time in the country of the other, and, moreover, having previously made several important individual contributions to the study of violent crime. It is from this background that they try to define such basic concepts as culture, subculture, and the underlying norms and values. As a preliminary to the more detailed analysis of the literature on homicide presented in Chapter IV, they are here concerned with certain principal trends, as, for example, the Freudian theory of aggression, the frustration–aggression hypothesis, the effect of the media of mass-communication and of methods of child-rearing. There is also some interesting material, not easily found elsewhere, on certain areas distinguished by exceptionally high rates of violence such as Sardinia and Colombia. The chapter ends with a list of propositions on the concept of 'subculture of violence', but so far no final explanation of its genesis can be offered.

In Chapter IV the most painstaking survey so far in existence is given of the literature, covering every discipline that has contributed to it. Here, 'for the sake of clarity and parsimony of presentation', the various ways of studying the subject had to be kept separate, but an integrated approach still remains the ultimate aim. So we are taken on an extended tour through the biological, neurological, psychiatric, and psychological writings on violence on an international scale. In their analysis of motives of murder there is a brief reference to the 'motiveless murder', a concept of doubtful reality in which I have been especially interested.

Chapter V is reserved for social studies and questions of treatment and research, and the authors do not hesitate to extend their critical comments to the work of sociologists. Much of this research has been done by scholars who possess 'but little peripheral vision and inadequate communication among themselves', and investigations of such isolated variables as, for example, age, sex, race, or class of samples of offenders often remain as meaningless as the corresponding work of some biologists and psychiatrists. Special attention is paid in this chapter to the position in developing countries, and selected culture case studies are discussed to test the universal applicability of the theory of the subculture of violence. While the authors make no claim for such universal applicability, they have assembled sufficient material to show the presence of such a subculture in many different parts of the world.

As so often in such studies, the final section on control, prevention, and treatment of crimes traceable to a subculture of violence is the area in which further research is most urgently required. This is certainly not the fault of the authors, but is inherent in their subject. 'The methods and techniques, the procedural guidance to be exercised in the process of subculturally oriented theory can be commented upon only very briefly,' they write, 'for no direct experimentation using the notions of a subculture of violence, and obviously no evaluative results are available.' With equal, and perhaps even excessive, modesty they maintain that 'basic evidence for the existence of a subculture of violence is still missing and tautological', but they provide at least some invaluable guidance for future research. In their own fieldwork on the subject – at present being undertaken in Puerto Rico (briefly outlined, for example, in the *British Journal of Criminology*, Vol. 3, No. 4, April 1963, pp. 377–388) – they have taken the logical step to fill the existing gaps by empirically testing certain hypotheses emerging from the existing body of theory. The scientific and theoretical foundation for this research has been brilliantly provided in the present work.

HERMANN MANNHEIM

London, Spring, 1966

Preface

The authors of this volume first met in Italy in April 1958 when one of us had just published a book on homicide in which he had used the phrase 'subculture of violence'. Each of us had independent intellectual interests in homicide which quickly merged with a personal friendship, and the ensuing years have brought us together on many occasions. The present book represents the intimate collaboration of a psychologically oriented sociologist and a sociologically oriented psychologist. Each of us represents the traditional criminological training of his own native continent; the one being social and cultural, the other, medical and biological. Yet we have crossed our disciplines as well as the Atlantic by spending considerable periods of time in each other's country. By bringing our disciplinary perspectives together on topics of mutual concern, we feel that we have gained much from the intellectual inter-action, and we hope that the personal and professional *Verbundenheit* has been adequately reflected in this volume.

We have tried to show the extent of our synthesis by a critical review of literature from several disciplines that bears upon the problems of criminological research and theory, and upon our thesis of a subculture of violence. Integration is not 'mere eclecticism', for, while we have drawn upon different disciplines and would welcome scientific thought from others, we have directed our limited interdisciplinary perspective to specific problems. Crimes of violence may be associated with many factors, but we have purposefully avoided the 'market-basket' approach with which the shopper picks up any kind of data, without knowing how to digest them. We do not deny the advantages and products of single-disciplinary efforts in research and theory. But we believe that the study of criminal deviance has reached a point where representatives of two or more disciplines can successfully analyze a delimited area of common concern. Although the history of efforts to promote interdisciplinary cooperation in the behavioral sciences has not been blessed with outstanding success, we firmly believe the efforts should continue. Our own experience has led us to be more than ever convinced that when the notions of one discipline are subjected to the sharp edge of critical comment by another discipline, the fuzzy layers of impression, inadequate methodology, incomplete theoretical models, and non-operationa hypotheses are quickly cut from core ideas that might be better reconstructed with integrated tools.

We begin this volume with a classic request for scientific collaboration and integration. We provide a relatively rigid definition of criminology and review recent research and theory in this field. We take up the problems of integrating not only different disciplinary perspectives but also theory with empirical research. A chapter is devoted to the problems of defining and measuring the elusive concepts of subculture and values. Using the former central concept as a basis for merging some of the major tenets of sociology and psychology, we focus on the criminal display of violence and formulate a set of propositions about a subculture of violence. Next, we summarize an array of studies and theories related to aggression and assaultive crimes, particularly homicide, and note briefly how these references contribute to our thesis of a subculture of violence. The bibliography presented in these chapters has been gleaned from many years of collection and reading by both authors and represents, we trust, a resource of some value to other scholars who wish to pursue the study of homicide and other assaultive crime in different detail or from another theoretical perspective.

Although it will be clear to the reader where studies in psychology are under review and where analyses in sociology are summarized, we wish to emphasize that our thinking and writing have been blended throughout the book. Variables and theories have sometimes been considered separately because they have been historically studied and developed in this way. But as we move through the spectrum from biological bases of aggression to socio-cultural studies of homicide, we have each contributed to the other's specialty and have tried to interpret existing knowledge by relating it to our main theory.

It is sometimes difficult for theorists to defend themselves against the attack that claims they have selected only those data which fit their theory. Our rebuttal to such a charge may be traditional and like the chicken–egg problem of induction–deduction, but it is an honest statement: the subculture-of-violence theory emerged from exposure to empiricism, from the collection of data about violent crime and analyses of homicide offenders. Some facts must always precede theory. The assembly of a large number of facts, consistent in content and collected in sophisticated detail from a variety of places, increases the probability of developing a theory that will bind the facts together into parsimonious abstraction. After a theory is formulated, the data are often re-examined in a style that is somewhat analogous to the procedure of the clinician who tries to capture in the life-history of his patient the meaningful and significant events that express the etiology of a current crisis. This kind of review of the facts is not a biased selection to 'prove' a theory; it is a return to data that have been somewhat randomly, irregularly, and independently arrayed, in order to arrange them into the framework of a meaningful and reasoned interpretation. The interpretation, which we ennoble into a theory, is like a sieve that picks up only relevant material; and we have tried to refine the mesh by an interdisciplinary weave that loses fewer data than would a single approach with a cruder screen. It is obvious, however, that any theory so formulated needs more than the backward glance at old data. Theories must be tested by new facts that are collected for the express purpose of confirmation or rejection. Both the central notion of a subculture of violence and the subsidiary inferences of prevention, control, and treatment that stem from it should be put to the test.

In acknowledging indebtedness, it is common practice for married authors to pay tribute last to their wives. Because of their uncommon assistance and patience, Lenora Wolfgang and Mirella Ferracuti deserve to be recognized first. They have done much more than take care of us and our respective children while we worked. They have listened to, read, and discussed the ideas expressed in this volume. Their mark is on many pages that have been reconstituted because of our discussions with them.

The Social Science Research Center of the University of Puerto Rico, first under the direction of Millard Hansen, and now of Raphael de Jesus-Toro, generously supported our work and made possible the regular and unscheduled times the authors could be together for joint writing. Our students at the University of Pennsylvania, the University of Rome, and the University of Puerto Rico deserve our thanks for listening and contributing to some of the ideas that found their way into the book. We are grateful to many unnamed colleagues who discussed with us some of our earlier papers on the subculture of violence. Thanks are due to Carmen H. Lopez, executive secretary of the Social Science Research Center, and her staff for their continuous assistance; to Jean Wilmot, administrative assistant of the Center of Criminological Research at the University of Pennsylvania; and to Shirley Murray, who prepared the index.

We are honored in having Hermann Mannheim provide the foreword, and are grateful for his regular encouragement of our work. The professional debts we owe Thorsten Sellin and Benigno Di Tullio are of such long standing and proportion that we respectfully dedicate this book to them as an inadequate but sincere gesture of our esteem and appreciation.
M. E. W.
F. F.

Acknowledgements

We wish to record our thanks to the publishers and others who have granted us permission to quote at length from published works, and in particular those listed below. The fullest possible bibliographical details of all works cited are given in the Notes and References at the end of each chapter.

Basic Books, Inc. in respect of *Toward a Unified Theory of Human Behavior*, edited by Roy R. Grinker; The Free Press of Glencoe in respect of *Essays in Sociological Theory*, by Talcott Parsons; Harper & Row, Publishers, Incorporated, in respect of the passage by Gunnar Myrdal from *Value & Social Theory*, edited by Paul Streeten; Harvard University Press in respect of *Toward a General Theory of Action*, by Talcott Parsons and Edward Shils; The Philosophical Library in respect of *Trends in Social Science*, edited by Donald P. Ray; Professor Clarence Schrag in respect of 'Some Notes on Criminological Theory' from *Conference on Research Planning on Crime and Delinquency (1962)*, edited by William R. Larsen; Social Science Research Council in respect of the passage by Thorsten Sellin from their *Bulletin*, 41, 1938.

1 · The Meaning of Integration

Owing to increasing specialization in the study of human behavior, there has been a lack of integrated scientific theory. All knowledge tends to be unitary, and disciplinary activities are only artifacts required because of man's limited grasp of the universe of ideas. But as specialization increases, scholars reach the point where they begin to ask significant questions that cannot be answered satisfactorily within their own framework. They seek knowledge and assistance from scholars in other areas who are usually asking questions that also require outside help for answers. Often, however, contacts and conversations between two or more disciplines reveal that the information sought is possessed by no one. The sociologist, for example, may have meaningful questions to ask the endocrinologist about endocrinal imbalances and their possible relation to deviant behavior, only to learn that the biologist is unable to provide adequate answers to his questions. The reverse, obviously, also occurs.

It is usually at such a point that tentative requests or firm demands have been made for interdisciplinary research or conferences. Almost blind faith in the assumed virtues and benefits of disciplinary cross-fertilization has characterized some of these demands. But many efforts in the past have failed to yield the desired results. Unless a single mind can absorb the accumulated substantive knowledge of two or more fields, the attempt to examine phenomena from several viewpoints usually breaks down because of personality conflicts or because communication of basic concepts and operational terms is lacking. If anything is produced from the combined efforts, it is often a disjointed, unrelated multidisciplinary display of separate knowledge reflecting each scholar's orientation, without much influence or effect from others. Perhaps fearful of diluting his own approach, each scientist sometimes becomes more tenaciously attached to his original framework. The psychiatrist has difficulty in convincing the sociologist that the clinical approach is a useful way of obtaining data or of verifying hypotheses. The statistically oriented sociologist or mathematically trained psychologist has difficulty in impressing the clinician that sufficiently large groups, representative samples, control groups, and association tests are necessary for the proper testing of hypotheses.[1]

Joint writing by two or more researchers, even in the same discipline, is difficult. Even slight differences of emphasis in orientation become magnified when two sociologists try to write something together. Differences of writing style, theoretical orientation, allegiance to the works of other scholars in their field, and so on can create difficult if not insoluble problems in doing joint research or joint writing of an analytical paper. But these problems are compounded when scholars from different disciplines try to work together. If there are lasting results, they reflect a splicing of separate writing or research and thinking rather than a synthesis.

Although there has been some success through interdisciplinary efforts,[2] few persons would disagree with the assertion that most creative theoretical and empirical analyses have come as segmental, limited accumulations of knowledge. Even 'team' research reflects separate writing by individual scholars, followed by editing from directors who were responsible for the entire program and who provided their own separate analyses. Perhaps this is the best, if not the only, way to proceed if different disciplines are merely to be represented and not interrelated on a research task.

We believe that, however empirical research and theory will be developed in the future, up to now there has been inadequate integration of knowledge already accumulated and reported in scientific literature. In no wise are we suggesting that interdisciplinary or multidisciplinary work should be discouraged. Quite the contrary. But whether our knowledge of human behavior increases through the efforts of individuals in separate disciplines working alone or through the efforts of multi- or interdisciplinary teams, integration of past and present knowledge and theory should be considered a *sine qua non* of these efforts.

We use the term 'integration' because we are suggesting that it means something different from interdisciplinary collaboration. *Integration in this context means bringing together empirical data, relative to the same phenomenon, that have been collected by independent disciplines and interpreted within their limited parameters of orientation so that an analytical synthesis becomes minimally the combination of the parts and maximally a new perspective.*

This process involves more than establishing a clearing-house of information to be shared. The function of such a clearing-house is to bring related research and theory to the attention of interested scholars. It is a collection agency but it cannot achieve integration.[3] Yet dissemination is not integration. Only the collation of material can be performed by the scholar who is searching for knowledge that has been collected to test hypotheses related to the phenomenon under his own investigation. Integration is described in *Webster's Unabridged Dictionary* as 'The act or process of making whole or entire . . . integrate: to form into one whole; to make entire; to complete; to round out; to perfect'.[4] It seems clear to many scientists that integration can most quickly proceed through experimental research plans that include two or more disciplines working together, but there is nothing to preclude ex-post-facto integration operations. Furthermore, although the common language of mathematics or standard symbolization may be convenient procedures for communication between disciplines, reductions to lingual homogeneity are not necessary for integration. Each speciality may use its own terminology without invasion or intrusion of the others, for in integration scientific sights are set upon a single focus that is multidimensional.[5]

It should be made clear that we are not proposing a modified neo-positivism or an extended and intensive eclecticism.[6] The positivist has a limited perspective and usually does not relate his multitude of unrelated data to a meaningful analytical thread. The eclectic has no explicit parameters and generally fails to discriminate the quality of data or the value of theoretical positions. He wants all of them without losing anything. His results are still characterized by the separation of fact and theory that were reflected in the original sources of his material. All of his data stand at equal attention but on distinctly different battlefields. The enemy of ignorance, or lack of knowledge, is attacked by the arrows from many bows, some finely hewed, others crudely created. The diffusive and divided effect is often of little value, like a phalanx of men each shooting straight ahead but with the common foe in the center directly in front of only one man. The splendid array of unrelated facts signifies diligent but ineffectual labor. As Donald Ray has said in a similar context, 'the interweaving threads which logically require connection in these various substantive problems are too frequently absent and this fact comprises the general interdisciplinary deficiency'.[7]

The collection of unlinked theories is no better than the collection of unlinked facts for promoting science, and serves only as a convenient catalogue of ideas, as a pedagogical device for learning what has preceded the present. Although there is recognized value in a broad eclectic view at the outset of integrated research, generally, in the past, eclecticism has denoted an indiscriminate means and an all-embracing end of research and theory. A wide-eyed vacuous appearance unstamped by any specialization and innocently setting up a multitude of interrogative hypotheses ('testable questions'), often ends a given search for knowledge with the same expansive expression – i.e. with all disciplines represented and with unrelated questions answered in unrelated ways. Although integrated research and theory begin with equal respect for all disciplined scientific pursuits of knowledge, there is also focus and delimitation, a search for various disciplined attacks on the same phenomenon in order to seek time and space verities of more universal dimensions.

Integration means that related questions and hypotheses will be answered and tested in related ways; that the same focal delimitation that directed the outset of research and analysis is maintained to the point of conclusion. Integrated research permits any discipline to be the initiator of a point of inquiry on a given topic so long as the traditional canons of scientific method and logic are maintained. Thus, for example, some synergistic effect can emerge through integration, whether an analysis of Leonardo da Vinci is begun by a psychologist, a sociologist, or an art historian. So long as we recognize that Leonardo was a personality, that he lived within a given culture context, that his art is an extension of his person or vice versa, we are simultaneously recognizing the need for and importance of an integrated approach. Integration requires more than a chapter on the psychology of Leonardo, followed by a chapter on the historical setting of the Renaissance, then by a chapter on the development of his art form. Each of these separate analyses might be made, of course, but an integrated perspective asks questions and formulates hypotheses that can best be examined by a blended interwoven analysis. These questions and hypotheses, we believe, are not merely on a higher level of complexity, requiring a kind of Comtian recognition of an hierarchical order of the disciplines; they are on a different level of significance. Through integration we are seeking meanings (*Verstehen*, in a Weberian sense) behind the concatenation of a multidimensional set of attributes and variables.

We agree with Parsons that 'the two central tasks [of science] are clearly empirical research on theoretically significant problems, and theory-building in the specifically technical sense'.[8] But progressive specialization, it is often argued, has contributed to an increase in more and more precise empirical research on less and less significant problems;[9] and 'the striving for unification of knowledge was left to the individual and no explicit attempt was made to accumulate knowledge concerned with the integration of diversified fields'.[10] We agree with Ruesch that with the increasing amount of technological information, the individual solution used by our disciplinary pioneers and predecessors is no longer applicable. A Pico della Mirandola could not exist in the twentieth century. 'Instead, various attempts at establishing a universal scientific language, at agreeing upon basic scientific assumptions, at developing generally acceptable theoretical systems and at constructing giant electronic brains can be interpreted as moves to build the foundation upon which a body of knowledge which deals with the *integration* of specialized scientific information can rest.'[11]

The movement toward integration, however, is slow. Even within a single discipline there have been factional disputes and atomization of thought and research. As a consequence, 'there is little systematic codification of empirical knowledge, hence little basis of cumulative development of the empirical organon'.[12] Theoretical generalizations that can emerge under these circumstances are likely to result in a pluralism of 'schools', and we have abundant evidence of such pluralism in criminology, which is the area of our special concern in this volume. We believe that the history of criminology and even the definition of its field reflect too much empirical eclecticism and theoretical pluralism, and that the moment has come for an attempt to integrate the diversities represented in this discipline. To this extent we are in accord with Parsons when he recently said, 'The beginning of the crystallization of science . . . tends to involve the dropping out of the "war of schools," especially at the level of the frame of reference. Beyond this will tend to emerge a common theoretical scheme, first of the definition of categories, then gradually more and more closely integrated generalized propositions. With this goes both empirical and theoretical critique of older empirical generalization and the gradual codification of available empirical knowledge.'[13]

In the present study we are focusing on a relatively delimited subject, violence, especially as it is manifested in criminal homicide. We have deliberately chosen to restrict our analysis in order to perform some of the tasks of integration within a manageable framework. Moreover, we cannot hope to integrate all knowledge regarding homicide, for our orientations represent only some disciplines, namely, sociology and psychology (and, to a limited extent, biology). The ultimate end of integration is grandiose and ambitious but worth the candle. Our immediate goal is to examine the techniques of scientific integration and to demonstrate its application by collating data and theory from sociology, psychology, and biology relative to a major form of deviant conduct. In essence, we are asking, as does Roy Grinker in the symposium *Toward a Unified Theory of Human Behavior*, 'What does one discipline need and what can it accept and use of the assumptions and concepts of another, and, at the same time how can that discipline communicate its own concepts and assumptions to another.'[14]

Throughout this review we shall emphasize the interdependency of the branches of science. Our efforts, whether or not successful, imply that 'one of the foremost problems surely is the trend toward overspecialization or the atomization of the social sciences, and conversely, the underdevelopment of the generalist approach'.[15] We agree with Tyler that 'the assumptions on which an individual discipline is based may be matters of doubt or may even be empirically improbable when treated in a different context. This does not invalidate a discipline as a science but it limits its range of explanation and prediction. As these limitations are being recognized, efforts are correspondingly being made to develop interdisciplinary research endeavors which will help to test some of the assumptions on which the particular scientific constructs can properly be applied'.[16]

Through the vehicle of an intellectual analysis of violence we hope to bring diverse perspectives into logical integration, into a confluence of different ways of approaching the same phenomenon, into an integrated conceptual scheme that will maximize assimilation of the intellectual processes by which things become known. Criminology is in a peculiarly ripe position for this kind of integration because of the variety of scientific orientations that have contributed to its development. Sociology and psychology are perhaps the prominent disciplines in this respect. But we wish to emphasize that our integrative approach, like that suggested by Inkeles, should not result in 'the reduction of one discipline to another but the articulation of the two for certain specific purposes under certain specific conditions'.[17]

Furthermore, we are not yet prepared, even within the limited scope of our substantive framework, to suggest that there can be a completely unified theory. Integration, or 'interaction' theory, may be a start in the direction of a unified system, but integrated research and theory maintain respect for the separate and diverse perspectives while seeking to unite them at some point of mutual interest and interdependence. Lawrence Frank has also expressed an aspect of this position: 'Whatever exists actually . . . has a variety of dimensions, and each of our specialized disciplines is constructed upon observing, measuring and interpreting one set of those dimensions and more or less deliberately ignoring all others. We are struggling to gain a conception of a multidimensionality of human organism-personalities and to learn how we can deal with multidimensional observations without distorting or neglecting one or more of them or trying to warp all of them into a single dimensional system or framework.'[18]

Perhaps more than Frank we should like to emphasize that multidimensionality as it has existed thus far in criminology has been characterized by too much separateness and that we prefer the term integration because it recognizes the need for multidimensional observation while stressing the equal need for purposive concerted congruity. Relative to the integration of sociology and psychology, probably Inkeles and Merton come closer to our position. 'Our criterion,' says Inkeles, 'should not be disciplinary purely but, rather, the adequacy of our analysis. The central thesis . . . is that adequate sociological analysis of many problems is either impossible or severely limited unless we make explicit use of psychological theory and data in conjunction with sociological theory and data. Indeed, I would assert that very little sociological analysis is ever done without using at least an implicit psychological theory. It seems evident that in making this theory explicit and bringing psychological data to bear systematically on sociological problems we cannot fail but improve the scope and adequacy of sociological analysis.'[19] And in discussing the problem of asking meaningful questions as a means of initiating research theory, Merton notes that the sociologist often needs to seek answers from other disciplines, particularly psychology. As he points out in a paper on 'Notes on Problem-Finding in Sociology': 'One of the more wide-ranging examples of this type of problem involves the question of how to account for regularities of social behavior that are not prescribed by cultural norms or that are even at odds with these norms. It casts doubt on the familiar assumption that uniformities of social behavior necessarily represent conformity to norms calling for that behavior. It identifies a gap in that narrowly cultural theory of behavior that, expressly or tacitly, sees social regularities as culturally mandated. Yet many social regularities need not, of course, have this relation to culture.'[20]

In his discussion of personality and social structure, W. I. Thomas came close to the interactionist position that we wish to emphasize by our term integration.[21] Most social psychology today, as Inkeles suggests, is a grab-bag category and involves examination of a social situation in which an individual behaves, or examination of an individual as he behaves in a social situation. Unfortunately, there is little in contemporary social psychology that seeks to integrate sociological data and theory with data and theory about individual personality.[22] Inkeles appears to agree with Merton that uniformities and regularities of behavior do occur without the invariable presence of culture prescriptions, but goes further, to the point of asserting that 'all institutional arrangements are ultimately mediated through individual action. The consequences of any institutional arrangement, therefore, depend, at least in part, upon its effect on the human personality broadly conceived. The human personality system thus becomes one of the main intervening variables in any estimate of the effects of one aspect of social structure on another'.[23]

The integration towards which we are striving, consequently, emphasizes the fact that a full understanding of any social situation, its etiology, its ramifications and consequences, requires the knowledge of not only the main facts about the social structure (which is the domain of sociology) but also the main facts about personalities which function in that structure (the domain of psychology). 'What is required, therefore, is an *integration* or coordination of two basic sets of data in a larger explanatory scheme – not a reduction of either mode of analysis to the allegedly more fundamental of the other.'[24]

The history of the physical, biological, and social sciences reveals that study begins with orderless or poorly ordered descriptions of basic phenomena in the field; these descriptions are later classified and catalogued in ways that seem to make sense. But with understanding, as Everett Hagen points out, comes a system of classification more closely related to the functioning of interacting elements. 'Gradually, generalizations about functioning are reached which are useful in predicting future events. As the generalizations gain rigor, they take the form of analytical models of the behavior of the elements being studied.'[25]

We realize that the study of violence manifested through homicide is a narrowly defined point within the general social and biological sciences, but we hope to move toward generalizations that may aid in the construction of analytical models. As we have said, we are focusing attention on this relatively delimited area in order to interrelate elements from two major perspectives that examined the same phenomenon. Although we believe these efforts may contribute toward the building of a comprehensive theory, 'most of those engaged in interdisciplinary research', as Tyler asserts, 'are not focussing their efforts at this time upon the building of any single social science map but are rather seeking to relate some of the disciplines that deal with similar or related problems in connection with similar or related phenomena and in this way to bring an increasing interrelationship among these data, phenomena and conceptualisms'.[26]

There are several types of integration to which we have alluded and to which we shall refer throughout the rest of this study in ideas. These are the integration of:

1. disciplines in initiating and conducting research;
2. scientific theory and data within and between disciplines;
3. scientific theory and clinical practice in diagnosis and treatment.

Our efforts toward integration are part of the middle-range approach, and, because we are still in the early stages, emphasis is placed on the first two types mentioned above. Research on treatment strategies can, of course, proceed before causal relations are known, but development of theory underlying the collection of data on treatment must ordinarily precede the design of experimentation. The theoretical formulation we propose is an outgrowth of the past developments in criminology, which developments we shall briefly describe in the next chapter. The review of theories and empirical research that are related to our thesis and the substantive issues that it encompasses follow the formulation. An integrated model for research that recognizes the interactional character of the formulation is presented, but at this stage is best described as heuristic. Hence the suggestions for diagnosis and treatment can themselves be only tentative, for both the theory and the models must be considered to be in a developmental stage, open to review, critical analysis, and revision.

In 1951–1952 several behavioral science conferences on interdis-

B

ciplinary team research methods and problems met under the auspices of the National Training Laboratories of the National Education Association. The patterns of collaboration which were discussed and described by the delegates included the following:[27]

1. *Fusion.* In this approach, 'disciplinary loyalties are discarded and all researchers subscribe to an over-all theoretical system within which an attempt is made to handle all problems that are undertaken'.
2. *Multivariate Approach* – with a common focus. Members of a research team 'work together on the same central problem but use their own methods and stay essentially within their own theoretical framework'.
3. *Formal Integration* – within which the separateness of disciplines is maintained.
4. *Division* of problem into subinquiries with interdisciplinary collaboration.
5. *Collation.* This is the loosest kind of collaboration, 'a type of interdisciplinary research in which members of different disciplines, each with different theories, work in the same general problem area without any specific provisions for integration. They exchange information and data, but essentially each uses his own techniques to work on his own part of the research'.

It should be obvious from our previous discussion that we favor fusion in reference to interdisciplinary research. However, we do not believe it necessary to discard 'disciplinary loyalty' in the sense that one abandons intellectual attachment to concepts, theories, and findings if these have been fruitful in producing operational hypotheses and useful data. What should be discarded in fusion is a unidimensional perspective on the problems under investigation, for each team member must expand and accept the injection of concepts, theories, and findings into his own set of ideas so that integration can be achieved.

Finally, the outline of the characteristics of close collaboration presented by the aforementioned conferences is the result of many discussions and of case materials presented by leading representatives from anthropology, psychiatry, psychology, and sociology. We have used the items in each of the four categories as excellent guidelines for our own thinking, discussion, writing, theory-building, and research-designing.[28]

A. *From the standpoint of the research problem*
1. Focus on a single clearly defined problem.
2. Problem definition determined by demands of problem rather than by disciplinary or individual interests.
3. Formulation of the research problem in such a way that all participants can contribute to its solution.
4. Existence of collaborative potential as a result of previous work on the problem by more than one discipline.

B. *From the standpoint of theory*
1. Acceptance of a unified overall theory.
2. Acceptance of a common set of hypotheses and assumptions.
3. Agreement on definition of common concepts.
4. Agreement on operational definitions.

C. *From the standpoint of methodology*
1. Utilization of resources of all relevant disciplines in exploring possible methodologies.
2. Team agreement on most appropriate methodology, including research procedures, relevant variables to be measured or controlled, and methods to be used.

D. *From the standpoint of group functioning*
1. Selection of team members on basis of their ability to contribute to research objectives.
2. Approximate parity of influence exerted by the representatives of one discipline on another.
3. Acceptance of leadership regardless of disciplines from which leader and researchers come.
4. Flexibility of roles.
5. Development and use of a common language.
6. Free communication among all team members.
7. Free interchange of information about the research, with mechanics for facilitating such interchange when necessary.
8. Sharing of suggestions, ideas, and data among members from different disciplines.
9. Participation of all team members in joint planning of each step of the research.
10. Reciprocal teaching and learning among team members – a continuous learning process.
11. Problem-centered rather than discipline- or individual-centered team activity.

12. Minimum influence on research plans and operations exerted from outside the research team.

13. Willingness of participants to subordinate their own methods and interests to achieve project aims.

14. Publication of research reports by the group as a whole rather than by individual members.

Finally, we wish to stress the differential roles of theory construction and eclectic methodologies. Developing a model for analyzing a problem may – and often does – require a single or 'one-sided' theory; but the observational research strategies should be many-sided. Eclecticism at the outset and as a model for analysis sacrifices parsimony and tolerates too many ideas, often of weak or no merit.[29] While a theory from a single discipline may sometimes polarize theorists, as such procedures have done in the past, it is viewed here, as David Mechanic has expressed it, simply as a strategy of approach rather than a dogmatic assertion of priority.[30] Mechanic's quotation from Max Weber's essay on objectivity is used for clarification of 'one-sided' analysis:

'The justification of the *one-sided* analysis of cultural reality from specific 'points of view' – in our case with respect to its economic conditioning – emerges purely as a technical expedient from the fact that training in the observation of the effects of qualitatively similar categories of causes and the repeated utilization of the same scheme of concepts and hypotheses (*begrifflich-methodischen Apparates*) offers all the advantages of the division of labor. It is free from the charge of arbitrariness to the extent that it is successful in producing insights into inter-connections which have been shown to be valuable for the casual explanation of concrete historical events.'[31]

Our own comments are not really in disagreement, but they do supplement these by Weber. When the 'insights into inter-connections' occur from a 'one-sided' theoretical perspective, they require an integrated eclecticism to test them. We have no objection to a model or a theory that comes from one discipline so long as ultimately the many-sided aspects of such a theory are recognized, if they exist, and are accounted for and integrated in the research designed to predict or explain from the theory. A theory is revised and improved through cross-fertilization, and we shall urge throughout this book the use of an eclectic research strategy in collecting data to test theory. Thus, whatever efficiency comes from a focalized and delimited, or even a one-sided, theoretical statement, scientific pursuit to examine the proposition from several related disciplines satisfies our requirement for integration. *Theory should therefore generate an eclectic research technique, but an eclectic approach by itself is not theory.*

It is within this framework that we shall pursue the development of criminology in general and more particularly our analysis of crimes of violence.

NOTES AND REFERENCES

1. Paul E. Meehl's *Clinical vs. Statistical Prediction*, Minneapolis: University of Minnesota Press, 1954, is still one of the most useful discussions of these and related problems. The subtitle of this book is especially revealing of the scope of its contents: 'A Theoretical Analysis and a Review of the Evidence'.
2. For an encouraging summary of these efforts, see Ralph W. Tyler, 'Trends in Interdisciplinary Research', in *Trends in Social Science* (edited by Donald Ray), New York: Philosophical Library, 1961, pp. 137–151.
3. Certainly much sharing of ideas is served by such publications as *Excerpta Criminologica* and the organized efforts of the National Council on Crime and Delinquency; the lacunae of communication are filled by their existence. This kind of collecting, abstracting, and distributing service aids the scholar in a single discipline to know what is being done outside his own orientation. The help to bibliographical construction is almost unlimited, and, as we shall see, it is of considerable value in the move toward integration. *Excerpta Criminologica* is a commendable effort to bring in abstract form the most important criminological research and theory from all over the world to the attention of interested scholars. The official language is English and the publication is printed in The Netherlands. It is prepared and published by the Excerpta Criminologica Foundation in cooperation with the National Council on Crime and Delinquency.
4. *Webster's New International Dictionary of the English Language*, Second Edition, Springfield, Mass: G. & C. Merriam Company, 1957.
5. We should add that different foci on the same phenomenon are also desirable. As Laura Thompson has said: 'It may be one of our goals in multidisciplinary research that we do not work alone each in our own science, but that perhaps as we continue working together in multidisciplinary teams, we shall be able to observe multiple foci.' (Laura Thompson, discussant in Jurgen Ruesch, 'The Observer and the Observed: Human Communication Theory', *Toward a Unified Theory of Human Behavior*, edited by Roy R. Grinker, New York: Basic Books, 1956, pp. 39–40.)
6. Nor does our use of the term integration have any relationship to Sorokin's reference to 'integral truth', which he refers to as 'three-dimensional' because its sources are intuition, reason, and the senses. Claiming that his 'integralist sociology' has produced a profound revolution in the social sciences because the integralist method contains all the methods of ascertaining 'truth' and is more adequate than any of them taken separately, Sorokin seems to assert that his integral truth is closer to the absolute truth than any one-sided truth. See

Pitirim Sorokin, *Social and Cultural Dynamics*, Vol. 4, New York: 1941, pp. 677–693.

However, when Sorokin talks about integration as being more than spatial adjacency and as indicating that there must be some kind of connection that is logical or functional in the integrated analysis, there are aspects to his 'logico-meaningful integration' which connote some of the things we have been referring to in our use of the term integration as a methodological procedure leading to a collation of data and theory. For example, Sorokin says: 'A study of any purely spatial and mechanical congeries cannot give anything but a mere descriptive catalogue of the parts. Since these are not united causally no formula of causal uniformity, no causal or functional generalization, can be made of them.'

'In a study of cultural syntheses the parts of which are united causally or functionally, the causal–functional method with its more or less general causal formulas provides the proper procedure . . . The essence of the logico-meaningful method of cognition is . . . in the finding of the central principle . . . which permeates all the components, gives sense and significance to each of them, and in this way makes cosmos of a chaos of unintegrated fragments' (Pitirim Sorokin, *Social and Cultural Dynamics*, Boston: Porter Sargent, 1957, p. 14).

7. Donald P. Ray (ed.), *Trends in Social Science*, New York: Philosophical Library, 1961, p. 6.

8. Talcott Parsons, 'Comment' to L. Gross, 'Preface to a Metaphysical Framework', *American Journal of Sociology* (September, 1961) 67:139.

9. Sorokin is especially acrimonious on this topic. See his *Fads and Foibles in Modern Sociology and Related Sciences*, Chicago: Henry Regnery, 1956.

10. Jurgen Ruesch, 'Introduction', *Toward a Unified Theory of Human Behavior* (edited by Roy R. Grinker), New York: Basic Books, 1956, p. ix. Ruesch does state, however, that '. . . ultimately the information derived from a team of twenty people is to be integrated in one brain. We have no machine as yet that compares to the integrative qualities of man's brain' (Ruesch, 'The Observer and the Observed', *op. cit.*, p. 40).

A similar expression of this idea may be found in Roy R. Grinker in the same book: '. . . observations in all sciences are derived by an individual who has a position in relation to his object. He receives and transmits information which is limited by his position. This may be at an inner or an outer boundary but never both at once. Each set of observations may be complementary to one another or an oscillation process may facilitate a fusion of separate observations. Not even multiple observers in multidisciplinary research can achieve more, since the data requires integration in the mind of a single scientist. Hence, natural events are viewed, not in terms of the reality of the matter, but through the eyes of an observer who is part of the communication system' (*op. cit.*, p. 53).

11. Ruesch, 'Introduction', *op. cit.*, p. ix. Emphasis added.
12. Talcott Parsons, 'Comment' to L. Gross, 'Preface to a Metaphysical Framework', *American Journal of Sociology* (September, 1961) 67:137.
13. Talcott Parsons, 'Comment' to L. Gross, 'Preface to a Metaphysical Framework', *American Journal of Sociology* (September, 1961) 67:138.
   We can find no particular argument with Llewellyn Gross's desire to conceive of science as a continually self-corrective system of thought, but we can find no particular need for the 'metatheoretical framework' which he describes as 'neodialectic'. Gross contends that 'neodialectic's central premise is that every viewpoint, including its own, must consider an indeterminant number of opposite, complementary, and synthesizing principles'. It is true, of course, that science on all fronts has proceeded by seeking out the contradiction and attacking it and that insufficient complementarity and synthesization have characterized developments in sociology in general and criminology in particular. But we are inclined to agree with Parsons that 'sociology entered this stage [dialectical] in the generation which spanned the turn of the century and ended about 1935. During that period the "war of schools" drastically diminished' (Parsons's Comment on Gross, *op. cit.*, p. 138). Moreover, continually confronting alternatives at each level of analysis is destructive of a developing theoretical system. The objective scientist presumably seeks out information and data which challenge his position and he deals with them either implicitly or explicitly in his textual development throughout his analysis.
14. Roy R. Grinker, 'The Intrapersonal Organization', *Toward a Unified Theory of Human Behavior*, p. 3.
15. Donald P. Ray, *op. cit.*, p. 3. This author none the less has some cogent remarks about the specialist: 'The usefulness of the specialist in ever increasingly complex societies should not be discounted. But the similar usefulness of the generalist requires advancing recognition. The adaptation of both, especially in group research, should be encouraged. Most social scientists seemingly wish to be recognized as a specialist in one area or another and this attitude perhaps defines the id. As the scholar matures frequently his interests broaden, but in most cases this phenomenon occurs at a later rather than at an earlier period. In the interests of more productive research, there remains a need to develop generalist tendencies during the earlier and more fruitful years of the researcher so that such tendencies might enrich his specialization. . . . But in organizational work as well as in substantive research the concept of more integrative and interdisciplinary undertakings provides a new frontier for social science. The specialist fortunately will not be lost since the specialist by his very nature will endure. The organizational factor in interdisciplinary research will require attention, and there is opportunity for innovation in this respect' (*Ibid.*, pp. 3–4).

16. Ralph W. Tyler, 'Trends in Interdisciplinary Research', in Donald P. Ray (ed.), *Trends in Social Science*, New York: Philosophical Library, 1961, p. 140.
17. Alex Inkeles, 'Personality and Social Structure', *Sociology Today*, New York: Basic Books, 1959, p. 272.
18. Lawrence K. Frank, discussant in Jurgen Ruesch, 'The Observer and the Observed: Human Communication Theory', *Toward a Unified Theory of Human Behavior*, edited by Roy R. Grinker, New York: Basic Books, 1956, p. 40.
19. Inkeles, *op. cit.*, p. 250.
20. Robert K. Merton, 'Notes on Problem-Finding in Sociology', *Sociology Today*, New York: Basic Books, 1959, p. xxxiii.
21. William I. Thomas and Florian Znaniecki, *The Polish Peasant in Europe and America*, Vol. I, Second Edition, New York: Dona Publications, 1950; see especially pp. 68–69.
22. Inkeles remarks along these lines: 'Although I do not urge that personality and social structure be considered an area of inquiry distinct from social psychology, I cannot easily reconcile the basic unity of the approach I have urged and the grab-bag generally called social psychology. Nor would I equate the approach I have stressed with much of the work done by psychologically trained social psychologists. In most of their work there is as little systematic use of sociological theory and data as there is of psychological theory and data in the work of sociologists' (Inkeles, *op. cit.*, p. 274).
23. *Ibid.*, p. 251. Roy Grinker also speaks of this interaction of parts of a system: 'Although anatomically and physically there may be some distinctions between two parts of a system, if we view the system functionally we may ignore the purely anatomical parts as irrelevant and the division into organism and environment becomes vague. Thus, a system is the whole complex of the organism and environment. Environment is composed of those variables whose changes affect the organism and which are changed by the organism's behavior. Thus, both the organism and environment are two parts of one system. By adding an environmental parameter to the variables that are significant for a system, then the system always has an extended environment. Reversing this, passing to within the boundaries of a system, what are known as system functions become environment, and the parts of the system become in themselves focal system under observation' (Grinker, *op. cit.*, p. 371).
24. *Ibid.*, p. 273. Emphasis added.
25. Everett E. Hagen, 'Analytical Models in the Study of Social Systems', *American Journal of Sociology* (September, 1961) 67:144.
26. Tyler, *op. cit.*, p. 141.
27. Margaret Barron Luszki, *Interdisciplinary Team Research Methods and Problems*, No. 3 of the Research Training Series, New York: National Training Laboratories, 1958. The bibliography in this volume is extensive and useful for more intensive examination of the problems involved in interdisciplinary research.

For another type of examination of how interdisciplinary methods may function and what kinds of problem in the behavioral sciences require empirical research and theoretical models of an integrative character, see the following volume sponsored by the Air Force Office of Scientific Research, which is a compendium of reports from the First Interdisciplinary Conference in the Behavioral Science Division, held at the University of New Mexico: *Decisions, Values and Groups*, edited by Dorothy Willner, with an Introduction by Anatol Rapoport, New York: Pergamon Press, 1960.

28. Luszki, *op. cit.*, pp. 135–136.

29. Albert Cohen has succinctly discussed the reasons for not considering the multiple-factor approach a theory. He says, for example: 'A multiplicity of factors is not to be confused with a multiplicity of variables. . . . Explanation calls not for a single *factor* but for a *single theory* or system of theory applicable to all cases. . . . A 'factor' as here understood is not a variable; it is a particular concrete circumstance. A multiple-factor approach is not a theory; it is an abdication of the quest for a theory' (Albert K. Cohen, *Juvenile Delinquency and the Social Structure*, Ph.D. Thesis, Harvard University, 1951, pp. 5–13).

30. David Mechanic, 'Some Considerations in the Methodology of Organizational Studies', pp. 137–182, in Harold J. Leavitt (ed.), *The Social Science of Organizations*, New York: Prentice-Hall, 1963, p. 171 cited. This entire book, but especially the perceptive chapter by Mechanic, is relevant to our discussion of the meaning of integration.

31. Max Weber, 'Objectivity in Social Science and Social Policy', in *The Methodology of the Social Sciences*, by Max Weber, translated and edited by Edward Shils and Henry Finch, New York: The Free Press, 1949, p. 71; cited by Mechanic, *op. cit.*, p. 167.

See also the provocative discussions of theory construction, philosophy, operationism, etc., in Melvin H. Marx (ed.), *Theories in Contemporary Psychology*, New York: The Macmillan Co., 1963. For an analysis of how these problems of theory and method arise and might be handled in social action and social research, see Leslie T. Wilkins, *Social Deviance: Social Policy, Action and Research*, London: Tavistock Publications, 1964; Englewood Cliffs, N.J.: Prentice-Hall.

II · Criminology as an Integrating Discipline

THE MEANING OF CRIMINOLOGY

THE SCOPE OF THE FIELD

The term criminology has been defined by almost every author who has written a text in the field. The varied content of criminology, as conceived from the beginning by writers like Lombroso, Ferri, Garofalo, Aschaffenburg, and other pioneers,[1] has permitted an extensive and confused use of this term for the many subdivisions of the subject. The multiform status of the teaching of criminology has not facilitated an academic definition of the field. Textbooks generally refer to a mixture of data on science, law, public administration, and morality; and the commonplace dichotomy into 'criminology' and 'penology' has been with us at least since the days of Parmelee.[2] Sutherland's definition has been standard for many years: 'Criminology is the body of knowledge regarding crime as a social phenomenon. It includes within its scope the processes of making laws, of breaking laws, and of reacting toward the breaking of laws. . . . The objective of criminology is the development of a body of general and verified principles and of other types of knowledge regarding this process of law, crime, and treatment.'[3] Webster's unabridged edition of the American dictionary appears to have incorporated part of Sutherland's perspective, for we read that criminology (L. *crimen, criminis*: crime + -logy) is 'the scientific study of crime as a social phenomenon, of criminals, and of penal treatment'.[4]

We believe that the term criminology should be used to designate a body of *scientific* knowledge about crime. This is essentially the basis for

Thorsten Sellin's introductory chapter of *Culture Conflict and Crime*,[5] which remains as one of the most pervasive and precise statements about the content area and theoretical structure of criminology.

This conceptualization of criminology is neither narrow nor confining. A scientific approach to understanding the etiology of crime may include the statistical, historical, clinical, or case-study tools of analysis. Moreover, there is nothing inherently quantitative in scientific methodology, albeit the most convincing evidence, data, and presentation in general sociological replications of propositions appear to be quantitative.[6] Probably the most fruitful source of analysis of empirical uniformity, regularity, and systems of patterned relationships can be found in the statistical studies of causation and prediction. However, interpretive analyses that may occasionally go beyond the limits of empirically correlated and organized data (but not beyond empirical reality) can be useful and enlightening. If description of the phenomena of crime is performed within a meaningful theoretical system, the methods and the goals of science are not necessarily discarded in the process but may be retained with all the vigor commonly attributed to sophisticated statistical manipulation.

We are contending that criminology should be considered as an autonomous, separate discipline and body of knowledge because it has accumulated its own set of organized data and theoretical conceptualizations that use the scientific method, approach to understanding, and attitude in research. This contention has recently been supported or at least examined by Vassalli,[7] Bianchi,[8] Grassberger,[9] Pinatel,[10] Pelaez.[11] Such a position does not negate the interdependence existing in the contributions to this discipline by a variety of other field specializations. Thus, sociology, psychology, psychiatry, law, history, biology, with such allied fields as endocrinology, physiology, physical anthropology, and biochemistry, may individually or collectively make substantial contributions to criminology without detracting from the idiosyncratic significance of criminology as an independent subject-matter of scientific investigation and concern. One need not adhere to a Comtian hierarchy of the sciences to realize the unity of all knowledge, or, especially, to appreciate the fact that a higher order of complexity of phenomena such as human behavior requires the use of disciplines devoted to specific aspects of this order. As the biochemist must use and rely upon research both in biology and chemistry in order to understand the functional interrelationship of physiological processes, and as the sociologist employs data from biology, psychology, and other disciplines to analyze the dynamic aspects of personality formation within a particular cultural milieu, so does the criminologist need and use related scientific information from different fields.

The argument may be made that there is no special separateness to criminology as exists in other disciplines, and that this fact, therefore, currently delays the existence of criminology as a distinct field. The histories of most scientific specialties follow similar developmental trends,[12] i.e. a branching-off from a larger, more inclusive area of investigation; next, an increasingly narrow, refined, and detailed analysis along 'idiographic' lines in order to legitimize devoted and disciplined concern with the special subject; and then a return to the 'nomothetic' and more enveloping universe of investigation that can embrace a variety of scientific specialties.[13] Thus, it appears that separate disciplines merge and develop in a way that is sympodial rather than unilinear.[14]

The early writings of Della Porta and Lavater on physiognomy and of Gall, Spurzheim, and others on phrenology were not principally concerned with criminal behavior, although references to the criminal occasionally appeared in their studies. Some historical continuity can be traced in medical literature from these writings on physiognomy and on craniology and from those of Pinel, Esquirol, and Rush, to Prichard, Ray, and Maudsley on moral insanity; from Despine and Morel on moral degeneracy to Lombroso on the born criminal and criminal type. Lombroso was primarily a physician and professor of psychiatry before acquiring a reputation as a criminal anthropologist. It was German materialism and French positivism, synthesized through the prism of Lombroso's medical training, that led to *L'Uomo Delinquente* in 1876 and to the shift of emphasis from the crime to the offender, from the classical to the Italian school. The new emphasis gave birth to the concentrated scientific study of crimogenesis that had long before been in embryonic state.[15] At least in part, the preoccupation with a medical approach to crime is still present in today's Italian criminology.[16]

But increasing specialization and delimited concentration *ultimately* lead to ever-wider areas of inquiry. By probing his subject-matter in depth, the scientist eventually reaches a point in his inquiry and hypothesis construction where he asks questions for which answers must come from more than one discipline. In more advanced stages of scientific inquiry, multidimensional and interdisciplinary approaches are almost inevitable. Although modifying but not abandoning his ideas of the atavistic criminal, Lombroso late in his career came to see (with the help of Ferri) the importance and necessity of examining the *social* 'causes and remedies of crime'.[17]

We thus see that maturity of a discipline involves increasing interdependence. The environmental approach in criminology, historically developing from roots distinctly different from Lombrosian precursors, eventually merged with the latter. Contemporary American criminology can be said to have an historical linkage with Guerry, Quetelet, and de Champneuf, who represented the cartographic school of the nineteenth century, as well as with Tarde's law of imitation, Durkheim's sociological determinism, and the environmental approaches of Ferri, Garofalo, Colajanni, and others.[18] The literature on crime, from an environmental perspective, may have grown from ideological bases quite different from those of Lombroso; yet the synthesis has occurred and is even now constantly reoccurring while inquiry and research proceed in both areas. From forensic medicine, clinical psychiatry, and anthropology, as well as from 'political arithmetic' and positivistic attempts at societal reconstruction, developed the sympodial branches of criminology, which today appears to be emerging as an independent discipline.

The diversity of present-day *approaches* to the study of crime and criminals can hardly be denied. Sellin has remarked in his introduction to the Swedish handbook of criminology:

> 'The sociologist studies crime as a social phenomenon and approaches this study with preconceptions, premises, frames of reference and techniques common to sociology, in which he is trained to do research. Psychologists, psychiatrists, endocrinologists, geneticists, and the representatives of many other disciplines similarly contribute to criminological knowledge only to the extent that they use their specialized training and funded knowledge in exploring problems of significance to an understanding of criminality. This is the inevitable result of the growing specialization of scientific work.' [19]

This diversity of approaches may lead some observers to believe that there is not a single separate scientific discipline of criminology. On the one hand, a macroscopic perspective views criminology as a study of crime that includes institutional patterns of law and the social reaction to crime in the form of adjudication and the integrated system of penal sanctions.[20] The analysis of crime from this institutional framework is well illustrated by Jerome Hall's[21] study of theft, by Radzinowicz's[22] review of the history of English criminal law, and by the general field of the 'sociology of law'.[23] On the other hand, microscopic analyses of criminal behavior or personality that attempt to measure significant differences between criminals and noncriminals take the form of biological, psychological, psychiatric, and sociological emphases. In the best sense of eclectic positivism, the Gluecks have generally proceeded in this manner in their abundant contributions to criminological research during the past thirty years.[24] It is commonplace in the field of criminology to refer to studies of organic diseases, identical twins, endocrinology, and somatotypes in the biological approach; to psychometric testing of intelligence, personality attributes, Freudian psychiatry in the psychological approach; and to ecological areas, differential association, culture conflict, role theory, and reference groups in the sociological approach.

Neither the definition of 'crime' nor that of the 'criminal' is standardized or universally accepted as a unit of criminological research. Perhaps more in the United States than elsewhere there are vital and critical differences in the conceptualization of these two terms. It is not merely that criminal statistics are subject to criticism there because of state variations in criminal statutes. The *Uniform Crime Reports* published by the Federal Bureau of Investigation under the auspices of the Department of Justice in Washington serve as a useful though not totally adequate basis for establishing a crime index for the nation.[25] The problem is deeper than this, however. The formal legalistic definition of crime as the unit of criminological research is posited against the broader concepts of conduct norms,[26] antisocial or deviant behavior,[27] and 'white-collar crime'.[28] The classic report of Michael and Adler,[29] the writings of Tappan,[30] and of Jeffery[31] suggest that the major perspective of crime should be a legal one. A similar position has been taken by many European legally oriented scholars.[32] Like Sellin and Sutherland, Gillin has emphasized the need for a wider, sociological unit for analysis by defining crime as 'an act that has been shown to be actually harmful to society, or that is *believed* to be socially harmful by a group of people that has the power to enforce its beliefs and that places such an act under the ban of positive penalties'.[33] The difference between these two approaches is, obviously, more apparent than real.

Can these diversities of approach and of operational definitions be considered as parts of a unitary whole? We think the answer is definitely in the affirmative. Analogy is not one of the strongest forms of argument, but it is often useful and convincing. If we examine other disciplines, we see similar diversities and problems of operational definitions. History is not only a methodological tool, it is a field of study as well. As such, history includes an obvious diversity of space-time dimensions to which politics, economics, medicine, technology, art, etc., contribute substantive data and provide theoretical insights.[34] Definitions and delimitations of historical periods still create problems for historians. Because the Middle Ages and the Renaissance merge 'like a trainwreck in time' there is no universal agreement about the designation for the period known commonly as 'the Renaissance'. Similarly with terms such as 'Classical', 'Romantic', 'Baroque', debates in historical analyses continue. The study of art can no longer be made on the basis of aesthetics alone, but increasingly requires knowledge of the culture milieu in which the artist and style were born and flourished, and even of psychological insights into the artist's personality.[35] Is the relatively new area of industrial sociology a contribution to an understanding of industry or of sociology? It is patently both. Does research with lysergic acid contribute to biochemistry or to psychiatry? Again, both. The cultural anthropologist who studies the law of primitive man[36] adds to the accumulated literature of anthropology, the philosophy of law, and criminology. We need not labor the point further, for differential approaches to the same subject-matter are manifestly present in all disciplines. The predominantly biological and legal orientation of some European criminology, which has a long historical tradition, and the American environment orientation that is equally linked to its own historical continuity are simply different approaches to the scientific study of crime and the criminal. So long as theory and research on crime, criminals, and social reaction to both are based upon a normative orientation that is *scientific* and whose goals constitute a description, measurement, analysis, or interpretation of patterns, uniformities, causal relationships, and probabilities, we may assert that such theory and research comprise the field and our meaning of criminology.

Finally, if all knowledge is unitary and separate disciplines are but artifacts of analysis, we should expect any single discipline to make contributions to other and especially to closely related fields. Specifically, criminology must be more than a recipient of empirical data and theory; it must also give something of substantial value to related areas of science. In this criterion of scientific specificity, criminology shows its weakest side. Probably because criminology is still a young science and temporally close to its nascency, it has not given as much as it has received. We cannot here engage in the polemics of measuring or reciting the quantity or quality of research and theory that freely flows to and from the field. However, despite its acknowledged indebtedness to other disciplines, criminology has made important contributions to the fuller understanding of deviant behavior, norms of conduct, personality formation, biological and psychological mechanisms of individual behavior, both normal and pathological, subcultural patterns of institutionalization, the structural-functional approach of social analysis, learning theory, class and status hierarchies, role theory, psychopathology, law, history, philosophy.[37] Moreover, criminology has used practically every particular tool of scientific research and has thereby strengthened and embellished these techniques through usage and experimentation. The statistical, historical, clinical, life-history, and experimental methods have been employed to advantage in every country where criminology has achieved the status of a university discipline. That teaching and research in criminology may be performed principally in schools of law or medicine in one country or region (as is the case in Europe) and mostly in departments of sociology in another country (as is the case in the United States) affects only the primary orientation of criminology. But differences in administrative localization also add to the diverse contributions that criminology may make. Increasingly in the future, criminology should be able to absorb disciplinary diversity and to provide more theoretical and empirical services to related disciplines, whether these areas be law, history, sociology, psychology, or biology. Several hopeful beginnings have been made both in Europe and America, but this interdisciplinary fertilization is still in its infancy.

We have said nothing thus far about penology. It is standard practice in America to include the subjects of probation, parole, imprisonment, and other treatment or punishment procedures in the field of academic teaching of criminology. May we legitimately include 'corrections' or 'penology' under our meaning of criminology? The answer should probably be negative if by 'corrections' is meant the social work activities of probation and parole officers, the organization and administrative functions of the police, or the management of penal institutions. The answer should be affirmative, however, if we mean, as previously indicated, the scientific analysis, measurement, and interpretation of patterns, regularities, causal or associational relationships and probabilities of the same subareas of criminology. If control and prediction in experimentation are integral goals of research, and, regardless of the substantive area, if analysis proceeds by means of the scientific method, then we may include within the scope of criminology any correctional research that embraces these goals and this method.[38] Matters purely of public or judicial administration may have peripheral interest but do not constitute a science of crime. Technical operations in the management of a police force or of a prison do not fall within our framework of reference to criminology. Historical studies that trace the evolution of punishment, if properly conceived and executed, may very well be included in the history of criminology. Various kinds of analyses of the police, judicial, and penal statistics are part of criminology, but the mere tabulation without scientific inquiry of a prison population certainly is not. Any study of the offender after the crime that seeks to understand the causal or treatment process and that employs a scientific perspective and method is contained within our meaning of criminology. Group or individual psychotherapeutic analyses and prison community or parole prediction studies should be included. Phenomenological studies of such crimes as homicide, embezzlement, and narcotic drug violations, and even taxonomic exercises establishing Weberian ideal types for purposes of analysis, are legitimate areas of criminology. Expert opinions on single offenders are certainly made in the area of criminology, their proper site being forensic medicine and forensic psychiatry. However, carefully conducted psychiatric studies of groups of offenders can be, and have been, part of criminology.

The question of whether it is necessary to divide the discipline into 'pure' criminology and 'applied' criminology is now rarely raised. The dichotomy into pure and applied sociology has been an issue in that discipline since the days of Auguste Comte and more especially in America since the writings of Lester Ward. A socially utilitarian end that directs the course and sets the framework for analysis in a research design has been considered applied research.[39] Practical and almost immediate application of research for preconceived administrative or clinical purposes would connote 'applied' criminology. If the research aided the police to make investigations or to collect evidence leading to the arrest of an offender or if it helped the probation or parole officers to work more effectively among those in their charge, it would appear to be 'applied' criminology. As Greenwood[40] has indicated, this original dichotomy between pure and applied research is breaking down today. Because an administrative organization designates the area of interest and thereby to some extent sets the limits to the number and kinds of variables to be measured or to the goals of research, this action does not per se reduce the 'purity' of scientific analysis. A public authority that offers direction to investigation may in fact be an encouragement to research; and whether or not the findings have practical applicability does not determine the scientific character of research.[41] Interference in the scientific process, public policy that alone dictates choice of research methods, or suppression, distortion, or falsification of data are among the things that destroy scientificity. These are the major considerations of consequence in so-called 'applied' criminology.

Rather than concentrate on 'pure' versus 'applied' criminology, the primary question is whether the process of application of criminological research findings should be labeled criminology. Our reply is negative and concurs with remarks made by Sellin.[42] Use of scientific findings in social-work relationships with clients (or, more precisely in this consideration, criminal offenders) may be highly desirable but does not constitute science, hence, is not criminology. The juvenile court judge who would make use of the 'Social Prediction Scale' devised by the Gluecks and suggested by them as an appropriate guide in sentencing, is not engaging in a scientific pursuit. What the Gluecks have done is criminology; what the judge does with the results of criminology is administration of justice.

Thus we see that application of scientific research findings is not criminology – with one obvious exception: if these research findings are used by another researcher in criminology, either in the form of a replicated study as documentary support or as propositions upon which new hypotheses are constructed, this form of application is manifestly for scientific purposes, is absorbed once again into the scientific process, and is quite different from application in criminal policy. Therefore, in slight modification of our original contention, we may say that application of scientific research *for* scientific research is criminology; whereas, application of research in nonscientific pursuits is not criminology.

THE DEFINITION OF A CRIMINOLOGIST

Having defined and described the meaning of criminology, we turn to our next task, which is to determine *who* is the criminologist. Generally speaking, we shall contend that a criminologist is anyone engaged in the pursuit of learning embraced by our meaning of criminology. A criminologist is one whose professional training, occupational role, and pecuniary reward are primarily concentrated on a scientific approach to, and study and analysis of, the phenomena of crime and criminal behavior.[43] However, because we have referred to the wide diversity of approaches to the understanding of crime, questions may arise regarding the designation of 'criminologist' when applied to specific individuals who contribute segmental information to the field from other disciplines.

A physical anthropologist who participates in an interdisciplinary research on delinquency or crime, and who makes anthropomorphic measurements of a control group and an experimental group of delinquents, is not, by reason of this isolated activity, a criminologist. Hooton's[44] excursion in 1938 with *The American Criminal* did not gain for him a high status in criminology, although there was no impairment of his reputation as a physical anthropologist. William Sheldon[45] likewise is not a criminologist because of his *Varieties of Delinquent Youth* any more than is Seltzer,[46] who aided the Gluecks in *Unraveling Juvenile Delinquency*. This is not to say that a physical anthropologist cannot also be a criminologist. Should the application of anthropometry be made principally and regularly in the pursuit of hypotheses regarding crime and criminals, and should the body of scientific knowledge accumulated in general criminology be absorbed by the anthropologist in his training, then he most properly may bear the mantle of criminologist.

Correspondingly, the psychometrician or clinical psychologist does not *ipso facto* become a criminologist because he administers a Wechsler Bellevue Test to criminal subjects or because he interviews 200 inmates in a prison. Application of the Rorschach test to 500 delinquents does not qualify the administrator as a criminologist. And the sociologist who teaches a single undergraduate course in criminology as his only professional contact with the field is a sociologist, but he does not meet the criteria we have adopted to describe a criminologist.

It becomes clear, then, that, regardless of the diverse nature of contributory professions to criminology, there is an independent discipline to be learned and a special professional role to be performed. Whereas, it is true that no criminologist can function as a 'pure' criminologist without some other type of training and orientation (sociology, psychology, psychiatry, the law, etc.), there is a unit of analysis, a framework of reference, and a body of collected, organized, and analyzed knowledge that are available and must be required learning before an individual can function as a scientific agent in any field of criminology. Probably no scientist exists who is unadulterated by the data or theory of some other discipline than his own. (Perhaps only the mathematician can be 'pure' in this sense, but then we might contend that mathematics is either a tool or, in its higher complexities, sophisticated artistry and not a science.) The student of criminology could conceivably be trained with so broad an eclecticism that no single disciplinary orientation would dominate his thinking, but the present pedagogic arrangements, both on the European continent and in America, would make such a person a rarity. Consequently our generalization must be that, although the criminologist usually has a simultaneous or antecedent training in some other discipline than that of criminology, the other discipline becomes the avenue through which he enters criminology. The orientation is that which he brings into play as he engages in study and research in criminology. Thus, the anthropologist, psychiatrist, psychologist, and sociologist who have *also* obtained mastery of understanding and knowledge of the body of information and research that are contained in the field of criminology, and whose professional roles are centered upon the study of and research into crime or criminal behavior, are all criminologists.[47]

At present the title of criminologist is indiscriminately used to refer to anyone whose professional activity is focused on criminals. The probation officer, the psychiatrist in a penal institution, the technician in a ballistics section of a police department, the lie-detector analyst, the investigator for the district attorney's office, and even the professor of criminal law have occasionally been referred to as 'criminologists'. It is our contention that none of these persons by reason only of his activity is a criminologist; and that none of these professional activities constitutes criminology. What, then, can we say about the police officer, the lawyer, the judge, the prison superintendent, the probation or parole officer, and persons engaged in similar tasks? There is, of course, no simple or categorical answer, but there is an answer consistent with our foregoing remarks about the meaning of criminology and the function of a criminologist.

If any one of these persons in pursuance of his occupational role is principally devoted to the task of *scientific* study, research, and analysis of the phenomenon of crime, criminal behavior, or treatment of the offender, his role is that of a criminologist. It is generally unlikely that any of the aforementioned persons is thus occupied. In most cases the closest they come to being 'scientists' is in the application of criminological research findings, but as we have elsewhere indicated this kind of application is not criminology. We may refer to them, as Sellin has earlier done, as 'technologists' and the work in which they are engaged as 'criminotechnology'.[48] Working with criminal offenders is not a sufficient criterion for designation as a criminologist. The role of a peace officer consists in preventing, detecting, and investigating crime, in arresting and interrogating criminals and making them available for judicial action. He may make use of scientific knowledge such as may be found in chemical analyses of bloodstains or in ballistics reports, but he is engaged in application, not in production, of scientific knowledge. He may be partially responsible for providing the raw datum to be later used in research, but obviously this activity (no more than that of the census enumerator) is not science.

Our conception of criminology cannot be so narrow that the study of criminal law, judicial process, and penal treatment of the offender becomes excluded. Thus, study, research, and analysis that proceed along methodological lines embraced by science can be made by the student of law, members of the judiciary, and administrators or executors of penal treatment. However, the practicing attorney, the sitting judge, and the superintendent of the prison, by reason of their occupational relationships *per se* to crime and criminals, are no more criminologists than the criminologist who does research on the sentencing power and functions of judges is a judge. That two compatible professional roles may be performed simultaneously is, of course, possible, so a prison administrator may also be a criminologist if he should design, direct, or supervise a criminological research program in his institution. By the same logic a criminologist may be administrative chairman of a university department of sociology; the two statuses are compatible and coexistent but distinctly different.

By now it should be obvious that probation and parole officers may apply knowledge accumulated from research in social work, psychology and psychiatry but that they are not criminologists. The art of working with people, of guiding, supervising, directing, operating upon or controlling others remains *an art* whether or not scientific principles are applied in such interaction. Similarly, custodial officers in a prison, though surrounded by and working constantly with prisoners, are not criminologists.

A logically consistent and circumscribed position results from the previous discussion: a criminologist is one whose professional role is devoted to criminology. Any definition of criminology inferentially sets limits to the role of a criminologist. Our definition of criminology, though wide in the scope of subject-matter contained within the field, is narrow in terms of procedural processes and purposive goals. There are differences of opinion among criminologists about the inclusion and emphasis of certain types of subject-matter in criminology. This is a substantive and theoretical matter for discussion and debate. However, it should be clear and unmistakable that criminology means the use of the scientific method in the study and analysis of regularities, uniformities, patterns, and causal relationships concerned with crime, criminals, or criminal behavior.

MAJOR RESEARCH TRENDS IN CRIMINOLOGY

Although criminology is a relatively new scientific discipline, in recent decades there has been such a plethora of books, monographs, papers presented before meetings, articles, special reports and analyses by bureaus of correction on national and local levels that a thorough review of research is impossible because of limitations of space. At this stage of development it is even difficult to determine which of the many studies in criminology will have lasting significance. Of considerable aid to research in progress are: (a) 'A Bibliographical Manual for the Student of Criminology,'[49] published by the International Society of Criminology; (b) 'The Criminological Research Bulletin,' published by the *Journal of Criminal Law, Criminology and Police Science*;[50] (c) *Current Sociological Research*,[51] by the American Sociological Association; (d) *Research Relating to Children*,[52] published by the Children's Bureau in Washington, D.C.; and (e) *Sociological Abstracts* and *Psychological Abstracts*, which include a special section on criminology; (f) a clearing-house of information on research programs, which the National Council on Crime and Delinquency has established in the United States; (g) the launching of *Excerpta Criminologica*;[53] and (h) the excellent bibliographies published regularly by the United Nations Social Defence Section, as part of the *International Review of Criminal Policy*.

CLINICAL CRIMINOLOGY

History and Development in Various Countries

An interesting development that should be discussed in some detail is represented by the congeries of activities which are referred to as clinical criminology. At present clinical criminology is best represented by, but by no means limited to, some of the applications of criminological knowledge to correctional and forensic problems in European countries. It has achieved a measure of independence, and different textbooks and papers have identified it as a separate trend in criminology. Briefly, it represents the joint and integrated application of criminological knowledge and diagnostic skills to individual cases for purposes of diagnosis and treatment. Historically, this trend leads back to the medical individualistic tradition in criminology exemplified by the early Lombrosian efforts, reinforced by broad generalizations by Ferri and Garofalo.[54] However, the first practical realization of clinical criminological work took place, as Pinatel describes, in Latin America. Already in 1907 José

Ingenieros had developed an institute of criminology in Argentina, which followed an explicitly stated policy of clinical criminology. Other important national developments took place in the United States. In 1909, William Healy inaugurated the activities of a juvenile psychopathic clinic, later renamed the Institute for Juvenile Research in Cook County and still active, in which concentration was mostly on psychological and psychiatric examinations.[55] In 1913 an American Association of Clinical Criminology was founded, but the subsequent developments of the sociological school of criminology came to dominate the organization.[56] Several European countries, at the beginning of the present century, institutionalized clinical criminological activities in different levels of the judicial and correctional systems, as these activities could be adapted to the local settings. We can only refer in this context to brief examples without any pretense of completeness.[57] In Belgium, the work of Verwaeck in 1914 initiated the practice of detailed case studies in the correctional system, soon followed in Austria and Germany by the Graz Institute with a strong criminalistic approach, and by the Society for the Study of Criminal Biology in Bavaria. In Scandinavia, the dedicated work of Olof Kinberg and others represented a concentrated effort unparalleled in other countries.[58] Kinberg's textbook,[59] recently republished, still constitutes profitable reading for any serious student in criminology. To him we also owe one of the best definitions of clinical criminology. In his view, all criminology is a clinical science, concerned with individual cases in order to give a causal explanation of the crime, conceived as a reaction of individual personality to a certain situation, in order to find a rational treatment in order to eliminate the causes of the criminal symptoms. The strong organismic bent which characterized Kinberg's work, and which was founded on the personality theory propounded by Sjøbring,[60] somewhat limits the popularity of this Scandinavian approach in a psychiatric world mainly dominated by Freudian psychoanalytic formulations. It remains, however, as one of the more consistent and better integrated systems in clinical criminology. The strong medical tradition prevailing in the Scandinavian countries is still very viable and finds its expression in the existence of well-articulated and encompassing medical criminological services. It has also sponsored some of the most daring applications of medical and surgical advances in the field of criminology. The work of Rylander in the application of psychosurgery in criminal cases and the use of castration represent examples of such a trend. In Denmark, clinical criminology found its best application in the work of the Institution for Criminal Psychopaths at

Herstedvester, under the direction of Georg Stürup.[61] In Holland, a well-known example of clinical criminological work can be found in the Psychiatric Observation Clinic connected with Utrecht University. There is also in that country an interesting and new existential approach to criminology, exemplified by the writings of Bianchi and the Utrecht group.[62] In France, the Centre Nationale d'Orientation at Fresnes exemplifies one of the few attempts at mass application of clinical criminological principles to the classification and diagnostic intake of criminals. Recent French legislation has extended the requirement of personality examination to most of the correctional population.[63] A number of international meetings have been focused on what appears to be the most immediate practical application of the techniques of clinical criminology, i.e. the personality examination of the offender.[64] Inevitably, the largest area of application of the tools proposed for diagnosis and treatment by clinical criminology, because of the legal problems connected with their implementation, has been in the field of juvenile delinquency. No major juvenile system in any Western country today lacks diagnostic facilities, and several have extensive treatment facilities. A good example in the juvenile field is the British borstal system. In the United States there are several well-equipped diagnostic centers, such as the Medical Facility of Vacaville, California, and the New Jersey Diagnostic Center in Menlo Park, among the better known. There are, of course, psychiatric clinics functioning as part of judicial systems in various parts of the country. A good example is the Bellevue Clinic attached to the Court of General Sessions, whose work has recently been summarized by Messinger and Apfelberg.[65] Moreover, the earlier work of Bernard Glueck,[66] Winfred Overholser,[67] Wilson and Pescor,[68] and others was instrumental in the development and use of psychiatry in court and correctional settings. Although modest, occasional expressions of interest in the clinical approach have been present in the American literature;[69] some of these 'pioneer' writings come from what was called 'clinical sociology'.[70] Manfred Guttmacher's work at the relatively recent Patuxent Institution established under the defective delinquent statute of Maryland is an interesting and new experiment in clinical work with seriously disturbed criminal psychopaths.

In Japan, the Association of Correctional Medicine was organized in the early 1950s. Masao Otsu, as president of this organization, and Akira Masaki, president of the Japanese Correctional Association, were much responsible for the development of clinical criminology in that country, and for sponsoring the first joint meeting of the Japanese Association of

Correctional Medicine and the American Medical Correctional Association headed by Ralph Banay, in Tokyo, 1960.[71] Clinical work in detention centers and prisons has apparently become fairly routine practice in the last decade in Japan.[72]

In Italy the strong biological tradition instituted by Lombroso was continued, after ideological conflicts between the extreme advocates of positivism and the conservative efforts of the idealistic classical school by the work of scholars like Ottolenghi, De Sanctis, and Di Tullio.[73] One interesting development that has taken place in Italy is the convergence of interest in the study of criminal behavior on the part of the schools of forensic medicine and the more generally medically oriented criminologists. This development did not preclude, from the beginning, an interest in sociological factors, as evident, for example, in the writings of Di Tullio.[74] The prestige of the medical profession and the wealth of empirical material put at the disposal of the practitioners in both these fields by their work as experts to the courts, have continued a medical focus in criminology in Italy. On the other hand, the slow and retarded development of the social sciences which followed the idealistic dominance prevented the emergence of a sociologically oriented criminology except in the person of Niceforo.[75] In psychology, the biological tradition and the academic and professional links between psychology and medicine, aligned the psychologists with medically oriented criminologists and forensic psychiatrists.[76] Di Tullio's work is best exemplified by his conceptualization of the 'criminal constitution'. He tries to reduce the Lombrosian overtones of this term by consistently stressing the need for the examination of the 'global personality', drawing completeness and closure both from an awareness of social factors inspired by the principles of the more positivistic sociology of England and America and from a recognition of the usefulness of the anthropo-phenomenological, intuitive methodology of classical German psychiatry.

In the correctional field in Italy, this approach is represented in the comprehensive and detailed case studies conducted at the Institute for Observation of Young Adult Offenders in Rebibbia, Rome.[77] The research that is performed is on the individual offender, but funds are not provided in the budget of the Institute for testing general hypotheses about crime causation or effectiveness of treatment. Sociology is not an integral part of the Institute, not because this discipline cannot make important contributions both in a general analytical way and in introducing its own concepts, but because this discipline in Italy has little status and is more social philosophy than empirical or hypothesis-generating theory.

The cases at Rebibbia are obviously selective, and the multiple-factor approach is evident in the methodology. But this approach, it should be kept in mind, is used in a clinical etiology-treatment process similar to medical practice and not as a method of testing generalized hypotheses about criminality in the same way as criminology proceeds to study crime and criminals *en masse*. In a sense, each offender at Rebibbia becomes a research project with a team of professional specialists assuming specific tasks that contribute to an understanding of the phenomena responsible for the behavior of the subject before them. Each technician has his own set of hypotheses to test. The more delimited area of some (e.g. endocrinologist, internist) and the more pervasive, diffuse areas of others (e.g. psychologist, psychiatrist) more frequently favor rejection of hypotheses of the former group and acceptance of those of the latter group.

The Main Approaches and Their Limitations

In this clinical setting, then, a multiple-factor approach has meaning and pragmatic use, whether or not multiple-factor studies produce valid general theories of crime causation. In the absence of a proved theory from any single discipline that is applicable to all or even most offenders, the clinical setting in fact has no alternative but a multifaceted perspective. However, this necessity does not preclude the testing of broader theories or the development of a theoretical system for promoting research that transcends clinical and individual analysis. The integration of sociology into this setting might be helpful in encouraging an interdisciplinary trend where only multidisciplinary approaches now operate.

In close keeping with similar trends in the field of psychology, the focus of interest in clinical criminology is the individual *per se*. This focus admittedly limits the activities of the clinician to the immediate and temporarily restricted solution of individual diagnostic and treatment problems. Diagnosis is considered as a much more detailed and complicated process than the single application of a diagnostic label. It is, in effect, a personality analysis and reconstruction firmly grounded on the biology of the personality itself but extended to embrace the social determinants and implications of behavior. The clinical process, by definition, must make use of widely divergent methodologies and techniques, often unproved experimentally and occasionally conflicting, as in the case of the coexistence on the same diagnostic team of a physical anthropologist and a dynamically oriented, orthodox Freudian psychiatrist. This inevitably limits the possibility that clinical criminology will achieve the more rigorous methodology of sociology, and the humanitarian ethos of the field precludes experimentation as an avenue of development. At the same time, it greatly restricts the likelihood that clinical criminology will ever offer an encompassing theory of criminal genesis and criminal dynamics. It is admittedly a limited approach to the problem of crime, focused on immediate individual needs, designed to fulfill an action-oriented and socially required activity of the scientist. Although it must be aware of its limitations, it cannot be replaced by the grandiose social programs now frequently propounded by social policymakers and community organization workers. Clinical criminology must follow a multidisciplinary approach open at both ends of the biosocial continuum of sciences. Its best hopes for the future lie in the transformation from multi- to interdisciplinary and in the constant awareness of scientific development in both the biological and the sociological sciences. In this sense, the clinical criminologist is more frequently a consumer than a creator of theoretical formulations and constructs. On the other hand, the scientist, particularly the sociologist, working at the macroscopic theoretical level must rely for proof upon the functions of the clinician working through individuals who ultimately are collected together as arrays of variables and attributes for statistical manipulation and analysis.

SOCIOLOGICAL CRIMINOLOGY

In the United States criminological teaching, training, and research occur principally within the framework of sociology. A survey of recent past research in criminology in that country appears in Marshall Clinard's two chapters on this topic, one of which is entitled, 'The Sociology of Delinquency and Crime', published in *Review of Sociology: Analysis of a Decade*;[78] the other is 'Criminological Research', in *Sociology Today*.[79] In the first of these two chapters Clinard reviews sociological research and writing during the past ten years under such topics as: the nature of crime, criminal behavior and society, behavior systems, the theory of differential association, personality traits, war and crime, the administration of criminal justice, prediction of recidivism, and research techniques. Other topics in the latter chapter include anomie, class structure, the problem of differential response, situational factors, delinquent typologies, gang research. Our purpose in the present section, therefore, is not to review in detail the past or present researches in the field, for these have been amply covered elsewhere. Our primary purpose here is to indicate in broad outline the present *trends* of research, their conflicts, limitations, and strengths.

Earlier Trends in Research

To understand current criminology in the United States it is necessary to recall briefly the sociological tradition within which criminology has emerged. Before the First World War American criminological ideas and studies were primarily a reflection of European criminology. Much was written on the social aspects of crime mostly by social workers and journalists who discussed the evils of urban living, ignorance, poverty, immigration, the influence of alcohol, immorality, and so forth, as causes of crime in a general way. The first work bearing the title of 'Criminology' was published in the last decade of the nineteenth century by Arthur MacDonald,[80] who had accepted Lombroso's conclusions and was satisfied with the presentation of these to the American audience. In 1904 a course in criminology appeared on the curriculum of Princeton University, but it was not until 1918 that the first textbook for students in criminology appeared, written by a sociologist, Maurice Parmelee.[81] This book had a strong European orientation and was mainly a restatement of data that were included in the same author's book published a decade earlier on criminal anthropology.[82] In the period before the First World War a number of classical works in criminology by Lombroso, Garofalo, Ferri, Tarde, Saleilles, de Quiros, Aschaffenburg, and Bonger had been translated and published by the American Institute of Criminal Law and Criminology, founded in 1909. During the same year the Institute initiated publication of the *Journal of Criminal Law and Criminology*, so that American sociologists were made familiar with foreign criminological studies which until that time had been largely unknown to them. The International Congress of Criminal Anthropology held in Europe before the First World War had rarely been attended by Americans.[83]

The first generation of sociologists were philosophers, systematizers, introspectionists, but after the First World War American sociology entered a new phase and became more empirically oriented. American sociology became increasingly different from European social sciences generally and sociology in particular, which were primarily concerned with a highly macroscopic interpretation of society's development.[84] In the United States the broad outline of society and its major values were more likely to be taken for granted, with an emphasis given to particular 'social problems'. There was concern with how actual situations deviated from values and here problems were associated with slums, rural life, immigration, and Negro–white relations. This kind of interest, says Parsons,[85] helps to explain why American sociology has been far less concerned with the borderline of philosophy than has European sociology. Like general sociology, criminology has stemmed from its applied interests. This concentration on less macroscopic problems had a special advantage, however, for it encouraged the development of a variety of techniques for empirical research, as, for example, the use of personal documents, interviewing, questionnaires, and participant observations. These technical developments coincided with a similar growth in statistical methods. In general, American interest in empirical matters and this technical emphasis became much more pronounced than in Europe and helped significantly to speed the development of criminology, carried along by sociology, as an empirical science.

On the other hand, the pinpointing of research, made necessary by the labor and time involved in securing data, resulted in research that was more and more restricted and that often involved relatively unimportant questions. An increasing concern with methods in research techniques sometimes produced studies without firm theoretical foundations, largely in the hope that the mere random assemblage of heterogeneous data might, when analyzed, yield something of value. To the theoretical system-builders came a negative reaction that took the form of extreme empiricism and blindly rejected the help of theoretical tools in general.[86] This headcounting, fact-finding, survey form of empiricism continued through the 1920s and 1930s until shortly before the Second World War, when empirical inadequacy was exposed to the necessity for theoretical reconstruction. Even with recognition of the inadequacy of mere fact-finding, little that was new in theoretical formulation occurred until after the Second World War. Attempts were made to integrate the biological, psychological, and sociological emphases that had factored out important variables in earlier research, but these attempts usually resulted in unintegrated formulations that included a biopsychological or biosocial approach referred to by Gillin[87] as the 'modern clinical' approach or by others as the multiple-causation approach. There has been practically no interdisciplinary research, and up to the present time multidisciplinary research has not produced an integrated theory of criminal etiology. In Europe, the different schools showed a similar lag for different reasons.

Although American criminological research reflects the trends of American sociology in general, criminology was stimulated also by

William Healy's *The Individual Delinquent* (1915), which not only contained the first extensive survey of European researches on criminal behavior made by an American scientist, but also was rich in carefully analyzed case-history data from the first psychiatry clinic in the United States, organized by Healy for the express purpose of studying delinquents in connection with the juvenile court in Chicago in 1909. Healy played a leading role in the development of psychological and psychiatric criminology in the United States, as we have noted, and helped found the American Orthopsychiatric Association and the *American Journal of Orthopsychiatry*. His work stimulated the emphasis on multiple causation, but did not entirely replace the predominant sociological themes of the ecological school, which was developed by Ernest Burgess at the University of Chicago and brought into criminological research by Clifford Shaw and Henry McKay.[88]

The complete history of criminological thought has yet to be written. Such a history would include a description and analysis of the development of ideas from classical, medieval, and early modern times that slowly contributed to the emergence of a science related to the study of the criminal process and criminal behavior. Criminological thought antedating Lombroso was diversified and disunited, but slowly became amalgamated into a growing body of literature that made possible the appearance of a Lombrosian perspective during the last quarter of the nineteenth century. The accelerated growth of criminological thought and research since Lombroso has resulted in an accumulation of such dimensions that it is becoming increasingly difficult for single individuals to absorb and integrate all the materials. The previous reference that we have made to the contributions from a variety of disciplines to an understanding of criminal behavior makes obvious the problems of integrating theoretical and empirical research. There are whole libraries of clinical data from psychiatrists, innumerable studies by psychologists and psychometricians who have worked with criminals, and an abundant number of independent studies by sociologists. Techniques of analysis have in the past fifty years become increasingly refined, and studies are often so esoteric or localized that it is difficult to project any conclusions or interpretations beyond the confines of the geographical or temporal dimensions of the initial research. We have passed through usage of a variety of special techniques, including the clinical approach found in Healy's *The Individual Delinquent*[89] and still active in Italy with Di Tullio[90] and his school; the ecological analyses growing out of the studies of Shaw and McKay up through the work of Mannheim[91] and

Lander[92] and Morris.[93] The use of analytical induction is exemplified in such studies as W. I. Thomas's *The Unadjusted Girl*,[94] Lindesmith's *Opiute Addiotion*,[95] Cressey's *Other People's Money*.[96] The anthropometrical studies from Lombroso's *L'Uomo Delinquente*[97] to Hooton's *American Criminal*[98] and more recently Sheldon's *Varieties of Delinquent Youth*[99] and the Glueck's *Physique and Delinquency*[100] stand apart as separate kinds of analyses. Psychiatric studies have also been generally separated from the anthropometric-biological and even the sociological frameworks of analysis.

In short, it is possible to trace the development of criminology along traditional lines of biology, psychology, and sociology without much overlapping or integration of any of these approaches. This categorization of disciplinary approach to the understanding of human behavior generally has carried over to an analysis of criminal behavior. These separate historical lines became artifacts created for purposes of delimiting areas of analysis and making easier the task of reducing the number of variables requiring analysis in any configuration of variables connected with the etiology of delinquency.

Recent Trends

In more recent times, within the last thirty years, this same kind of multiplicity of frameworks is still evident. As we have noted, the ecological approach, although diminishing in importance, has probably had more careful usage and has its own traditional framework from Shaw and McKay to Terence Morris. Social processes in behavior systems of crime have been scrutinized by Shaw in *The Jackroller*,[101] in *Brothers in Crime*,[102] Sutherland's *Professional Thief*,[103] David Maurer's *The Big Con*,[104] Sutherland's *White Collar Crime*,[105] Clinard's *The Black Market*,[106] and Cressey's *Other People's Money*.[107] Phenomenological approaches to crime, which involve detailed analyses of the processes and patterns and regularities of behavior, have included such studies as Gillin's *Wisconsin Prisoner*,[108] which examined both sex offenders and those involved in murder; Henry and Short's *Suicide and Homicide*,[109] Wolfgang's *Patterns in Criminal Homicide*,[110] and investigations of sex offenders. Unfortunately, there has thus far been inadequate attention and research time given to a full description and analysis of the specific forms of criminal offense types. Probably because of the seriousness of homicide and its high degree of social visibility (hence detection), this offense has received more attention than most other types of criminal offense from a phenomenological perspective.[111]

There have been many studies using a multidimensional perspective, among which probably the most prominent have been made by the Gluecks. Whether their point of departure was a follow-up of adult offenders released from a reformatory or of juvenile offenders discharged from child guidance clinics and grown up or an etiological analysis of variables and attributes associated with delinquency, as in *Unraveling Juvenile Delinquency*, the Gluecks have followed the tradition commonly referred to as Comtian positivism or neo-positivism. This tradition involves the collection of a variety of facts from available sources, regardless of how these data may explicitly fit into a particular theoretical framework. As a matter of fact, this multiple-causation approach, best exemplified by the Gluecks, uses whatever data are present for developing insights that will, it is hoped, emerge through inductive reasoning in the final analysis of the collated data. We must refer to these studies as multidimensional rather than interdisciplinary, for each of the disciplines contributing to the accumulation of facts still continues with a separate perspective and independent conclusions, without reference to the other disciplines that are making proportionately equal, greater, or lesser contributions to the study. While the ultimate aim of these studies may be to produce a multiple-factor analysis, thus combining un-integrated research, in their present form they continue to present to the field merely independent analyses of body structure, mental and emotional attributes, parental relationships, and environmental conditions. However mindful the Gluecks may appear to be of the need to integrate their abundant material, integration and theory have not yet emerged.

Criminological theory has been characterized by separateness or insulation from many of these empirical contributions. There is a body of literature in criminological theory that almost stands apart from the other references, tools of analysis, and types of study we have previously mentioned. It is concerned with a line of developmental thought that can be traced from Durkheim's study of suicide and social integration,[112] through Sutherland's 'differential association',[113] Merton's analysis of anomie and social structure,[114] Parsons's theory of social action and sex-age roles,[115] to the recent analyses of delinquent gangs by Cohen,[116] Bloch and Niederhoffer,[117] Walter Miller,[118] and, most recently, Cloward and Ohlin.[119] Criminological theory in the United States owes a considerable debt to Sutherland's 'differential association' and Sellin's 'culture conflict' and conflict of norms, for the present emphasis on subculture analysis that views delinquency and crime principally from a psychosociological viewpoint – and in terms of role theory,

C

reference groups, 'significant others', conduct norms at variance with the predominant (middle-class) society, and even or more especially by reference to the normal rather than to the pathological delinquent – is related to the works of these two creative theorists. There have been various extensions of both the differential-association and the conflict-of-norms approach through such refinements as Cressey's further elaboration of Sutherland's original formulations,[120] Glaser's 'differential identification',[121] Sykes and Matza's 'techniques of neutralization',[122] Cohen and Short's attempts to identify particular patterns of subcultural forms of delinquency,[123] and Cloward and Ohlin's descriptions of the criminal, conflict, and retreatist subcultures,[124] by using as their point of departure for analysis elements of the taxonomy presented by Robert Merton.[125]

It is not our purpose here to examine in detail these studies or theories of criminality, or to embark upon a careful critique of any of them. We have made reference to a variety of significant studies and theories in order to indicate very clearly the isolatedness and the insularity of criminological research and thinking that occur even within the provincial confines of American criminology. Criminological theory has proceeded almost as if completely ignoring the abundance of empirical data that have been collected in support or rejection of delimited hypotheses. Theory without data is speculative and at best heuristic; data-collection without theory is heterogeneous fact-finding. Isolated, independent, and unilateral research that fails to relate findings to other research closely connected to the instant focus of attention simply compounds the isolarity of the analysis and interpretation.

But whether psychological, sociological, or psychiatric studies of criminal behavior – combined with their allied fields of biology, anthropometry, endocrinology, and so forth – can be integrated into a unified approach to the understanding of criminal behavior is an issue which criminologists have not entirely ignored.

The issue is primarily between those who advocate a positivist eclecticism or multiple-factor approach and those who demand or require a generalized theory of criminal conduct for purposes of analysis. The conflict, which sometimes results in vitriolic denunciations of the other's position, reveals the ambiguity and ambivalence of contemporary criminological thought. Most American textbook writers, including Gillin,[126] Tappan,[127] Caldwell,[128] Reckless,[129] Taft,[130] and Barnes and Teeters[131] assume the necessity for a multidimensional, eclectic multiple-factor approach to an understanding of crime, criminal process, and criminal behavior. Clinical criminology is certainly a manifestation of the multiple-factor approach, for relative to criminogenesis this school suggests that the criminal is the product of his biological inheritance conditioned in his development by the experiences of life to which he has been exposed from early infancy up to the time of the commission of the crime. In studying the criminal, therefore, its methods represent an approximation to the processes of modern medicine. Crime is looked upon not as some sort of abstract entity but as a kind of conduct that grows out of the response of a certain kind of biological organism to certain kinds of experience.

The multiple-factor approach and its critics

Representing the multiple-factor 'thesis' and the eclectic approach to causation, Sheldon Glueck recently stated that '. . . reliable researches, with their solidly verified factual foundations, indicate much more pointedly and specifically [than sweeping generalizations] the how and why of participation of community institutions in delinquency prevention programs and in addition indicate the role of various forms of psychotherapy and group therapy in a preventive program, as well as other approaches *relevant to the facts* revealed in the intensive study of several samples of delinquents and criminals and nondelinquents'.[132] The Gluecks, along with other scholars such as Mabel Elliot, Francis Merrill, Ruth Cavan, and Caldwell, insist that crime is a product of a large number and great variety of factors and that these factors can be organized into general propositions. As previously indicated, Healy was probably among the first to emphasize multiple causation in the cases of individual delinquents at a time when many persons were seeking to discount the biological and physical explanations of crime. Healy was determined then, as the Gluecks are today, that no theoretical orientation or preconception could influence his findings and that he would simply observe *any* causal factor that he found. As Sutherland and Cressey[133] point out, the consequence of his (Healy's) 'crass empiricism' was the discovery of no less than 170 distinct conditions, every one of which was considered as conducive to delinquency. The difficulty with locating factors, say the opponents of the multiple approach, is that these factors are usually arrayed in such a way that each is given equal importance; or, if they are not assigned equal weight in the contribution to crime, then attempts are made to distinguish degrees of importance and often the result is as much ambiguity as before. The adherents of the multiple-factor approach generally agree on the virtue of an integrated theory, and usually suggest that such a theory can develop out of the accumulation of factorial information over long periods of time and under diverse circumstances. They usually have a self-image of being data-collectors and of having the strength of empiricism behind them. Whether a homogeneous set of factors or a multidisciplinary, heterogeneous collection of factors forms the basis of their research, some of them have become increasingly sophisticated statistically, and perhaps the current prestige of this approach is reflected in the greater amount of statistical analysis now occurring in criminological research.

Hartung,[134] in his 'critique of the sociological approach', attacks the multiple-factor approach by suggesting that 'no conceptual scheme is provided by which the different disciplines could be organically unified into a single discipline or into a single theory (*not* a single factor)'.[135] The Gluecks, Weinberg, Tappan, Cavan, and Caldwell are among those who have expressed multiple-factor ideas regarding criminogenesis and who fall under Hartung's attack.[136] Cavan,[137] for example, states that no special theory is needed to explain criminal behavior, in the sense that it is unnecessary to posit criminal instincts, physical anomalies, or inborn mental quirks. She suggests the necessity for a correlation of the two major approaches, one being the sociological, which emphasizes social experience, and the other the psychiatric–psychological, which emphasizes individual and mental factors. Hartung takes her to task for making 'a facile statement' and conveying the impression of attempted fairness to each discipline without attempting to specify legitimate limits for either. But strong and explicit in his rebuttal of this kind of attack, Sheldon Glueck says: 'The multiple factor approach is much more illuminating and much more in accord with the variety of original natures involved in crime, the variety in kind and intensity of human and physical environmental influences involved in crime, the variety in behavior patterns of the acts and mental states and mechanisms embraced in the single legal concept of "crime." For this not only recognizes the evident fact of a wider variation in influences, weights and combinations of traits and factors in crime causation; it recognizes, too, that while there is a "core type" of offender there is also a variety of subtypes or fringe types.'[138]

Albert Cohen[139] has provided one of the most insightful critiques of the multiple-factor approach. He suggests, first, that there has been confusion of explanation by means of a single theory or system that could be applied to all cases. A single theory cannot explain crime in terms of a single factor for it is often concerned with a number of variables. A variable is a characteristic with respect to which something may vary, or a characteristic the value of which may vary either absolutely or in relation to some other characteristic. But neither a statement of a single factor or one fact, nor a series of such factors or statements about crime, is a *theoretical* explanation of crime. A single theory or a theoretical explanation attempts to organize and relate the known variables, and consequently is an abstract statement about the variations in the values of one variable related to known variations in the values of other variables.

Second, 'factors' are confused with 'causes', although each factor is also assumed to contain within itself a capacity to produce crime; in short, a factor is considered to have a fixed amount of criminogenic power. A statistical correlation between a factor and crime rates (for example, poor housing and crime rates) often leads a multiple-factor investigator to assign some kind of causal power to the factor. In view of the reluctance of criminologists today to follow a unifactorial approach, multiple factors are implicitly or explicitly assigned some kind of causal power when statistically associated with high rates of crime. Whether each factor is assumed to be independent of all other factors and therefore to operate independently in the (biological) predisposition to or in the (environmental) precipitation of crime, or whether each factor is assumed to operate in unknown ways or in statistically computed, related, and known ways (which may be determined, for instance, by factor analysis), the absence of any integrated explanation fails to satisfy the advocates of a generalized theory of criminal behavior. As Hartung remarks, 'Sociologists have been admonished to abandon their paste-pot-and-scissors eclecticism and to try to develop a generalizing theory that is in keeping with the philosophy of science'.[140] Or as Sutherland and Cressey rather bitterly observe, 'The principal argument . . . is that the multiple-factor theory, defined as a mere enumeration of the series of factors related in some manner or other to criminal behavior, is not adequate. The pride which some criminologists take in this multiple-factor approach is entirely misplaced. This "theory" should be recognized as an admission of defeat, for it means that criminological studies must always be "exploratory".'[141]

Theory as a guide to research

Criminologists concentrating today on the development of theory seek to legitimize their generalizing by frequent reference to the incisive writings of Parsons and Merton. (Most of the theorists in criminology have at one time or another engaged in some empirical, quantitative, or statistical research, but we are referring to writers whose most recent and important works have been in theory rather than in the collection of data.) In forming his own structural-functional theory of social systems in 'Position and Prospects of Systematic Theory in Sociology', Parsons examines the 'factor' approach:

'Not the least deleterious effect of the "factor" type of theorizing . . . is the division of the field into warring "schools" of thought. On this basis every school has some solid empirical justification but equally each, as a result of the need for closure of the system, involves insuperable difficulties and conflicts with other interpretations of the same phenomenon. . . . In such a situation it is not surprising that theory as such should be discredited and many of the sanest, least obsessive minds become disillusioned with the whole thing and become dogmatic empiricists, denying as a matter of principle that theory can do anything for science. They feel it is, rather, only a matter of speculative construction which leads away from respect for facts, and thus the progress of science can consist *only* in the accumulation of discrete, unrelated, unguided discoveries of fact.'[142]

A broad conceptualization to which is applied Mills's creative 'sociological imagination'[143] is implicitly viewed by the theorists as superior to what they consider random data-collection by the 'multiple-factor empiricists'. The 'data-collectors' suggest that they are engaging in fundamental research upon which – and only upon which – criminological theory can be based. Unless adequate data are amassed and arrayed in a methodologically sound way, no significant and lasting theory can emerge. Theory on a broad macroscopic scale may be desirable ('differential association', 'culture conflict', 'subcultures', etc.), but theory of this sort, they contend, should result *from* research on less pretentious, more modest levels of inquiry. This argument is more than a call for the use of Merton's 'middle-range' theory approach, for Merton's suggestion involves a reduction of abstractionism to researchable dimensions but still requires that the middle-range investigator should function within the framework of commitment to some broad schema, paradigm, or theoretical system. Hypothesis-formation, according to this suggestion, is a function of theory that generates testable assumptions. Hence, recent studies, such as those by Short[144] and others, that seek to measure by sociometric and other techniques the intensity, frequency, duration, etc., of Sutherland's differential association or that by Jayewardene,[145] which attempts to provide an index of the conflict of norms described by Sellin, fall within this range.

The multiple-factor data-collector may find this kind of research less noxious because, after all, data (of some kind) are being collected and there is evidence of allegiance to empiricism. On the other hand, the multiple-factor school feels uneasy about the fact that research of this kind is limited in scope, is restricted or 'walled in' by the confines of a theoretical perspective that does not truly and freely allow significant facts outside the range of the theory to have an equal chance of being considered, collected, and counted. The *a priori* assumptions, they could contend, restrict and predetermine the *a posteriori* interpretations; and the incidence and frequency data become merely the convenient luxuries of quantifying a theoretical position assumed in advance. If theory can be written without data, then data collected to test hypotheses generated by the theory are data selected too narrowly, and, even if some of these hypotheses are rejected, the theory may still stand unmodified. Eventually and almost inevitably, supported and confirmed hypotheses accumulate to buttress the theory no matter how great may have been the mortality of hypotheses growing out of the theory. Theory without data for establishing testable hypotheses is, therefore, viewed as premature, for it puts blinders on the investigator and excludes or understates facts that fail to fit into the preconceptions of the theory. The observations remain, then, 'thin' or 'skeletal'.

Remarks similar to these have been leveled at the previously mentioned recent and stimulating 'theories' of Cohen, Bloch and Niederhoffer, Miller, Cloward and Ohlin, *et al.* Cohen's emphasis has been discussed in relation to class structure, cultural change, and role-playing. He sees the development of a delinquent subculture as a process that builds, maintains, and reinforces a code of behavior that is virtually an inversion of the dominant (middle-class) values. The delinquent subculture is held to be developed and maintained as a solution to the problems confronted by the lower-class youth that relate to status. Middle-class male delinquency, Cohen suggests, is a consequence of the adolescent boy's anxiety concerning his masculine role.[146] The position of Cohen has been reviewed, magnified, expanded, and somewhat revised by Cloward and Ohlin. Currently associated with the theoretical viewpoints of these three authors is the description of a delinquent subculture that emerges from the socially structured division between the aspirations of lower-class boys and the means ('opportunities') available to them to realize these aspirations. Lower-class socialization does not prepare boys to perform according to the requirements or expectations of middle-class institutions such as the school, and, consequently, the lower-class boys suffer 'status deprivation' and low estimates of self. The interaction of a large number of such boys in an urban area leads to the establishment of a set of values held by them as a group, and the group values provide opportunities for the boys to recover their loss of self-esteem and neutralize them against further 'status punishment'. The status deprivation then provides the motivation from which the lower delinquent subculture emerges. Equally important is the 'status punishment' that is concentrated among lower-class groups who are at the same time residentially concentrated in certain parts of a large urban community. Once a delinquent subculture is formed, individuals may join for reasons that have little to do with the original motivation and creation of the subculture.[147]

Another theoretical position somewhat different from, and opposed in part to, the Cohen–Cloward–Ohlin views is that represented by Bloch and Niederhoffer.[148] This view stresses the element of age and differential access based upon age to various material and prestige goals in society. The juvenile gang arises in an attempt to create and maintain a set of status symbols that will help the adolescents to gain access to the rights and privileges of adults. Thus the hiatus in social structure between childhood and adulthood is partially reduced. The conferring by the gang on its members of a variety of symbols, including tattoos, uniforms, and group names, serves the same psychosocial function as the *rites de passage* found among many tribal societies.

Walter B. Miller,[149] in an article entitled, 'Lower Class Culture as a Generating Milieu of Gang Delinquency', posited that the delinquency norms found in some sections of modern cities are simply the adolescent version of 'lower-class culture'. It is this culture system that itself places high values on masculine toughness, 'sharpness', and other traits commonly found in gang life. Miller's position opposes the notion that the street gang or delinquent subculture arises from a reaction to the demands of middle-class culture. He emphasizes the view that the lower-class culture is a systematized body of beliefs, values, 'focal concerns' that exists in its own right and has done so for generations. From this perspective, the lower-class culture which is at variance with the dominant middle-class culture is not considered as a reaction to the beliefs, norms, and values of the middle class. It is one of many subcultures that develop around social variations of age, sex, class, etc. This culture is characterized by a distinctive set of values and by the 'female-based family' as a household form. The children may be illegitimate and even have different fathers, but most critical is the fact that this household system does not require the presence or regular economic support of a male for its survival. The women take turns caring for the children of those who are working, and public welfare payments are viewed as a routine source of income. Cross-sex association tends to be limited at all ages, and the same-sex peer group, says Miller, comes to fulfill crucial functions throughout life. However, there are special psychological problems arising for young males in such a social system. From birth through early adolescence, boys are raised in a predominantly female environment, and distinct sex-role identification models are generally absent. The desire to prove one's masculinity, added to the desire to become a successful male adult member of the lower-class culture, requires adolescent 'rehearsal' of the heavy drinking, toughness, and quick aggressive response to certain stimuli that are characteristic of the lower-class adult male. Such rehearsal involves activities not necessarily delinquent but often involving participation in conduct that is defined as delinquent by the authoritarian representatives of the middle-class culture. Thus, from Miller's point of view, the lower-class culture has its own value system and prescriptions of conduct that promote within that framework a normal delinquent child. This value system is viewed as positive rather than as an absence or negation of some other set of values. The areas that Miller describes appear to resemble certain 'lower-working-class' slums in England, where delinquency is a common feature of adolescence even among boys who regularly frequent the settlement house, as is reported by John Barron Mays[150] in *Growing Up in the City*.

Current Developments in Theory and Research

More recently, between 1960 and 1965, new statements on criminological theory and new research related to these major theories have appeared. Refinements and revisions come from research and reflection on basic problems and questions. Cressey,[151] in *Delinquency, Crime and Differential Association*, has embellished and enlarged Sutherland's differential-association theory and has thereby added clarity to the conviction which he holds for this approach. His exegesis is thorough and should provide new opportunities for research to test the theory as well as to apply it in clinical situations involving prevention and therapy. It is not our task to describe and criticize the theories and researches in the present review; but we suspect that Cressey's new statements on differential association will lead to further lively discussion and application.

It should be noted that Cressey also has an insightful chapter in this new work entitled 'Some Obstacles to Generalizing in Criminology', which coincides with much of our own thinking about the multiple-factor approach contrasted to theory-building. Moreover, Cressey asserts, as we have, that theory in general, rather than crass empiricism, will generate integration of the facts that are known about crime and must be accounted for in any explanation.

We have referred above to the use of the differential-association model by James Short and his associates working in Chicago. Recently, A. J. Reiss and A. L. Rhodes[152] made an empirical test of this theory to determine whether boys in close friendship groups have the same specific patterns of delinquent behavior. The data did not strongly indicate that differential association was an appropriate explanatory model, but they did support the subcultural theories of Cohen and Walter Miller. As Reiss and Rhodes remark, 'Delinquency among middle class boys, particularly for the more serious delinquent offenses, is independent of friendship choices, while among lower class boys the probability of committing any kind of delinquent activity is related to the delinquent activity of one's close friends.'[153] In general, this study emphasizes the difficulty of testing inferences from differential-association theory and the need to operationalize the hypotheses in order to test the meaning of friendship and other relationships over time.

In a multiphased study of anomie and class values in American life, Mizruchi[154] systematically assesses and utilizes Durkheim's and Merton's theories of social structure. In *Success and Opportunity*, his empirical research and conceptualization take him through an analysis of culture goals, alienation, and the meaning of success. As an alternative to that of Merton, he offers his own typology of 'structural strain' to explain deviance and suggests that the lack of social-class identification is not itself responsible for 'working-class apathy' but that it is the specific quality of the American dream itself. His research appears not to be built upon the Cohen or the Cloward–Ohlin theses but to derive directly from Durkheim and Merton. Among his studies are an assessment of the disparity between earlier occupational aspiration and current achievement, which finds, as expected, that the disparity is greatest in the lower classes. In addition, he isolates four sources of 'structured strain' in the social-class system: (1) the external limits imposed on the lower classes by the middle classes, which impede attainment of culturally prescribed goals; (2) the disparity between the success ideology and the objective conditions of American life, which limit success and achievement to a relative few at each level of the class structure; (3) the disparity between the lower-class value system and the requirements for attainment of success in American society; (4) the distinction between achievement and success.

Directly based upon Cloward and Ohlin's approach is Spergel's *Racketville, Slumtown, Haulburg: An Exploratory Study of Delinquent Subcultures*.[155] In a comparison of different neighborhoods and their characteristic patterns of delinquent conduct, Spergel analyzes the physical aspects of the areas, their ethnic composition, family life and interaction between children and parents, occupation and income, and variations in the patterns of aspirations and expectations of success among both adults and children. In accordance with the scheme that is becoming increasingly typical of much current analysis, critical aspects of the legitimate–illegitimate opportunity structures and their impact on individuals for achieving aspirations form part of his subject-matter. Spergel argues that both delinquent and conventional individuals are governed by the same culturally induced motivations for obtaining social status; the conditions for satisfying these aspirations, however, are not equally accessible to all persons. Up to this point, Spergel has added nothing new to the earlier formulations. He does make a modification of Cloward and Ohlin's assumption of a unitary criminal subculture, however, by dividing this subculture into *racket* and *theft* subcultures. But perhaps the major contribution of this work lies in the direct contact with representatives of the subcultures, established by various means including formal interviews. Moreover, it contains an interesting 'index of dysfunction' based on the level of job aspirations and job expectations and a section explicitly designed to present proposals for a program of social action.

Socio-psychological studies

In *Status Forces in Delinquent Boys*,[156] Martin Gold reports his findings from empirical research that is built upon more than the unilateral perspective of opportunity systems, and is characterized by a concentrated effort to employ a socio-psychological approach. First, Gold uses Lewin's field-theory approach[157] to understanding behavior. In this perspective, the individual is viewed as behaving in a dynamic field of forces and his behavior is conceptualized as movement toward or away from his goals. Deviant behavior is schematized with field-theory diagrams that depict forces representing either motivations of the individual or environmental pressures that drive and restrain the individual's movement in certain directions represented by means and goals. Then, in addition to raising and briefly examining certain theoretical issues in the writings of Albert Cohen, W. B. Miller, and Bernard Lander, Gold moves into a discussion preliminary to his own theoretical socio-psychological model. Although he takes certain cues from Lander's reference to anomic neighborhoods, based partly upon the correlation between high rates of delinquency and a low proportion of home-ownership, Gold claims that Lander has not specified whether community factors operated through small groups or directly upon individuals in a fashion more psychological than social-cultural. It will be recalled that, after relatively sophisticated multiple correlations and regression equations, Lander rather abruptly concluded his Baltimore study with a reference to the normless attribute of anomie. The bridge between his empirical data and his conclusion, or explanation, was inadequately built.

The early statements of Reckless, Dinitz, and Kay[158] are also used as reference points in the development of Gold's theoretical formulation. Reckless et al. have offered a theory that seeks to explain delinquency on the basis of weakened controls, and consequently stands somewhat apart, as a socio-psychological statement, from the more prevailing and more dominating theories of delinquent subcultures. Reckless has been concerned with a psychological factor, the self concept, i.e. the boy's description of himself. In accordance with this, youngsters who view themselves as 'good boys' because they are rewarded for being good at home and among their peers are not likely to become delinquents. Even in neighborhoods characterized by high delinquency rates, a positive self concept, it is asserted, insulates boys from becoming delinquent themselves. However, if they are not rewarded for 'being good' and if, on the contrary, they are rewarded by parents and peers for destructive and antisocial behavior, they will develop self concepts more conducive to delinquency. Thus, sixth-grade boys nominated by teachers as 'potential delinquents' more often had negative self concepts than had boys nominated as 'potential non-delinquents', according to research conducted by Reckless and his associates. Gold objects to the fact that an inadequate explanation is given of how a negative self concept develops and how it might be linked to social status.

Finally, as part of his socio-psychological background for theory construction, Gold refers to Albert Reiss's 'Delinquency as a Failure of Personal Social Controls'.[159] Reiss had argued that the major sources of personal control lie in the social controls of the community and its institutions, in primary groups, and in the personal controls of the individual through a strong ego or superego. Reiss found that the best predictions of recidivism from the strength of these three levels of control could be made from personal controls of the individual and his relation to social controls in terms of acceptance or submission. This conclusion of Reiss is integrated with the assumptions made by Gold in his own study, namely, that 'the causes of delinquency, as with any other behavior, must be understood in terms of the forces operating psychologically to provoke or control it'.[160] Gold avers further 'that an important determinant of one individual's control over another or the control of a group or social organization over an individual depends heavily on the *attractiveness* of the controlling individual or social organization to the control target. To the extent that an individual wants to have a positive relationship with another individual, group, or social organization, he will submit to their influence, agreeing with their standards and behaving as they would like him to behave. If such attraction does not bind the person to another, control or influence of the other over him is apt to be weak.'[161]

Although *Status Forces in Delinquent Boys* was published two years after *Delinquency and Opportunity*, Gold makes no reference to Cloward and Ohlin. None the less, because of the linkage to Cohen's *Delinquent Boys*, much of Gold's research is concerned with some of the same issues of achievement and aspiration, means-ends schema, and so on that appear in Cloward and Ohlin. However, Gold probes into the psychological dimensions of the individual and into the interrelationships within the family in an effort to 'get behind' the social system and opportunity structure. Forces relevant to delinquency, he suggests, may be classified as controlling or provoking. Controlling forces are hypothesized as consisting of attractions to norm-supporting individuals and organizations; the greatest potential for control is assumed to attach to the family group and, within it, the 'attractiveness' of the father is deemed to be most crucial. 'Attractiveness' of the community as a basis for social control, especially in terms of recreational and educational facilities, was also investigated. The provoking force leading to delinquency is hypothesized as being status deprivation, and Cohen's theory is employed to round out the operational framework of the study. It was found that the families, and especially the fathers, of delinquent boys were perceived by them to be less attractive than was the case with higher status and nondelinquent boys. 'Perhaps the most important implication of the study', says Gold, 'is that delinquency among higher status boys seems to follow upon the same set of provocative circumstances; but delinquency occurs less often among higher status boys because fewer of them are subject to such status problems.'[162]

There have been other recent works that have partially bridged the relation between the social structure and individual personality factors, such as John Ball's *Social Deviancy and Adolescent Personality*,[163] but substantively interesting as they may be, they have offered little new as findings or as means for buttressing (or even rejecting) theory. Ball's study, for example, is a carefully designed analysis of school children and delinquents, using mostly the Minnesota Multiphasic Personality Inventory. We are told in conclusion that 'the major findings with regard to delinquency support the interpretation that personality maladjustment is associated with this type of deviant behavior', and that 'MMPI profiles of the high school boys with records of delinquency were similar to those of their classmates who had not committed illegal acts'.[164] There are other similar studies of this sort, most of which may be found in the excellent annotated bibliographies by Gottlieb and Reeves[165] and by Denis Szabo.[166]

Through an extension of the ideas first introduced by Matza and Sykes in an article cited earlier, David Matza, in *Delinquency and Drift*,[167] reintroduces the component of free will; proposes that there is a subculture of delinquency (not a delinquent subculture as Cohen and others seem to suggest); argues that the bulk of delinquents really subscribe to the legal order and its basic prescriptions; attempts to show that distorted conceptions of one another's conceptions in an adolescent group lead to a condition of 'pluralistic ignorance'; convincingly contends that the subculture of delinquency is a reflection of, or is based on, many of the standards of the conventional order that are inconsistent and vulnerable to subcultural attacks. Often confirmed by society's labeling and police and judicial handling, the juvenile drifts into delinquency that may become a pattern, a career, a life style. Matza's position is not strongly at variance with the prevalent theories of delinquency and subcultures; it is more of an offshoot that sheds light on many of the social-psychological aspects of perception as well as on the social system, which is interpreted as having a kind of self-generating, inherent subsystem of deviancy as part of the normal functioning of the present American society.

Mathematical and statistical models

The Cloward and Ohlin thesis has generated another set of postulates and interesting refinements in the work of Leslie T. Wilkins.[168] In

Social Deviance, Wilkins integrates not only social policy, action, and research, but information theory, mathematical models, and the sociology of delinquent subcultures. After rejecting the claim of multiple causation to the status of a theory, Wilkins examines differential association, the views of Cohen and the critique of them by Kitsuse and Dietrick,[169] and the contributions of Cloward and Ohlin. He then attempts to incorporate these elements in a complex theory, and presents his own postulates as follows:

'1. People tend to behave with respect to situations and things as they perceive them to be.

2. Distinctions between what is legitimate and what is illegitimate are made culturally.

3. Legitimate and illegitimate opportunities can be distinguished, and the *balance* between the two types of opportunity presents an important variable.

4. If the balance between legitimate and illegitimate opportunities remains constant, the amount of crime will tend to vary according to the total number of opportunities. Hence it follows that the disturbance of the balance will modify the crime rate, if the rate is considered in relation to the opportunity structure.

5. Since perceptions influence behaviour, the definitions (perceptions) of the culture have an influence upon the members of the culture and the subcultures as perceived and defined by the culture itself.

6. Human decision-making skill (information-processing) is influenced not only by the nature of the information, but by the 'channel' through which it is received.

7. Information which is perceived as irrelevant (orthogonal) to the dimension of action is treated as no information.

8. Systems in which information regarding the functioning of the system is fed back into the system present different characteristics from systems where such feedback information is lacking or is minimal.

9. People do not play 'expected values', thus actual odds do not explain behaviour; even perceived expected values may not provide a sufficient basis for prediction of behaviour since small probabilities are not treated in terms of pay-off maximization.

10. Norms are set for the culture, but different sections of the culture will experience greater or less difficulties in achieving success within the norms.'[170]

Applying a 'general dynamic model' of how the distribution of information in a society occurs and affects attitudes mentioned in the above postulates, Wilkins suggests in eight steps that, as certain types of information in certain social systems increase, more acts will be defined as deviant; and more information about the behavior of deviants received by a conforming group will lead to more acts being *defined* as deviant and to more stringent action against what he calls the 'outliers' (outlaws). And in concluding his chapter on 'a general theory of deviance', Wilkins makes certain suggestions about social action based upon his postulates and integrated model. Among other things, he seems to suggest that, as a society becomes more flexible and tolerant of deviations, definitions of deviance will change and consequently the number of presumably criminal or at least dysfunctional acts will decrease and social control will become more secure. He says, for instance, 'Control of deviants can, it seems, be achieved by a society if the deviants are retained within the general value systems of the culture. If deviants could be integrated into the society before their deviance reached a level where it is impossible to deal with it without a definition as "outlier" ($X\sigma$ greater than a critical level) there would be fewer dysfunctional acts'.[171] Wilkins here seems to represent an integration of a socio-psychological orientation combined with communication and information theory models and application of mathematical and probabilistic statistics. The many provocative insights on the role of the scientific researcher and his relationship to action research, administration, and decision-making in policy-forming organizations are themselves important contributions. The extent to which his integrated set of postulates will be useful in generating hypothesis-testing research still remains to be seen, for it is too early to judge. Whatever the outcome, Wilkins adds to the current scene of theory construction an operational rigor that heretofore has been lacking.

There have been some interesting efforts, unfortunately few in number, to integrate the substantive field of variables and theories in criminology with mathematical models, set theory, psychophysics, mathematical and probability statistics. The descriptive and analytical studies to which we refer are usually something more than sophisticated applications of techniques; for the sociological or socio-psychological aspects from criminology can be intricately intertwined with the research instruments so as to produce contributions to both the field and the tools. We can do little more here than catalog some of these works as a means of drawing attention to this type of development and this kind of integration.

Thus, for example, Fararo and Sunshine in *A Study of A Biased Friendship Net*[172] provide a new analysis of Sutherland's thesis and reflect the kind of empirical research which differential association can inspire. In this work, the authors apply set theory and a mathematical model of sociographic analysis to the friendship choices and contacts in a junior high school. Mannheim and Wilkins[173] employed the most elaborate and refined probability statistics to expectancy rates in their study of *Probation Methods in Relation to Borstal Training*. Wilkins[174] has done the same with his carefully designed *Delinquent Generations* by applying these methods to a longitudinal cohort analysis. And he is currently developing information-amplification and diffusion models in a general theory of deviance within any social system. Moreover, his *Social Deviance*, theoretically and with related supportive empirical data, provides a set of postulates for social action by delineating target areas and establishing the most appropriate and rigorous means for achieving policy decisions regarding social goals.

Also in England, Greenhalgh[175] has published two special Home Office Reports on the use of correlation analysis and a preliminary correlation matrix when applied to the problems of measuring crime in a community. The first Report attempted to show that the rate of serious crime against property can be expressed as a complex mathematical function of eight out of twenty-nine demographic factors examined. The degree of correlation between the empirical mathematical function and serious crime was found to be very high; and the results of these correlations are suggestive, says the author, of how police operations might be more efficiently stationed in advance of crimes instead of relying retrospectively on the traditional simple data of the amount of crime known to the police.

In Sweden a research report by Georg Karlsson[176] on 'First-Time Legal Deviation as a Stochastic Process' provides a mathematical functional and dynamic model for estimating the probability of a number of individuals' becoming deviant. The population of any territorial unit 'is subject to a stochastic process which generates legal deviants at a certain rate – or rather, several different processes because we assume that the population is subdivided into several strata according to the different attributes that are influential in causing deviation'.[177] This model is based, like Greenhalgh's analysis, on demographic data about the age composition of the population and thereby provides another interesting link of integration with criminological research.

In New York City, Isidor Chein[178] has used similar, but not stochastic, models for computing rates of delinquency by census tracts. His monograph is more correctly an application of multivariate analysis to a measurement problem in delinquency, but both the techniques of use and his discussion of theoretical issues in rate computation should be considered creative contributions to this kind of integrated criminology.

One example slightly removed from the specific field of criminology may be cited in this brief review of efforts to integrate related variables and theory in a substantive field to mathematico-statistical models. Bernard Cohen, in *Conflict and Conformity*,[179] uses a mathematical model of the Asch[180] type of experimental situation which assumes that the process leading to conformity or to deviance is a four-state Markov process. While the copious details of this analysis are intricate, it is perhaps revealing to relate that Cohen uses data to determine the agreement with his model, that he uses the mathematical psychology of Bush and Mosteller[181] and others but does not once refer to any of the sociological or other forms of criminology in this study of deviance. The field of reference is entirely psychological.

Finally, within this context, Sellin and Wolfgang's research on crime index construction, reported in *The Measurement of Delinquency*,[182] uses, develops, and adds to the literature in psychological physics. The theoretical model for scaling the seriousness of law violations adopts the approach refined most fully by Stevens,[183] Galanter,[184] and others. General measurement theory is applied to the problems of establishing a more valid instrument for measuring the amount and types of delinquency in a community. In this study Sellin and Wolfgang directly interrelate material from criminological thought and research with what they consider the most appropriate scaling tools for deriving mathematical weights which have the benefit of a ratio scale and the principles of additivity in measuring police-recorded deviance. In forthcoming publications these authors hope to present new forms of ecological analysis of delinquency, using such concepts as 'random walk' and 'target nodes' from the mathematics of regional science.

Multiple Factors or General Theory: two approaches in search of a synthesis

These are some of the theories with their related research and some of the examples of integration current in the field of delinquency. We are not here evaluating these theories or analyzing them in detail. We have briefly alluded to them in order to show what is being done and to indicate the principal points of argument raised by some of the more empirically oriented multiple-factor scholars in the field. At a conference in 1960 on 'Sociological Theories and Their Implications for Juvenile Delinquency', held by the Children's Bureau under the aegis of the United States Department of Health, Education, and Welfare, David Bordua summarized some of the discussion of theoretical issues and disagreements raised at the conference. Below are some excerpts from this summary which focus attention on the problems most likely to be raised by the 'data-collectors':[185]

1. What population segments carry 'lower-class culture'? . . . It is perhaps unfortunate but nevertheless true that the use of a term like 'lower-class' even by professional social scientists may not be accompanied by careful specification of the referent of the term. The difficulty is compounded when a complex system of values, beliefs, household form, sex role patterns, and so forth, is attributed to a rather *unclearly specified segment* of the population. . . .

2. How isolated from the values of middle-class America are these lower-class boys? . . . ultimate resolution of the issue was a general agreement that more information was needed before further argument would be fruitful. . . . Over and above the *lack of empirical data* on the question, there was considerable lack of consensus concerning the real meaning of the question itself and the appropriate terms of reference for attacking the problem theoretically. . . .

We are still faced, however, with the *empirical problem of determining exactly* what components of the dominant culture are communicated to which lower-class boys and with what effect.

3. What is the relative value of the different theories in accounting for *variations* in delinquent subcultures? . . .

4. What are the sources of lower-class culture? . . .

None of the viewpoints pays as much *systematic attention* to this problem as it perhaps warrants.

The arguments of the generalizers, or the current theoretical school, are traditional ones in the history of science; i.e. without a guiding theory, which should be made explicit, the whole cosmic, organic, psychic, and sociological universes of variables are presented in unmanageable form to the investigator. Parsons has most lucidly stated the case for theory:

'At the very least, then, general theory can provide a broadly orienting framework. It can also help to provide a common language to facilitate communication between workers in different branches of the field. It can serve to codify, interrelate and make available a vast amount of existing knowledge. It also serves to call attention to gaps in our knowledge, and to provide canons for the criticism of theories and empirical generalizations. Finally, even if they cannot be systematically derived, it is indispensable to the systematic clarification of problems and the fruitful formulation of hypotheses.'[186]

However, Sutherland's general theory that purports to explain criminality as the result of an excess of 'definitions favorable to violation of the law over definitions unfavorable to violations of the law',[187] also has some indications of a broad universe of variables. For example, in one of the logical statements connected with this theory, we see the expanse and scope of the problems of investigation: 'The process of learning criminal behavior by association with criminal and anti-criminal patterns involves all the mechanisms that are involved in any other learning.'[188] And in another place, Sutherland states that 'differential associations may vary in frequency, duration, priority, and intensity'. But, as Sheldon Glueck points out in his critique of the differential-association theory: 'In the first place, has anybody actually counted the number of definitions favorable to violation of law and definitions unfavorable to violation of law, and demonstrated that in the predelinquency experience of the vast majority of delinquents and criminals, the former exceed the latter?'[189] (Actually, James Short and others, as we have mentioned, have made some interesting attempts to produce the kind of counting questioned by Glueck.) Recognizing that the multiple-factor method has been criticized for not having a theoretical framework, Glueck suggests that 'this approach is unquestionably more realistic and revealing of etiologic involvements than is the cloudy adumbration of a "theory" the proponents of which are so eager to establish the pre-eminence of nurture in the causal complex as to leave out of account fundamental variations in nature'.[190]

Our point, in any case, is that even the presumed guiding theory of differential association, whether 'adumbrated' or not, still allows for a multitude of variables that require much manipulation and restriction before integration of them can occur. And even in his stimulating discussion of culture conflict in crime, which has provided much of the underlying and sometimes unrecognized basis for contemporary criminological theory regarding subcultures and conduct norms at variance with larger society, Sellin leaves relatively untouched and unrestricted the vast multitude of both endogenous and exogenous factors that might contribute to criminality. In one of his oft-quoted statements from the essay on 'The Norms as a Personality Element', we read: 'Ultimately, science must be able to state that if a person with certain personality elements in a certain configuration happens to be placed in a certain typical life situation, he will probably react in a certain manner, whether the law punishes this response as a crime or tolerates it as unimportant.'[191] In the same section Sellin says that 'an important function of etiological research is, therefore, the formulation of generalizations which permit us to differentiate the violator from the conformist in terms of personality structure or growth process.'[192] Even if 'personality elements' are conceived in terms of norms that are incorporated into personality, the 'particular nature of the person who receives it [the norm] undoubtedly gives it at times an individual interpretation. . . .'[193] Again, as in the case of Sutherland's theory, Sellin's emphases on the normative structure and culture-conflict do not really exclude any variable in the biosocial environment that might predispose or precipitate criminal conduct.

In the ongoing and prevailing arguments between proponents of general theory and of the multiple-factor approach, the basic issue is: which provides for greater efficiency in the pursuit of adequate applicable knowledge and which is more consonant with a sound philosophy of science – (a) To start collecting data relevant to the general topic in the hope that some meaningful insights will emerge inductively and will permit limited hypotheses to suggest specific data-collection and factor analysis, and that through accumulation of significant factors a meaningful theory of delinquent behavior will develop; or, (b) to begin research with a meaningful general theory of delinquency so that separate testable hypotheses directed by and toward the theory may reduce the number of variables (factors) to manageable size for an analysis that will test the validity of the hypotheses and indirectly of the general theory, so that in time the theory will mature by embracing a body of confirmed researches that are based on data-collection? It is further suggested that every study undertaken with the multiple-factor approach must limit the known universe of variables by *some* criteria of judgement, albeit implicit and without theoretical formulations. If the search for data is a function of time, staff, or financial resources (as is all research) or simply the availability of kinds of data, some selective operation must occur. The limited selected factors collected, therefore, are prejudged to have some significant bearing on the dependent variable, delinquency. *A posteriori* interpretation without a preceding, guiding theory is, of course, much more random and faced with more alternatives than is interpretation of data collected in conjunction with hypotheses derived from a general theory. In any case, as Cohen has suggested, the collection of multiple factors is not *per se* theory; but the selection of a limited number of factors for analysis involves implicit assumptions.

The two positions, when viewed in this perspective, are not, in fact, so far removed from one another that resolution of differences is impossible. Multiple-factor adherents should:

1. state more explicitly the reasons for their 'choice' of particular items for analysis;

2. attempt to arrange these reasons for delimited factor choice within an integrated and meaningful relationship of factors, for factors that remain outside the framework of the rationale for selection are meaningless even if correlated with the dependent variable;

3. seek to link previous unintegrated but highly correlated data to existing theory; and

4. produce new theory which their integrated efforts may provide.

The generalizing theorists should:

1. examine and make more extensive use of analyses of data already collected by the multiple-factor approach in order to produce theory more closely linked to existing research;

2. specify more explicitly the range and parameters of their conceptualizations;

3. employ wherever possible the full complement of operational concepts in the theories so that data may be gathered to support the theories directly;

4. provide wherever possible operational hypotheses that flow directly from the general theory;

5. suggest the best sources and levels of quantitative and qualitative data that could be used to examine the specific components of the theory.

It is unlikely that either of the two broad approaches – theory-building and the multiple factor – outlined above will be abandoned, but the time and development of the history of criminology and the study of deviance are certainly ripe for the two positions to come together. We agree that it is possible 'that no one theory of criminal behavior will explain all criminal behavior', and that it would be 'desirable to define the areas to which any theory applies, so that the several theories are coordinated and, when taken together, explain all criminal behavior'.[194] We also agree with J. A. Mack's criticisms about delinquency research: 'The trouble about this comprehensive system of comparison [of delinquents with nondelinquents] is the immense number of distinctive personal and social factors which are relevant to delinquent behavior. The total of possible factors which may be specially connected with delinquency is limited only by the patience of the investigator and by the number of methods extant and professionally favored at the time of investigation. . . . The social and personal deficiencies revealed by any large sample of young offenders are so many and various that any thoroughgoing attempt to get behind the delinquents to the background forces at work leads in every direction and to every extremity and corner of the universe of social and personal life.'[195] If we are to get on with the business of scientific research in criminology, we must encourage the proponents of both approaches to get together at conferences and in the literature on international, national, and local regional levels in order to integrate the resources and contributions of both groups.[196] Scholars in each group are generally aware of the work being done by their colleagues in the other group. It is not ignorance but the ignoring of one another which causes the lack of coordinated research and of mutual cross-fertilization.

Theory, we believe, is necessary for the collection of multiple factors to be meaningful; and if eclecticism is viewed as a methodological approach, it can be used in conjunction with theory. While some researchers contend that we must first have a problem to be examined, and that examination of the problem can be pursued by a multiple-factor approach, the formulation of a problem and the components that are assumed to vary constitute the statement of the theoretical proposition. Merton, for example, distinguishes three principal components in the progressive formulation of a problem, and in doing so argues both for the need for empirical data and for the development of a theory to govern the collection of such data. He suggests that the first component is the originating question, i.e. a statement of what one wants to know. Second is the rationale, or statement of why one wants to have a particular question answered; and third are the specifying questions that point toward possible answers to the originating question in terms that satisfy the rationale for having raised it.[197] Empirical materials are of course necessary to answer the questions raised by the problem; and sometimes, only after fact-finding investigation has begun, do these data take on strategic significance in some kind of happy serendipital pattern.

More often, the strategic character of the data results from the strategy of design in theory. Obviously, sound facts are needed to support theory, and, as Merton suggests, 'fact-finding' should not be prefaced by an adjective of disparagement ('mere').[198] It is unfortunately true that impatience to arrive at explanation often produces faulty ideas based on pseudo-facts; but this is a criticism of the scholarly inefficiency, not the value, of a theoretical model.

A theory of deviance, or a criminological theory, like any other theory, consists of a logically integrated set of propositions about the relations of variables. These relations are conceptual abstractions that should be systematically connected to one another and should provide guides for the collection of data and interpretative meanings for empirical problems. The various assumptions, propositions, and hypotheses included in a theory should have logical compatibility; each subset should support the set from which it is derived in the theoretical structure, and inferences should be possible from one set to another. Throughout his many writings in sociological theory, Talcott Parsons has consistently asserted that the principal criteria of good theory are conceptual clarity, precision, and logical integration.[199] Other criteria, of course, are necessary for the development of good theory, and perhaps no more succinct and clear statements have been made about these criteria than those by Clarence Schrag in a recent discussion of criminological theory:[200]

'Theories are sets of interrelated assumptions that meet certain operational, logical, and empirical criteria. For example, the operational adequacy of a theory depends upon its *testability*. If the concepts employed cannot be related in some way to the data of observation, the theory must remain untested. Before theory can be used in prediction and explanation, it must be given an empirical interpretation by operational definitions or rules of correspondence.

'*Logical adequacy*, again, depends upon the theory's internal structure – the nature, scope, and consistency of its implications. *Generality* refers to the different kinds of phenomena with which the theory is concerned. *Comprehensiveness* is determined by the number and relevance of the variables included. If the theory fails to take into account a number of factors that have an important bearing on the phenomenon investigated, its comprehensiveness is limited. *Informative content* depends on the variety of claims the theory makes. Theories having high content make numerous claims that can be tested in various ways. *Fertility* indicates how well the theory is adapted to mathematical and logical operations. The most fertile theories are usually expressed in abstract mathematical notation and are subject to a variety of logical transformations. *Parsimony* aims at the elimination of redundancy and the establishment of a minimum number of theoretical concepts.

'Empirical criteria deal with the relationship between the claims of a theory and the relevant observable evidence. *Credibility*, for instance, reflects the degree of congruence between claims and observed evidence. *Predictability*, on the other hand, estimates how well the claims will hold true for future observations. Finally, the *significance* of the theory is measured by the capacity for solving the problems that initiated a research inquiry. It is sometimes easier to shift objectives during the course of an inquiry than it is to solve the initial problems.'

In criminological writings, our 'theories' are often little more than statements of well-known and often unrelated facts; or they are speculative suggestions seeking closer ties with empiricism. As Gunnar Myrdal has said in another context, but one that would be applicable to criminology, 'In our present situation the task is not, as is sometimes assumed, the relatively easy one of filling "empty boxes" of theory with the content of empirical knowledge about reality, for our theoretical boxes are empty primarily because they are not built to hold reality. We need new theories which, however abstract, are more realistic in the sense that they are more adequate to the facts.'[201] Moreover, if criminology is to avoid the lower order of theory construction involved in such statements as 'crime rises as the size of the city increases', the field must experience more analytical theory construction, which makes an effort to introduce an intellectual strengthening and abstraction of a greater number of related variables of social significance.[202]

Because the major developments in American criminology have been sociological, and because American criminology has tended in the post-war period to dominate criminology generally through prolific publication of both empirical studies and seminal theories, the interrelatedness of the individual and the social system in which he operates has often been neglected. Psychological theory and data are often ignored or relegated to a small part of a large-scale empirical research. At best, as Jeffery has stated, 'in current criminological literature it is customary to regard as separate processes the psychological process leading to criminality and the sociological process leading to criminality. This has been a major obstacle to the development of a theory of criminal behavior, since any separation of the individual from society is false'.[203] Thomas and Znaniecki's dictum of a generation ago should not be forgotten in the search for and development of new criminological theories: 'The cause of a social or individual phenomenon is never another social or individual phenomenon alone, but always a combination of a social and an individual phenomenon.'[204] It was recognition of this interactional perspective that led Alex Inkeles to comment on the Gluck's *Unravoling Juvenile Delinquency* as a study that showed how 'community disorganization was meaningfully linked to delinquency rates through the intervening variable of the personality types typically generated under such conditions of disorganization'. And, he added, such studies enable us 'to see why the previously noticed social conditions in delinquency areas produce the delinquent act, by revealing the creation of response propensities toward delinquent acts in the personalities subjected to those special conditions'.[205] That the interrelation between the delinquent propensity and the social structure may not be fully or adequately demonstrated to the satisfaction of many critics is clear; but the issue which Inkeles raises is one which should not be ignored, as it too often is, in current criminological theory.

In summary, the problems we have tried to delineate in contemporary criminology are certainly not unique to this field of inquiry. Rather, they are common to the behavioral sciences in general. But if deviance is to be more than a recognized fact, and if facts about deviance are to constitute a logically coordinated system of thought, then advances must be made in the development of theory and theoretical models or schemes. In addressing himself to problems of methodology in general, Myrdal states our position well:[206]

'Theory, therefore, must always be *a priori* to the empirical observations of the facts. Facts come to mean something only as ascertained and organized in the frame of a theory. Indeed, facts as part of scientific knowledge have no existence outside such a frame. Questions must be asked before answers can be obtained and, in order to make sense, the questions must be part of a logically coordinated attempt to understand social reality as a whole. A non-theoretical approach is, in strict logic, unthinkable.

'Underlying and steering every systematic attempt to find out the truth about society, there is therefore always a theory: a vision of what the central facts and the causal relation between them are. This theory which determines the direction of research should be made explicit. The danger of keeping the theory implicit – as unstated reasons for asking the particular questions that are asked, and of organizing the findings in the way they are organized – is, of course, that it escapes criticism.

'If theory is thus *a priori*, it is, on the other hand, a first principle of science that the facts are sovereign. Theory is, in other words, never more than the hypothesis. When the observations do not agree with the theory, i.e. when they do not make sense in the frame of the theory used in carrying out the research, the theory has to be discarded and replaced by another one which promises a better fit.

'Theory and fact-finding research should thus be continually readjusted to each other, on the principle, however, that in the final analysis the facts are decisive. As the theory is merely a hypothesis, the criterion of its truth can never be anything other than the pragmatic one of its usefulness in bringing our observations of facts into a meaningful and non-contradictory system of knowledge. And so scientific progress can be expected to result from a process of trial and error.'

To Myrdal's statement we must add that theories generated by different disciplinary perspectives need to be integrated if the desired higher order of intellectual abstractions, with mutually supportive and logically compatible inferences and empirical realities, is to be developed into a sound scientific criminology.

CLINICAL V. SOCIOLOGICAL CRIMINOLOGY

Among the different trends that exist in the broad, ill-defined field of criminology, it is relatively easy to identify two diverging approaches. On one side, the 'cold', abstract, theoretical search for regularities and 'laws' in the congeries of behaviors that existing statutes define as criminal is generally thought of as *sociological criminology*. On the other, by some analogy with practice-oriented efforts in medicine and psychology, the efforts leading to diagnosis, prognosis, and treatment of the specific criminal individual are often referred to as *clinical criminology*. Both have ancient roots and can be traced to very early stages in the development of the scientific concern with crime and the criminal. Nowadays, they have acquired further specifications and connotations which tend to identify sociological criminology with 'scientifically oriented' studies and, at least in the Anglo-Saxon countries, with academic teaching. Clinical criminology tends to be identified with penological practices, observation centers, treatment programs, etc. Confusion arises when very specialized forensic work performed on criminals is erroneously identified with (or as) clinical criminology, as, for example, medico-legal work on insanity questions.

The Clinician and The Scientist

Clearly, the clinician needs knowledge about general laws in his adopted field of action, and the scientist in the human behavior field needs control and confirmation from the laboratory provided for him by existing living problems and 'cases'. It is equally true that daily work preoccupations, occupational habits, different criteria for success and reward tend to separate the 'clinician' from the 'scientist' within any field of knowledge. However, most disciplines can preserve their identity and keep open the paths of communication between practice and general scientific knowledge through a common framework of professional training, a common methodological ground, a status unity. For example, the clinical psychologist has to undergo a training in general psychology and is exposed to laws, methods, values, which more properly belong to the general, academic psychologist in teaching and research.

Unfortunately, this is not the case in criminology. The 'general' 'scientific' criminologist tends to be a sociologist, the 'clinician' a psychologist, a psychiatrist, or a social worker. These different roles have facilitated a split between practice and science. Moreover, of the different disciplines working in the field of criminology, medicine, psychology, and social work have taken up the 'practical' end of the continuum while sociology has dominated the 'science' end. Exceptions can be found, but the somewhat overstated generalization probably portrays much of the reality of our field. The split has been increased and aggravated by the ensuing problems of terminology. The clinical criminologist has developed into an intuitive, client- (or patient-) oriented clinician, more and more indifferent to and ignorant of basic research in criminology. The broad (and often unconfirmed) theories of the sociologists have little meaning for him unless he can translate them into useful bits of information in his daily contact with 'cases'. He tends to rely more and more on his intuition, his 'clinical ability', his insight, his previous experience, the accumulated 'common sense' given him by prolonged contacts with other human beings. The scientifically oriented criminologist looks in vain for confirmation from the clinician. When he obtains it, it is impressionistic, hurried, clouded in unscientific terms such as 'degree of maladjustment' and 'amount of resocialization'.

Although from a clinical viewpoint it may be true that an adequate understanding of any one individual, or personality, derives from much knowledge about that individual, apart from this nomothetic interest, it is difficult to see how basic scientific value can be related to such individualized knowledge. Melvin Marx[207] has expressed this opinion in a recent discussion of this issue and adds that 'scientific interests do not require information on any one case, *per se*, but on a type of case, or, in practically all instances, a relatively large group of cases'.[208] Citing

W. A. Hunt,[209] he points out that in connection with the application of probability theory to clinical practice, evaluation of a clinician is dependent not upon his ability to predict satisfactorily in any one case but instead upon his continuing efforts in a number of cases. Gordon Trasler[210] has pointed to these same problems in discussing the different roles of the clinician and the scientist, referring to the fact that 'the clinician is concerned with individual cases, not because they represent a crucial test of some theoretical prediction, but because he wants to do something about them – or at least to give some help to those who have to take practical action'.[211] In this same context, Paul Meehl[212] has, through careful study, shown that despite its convincing quality, 'intuition', as a means of explanation and as a method, is extremely unreliable as a basis of prediction or as causal explanation. We need not review his findings here, but they are well documented and have been well received. Leslie Wilkins has also discussed this problem of the relation between the clinician's focus on the individual case and the scientist's concern for groupings of individuals as a basis for diagnosis and prediction. The remarks by Wilkins are so cogent and compelling for criminology that a full quotation seems justified:

'If a case is unique what experience can the clinician use to guide him? If experience of the past is of any value at all then it can be applied only by observation of *similarities* not differences. It is not the uniqueness that concerns the clinician but the similarities between the particular case and prior cases in his or other people's experience. If this is so, then this is exactly the same as with the statistical procedures in the prediction method where experience is derived from the past and is analyzed and condensed systematically by known procedures rather than subjectively. Moreover statistical experience can be based on samples of the population which we know to be unbiased. A clinician has only his own sample to guide him with no guarantee of its lack of bias.

'Is this criticism reduceable to a claim that a biased sample assessed subjectively provides better guidance than the procedures of the statistical method? If so, there is no denying the clinician's right to make such a claim in the name of faith and hope but not in the name of science or technology. It is certainly not acceptable to claim in the same breath that the past is no guide ("the case is unique") and that it is experience that counts.

'But perhaps it may be conceded that when facts are being considered, statistical methods are acceptable, and stress might be laid on the importance of the "significant intangible features of personality frequently observed in the clinical situation." If these features are "intangible" how can we know that they exist? How in fact does the clinician take them into account? Can they not be described in words? If not, are they more than the prejudices of the observer? If they are describable they may be dealt with statistically (although the statistician would reserve his right to introduce the describer as well as the described as a possible source of variance.) How do we know that these intangible features (if they exist) do not so overlap with observable, objective features that there would be no point in including them? Indeed we cannot test this until those who maintain that they can deal with these intangible features can reduce their claim to a set of hypotheses of a kind which can be tested.

'Faith in intangibles, if coupled with a scientific attitude, is an essential challenge to further development. There is no wish to discourage faith but only to indicate that it is not a substitute for nor an answer to analytical methods. It might indicate where the next step forward in the scientific method might be made, and should stimulate effort towards further scientific endeavor, but not be used as a criticism of such endeavor. Science acknowledges the partial nature of knowledge and looks always for newer, better explanations, but cannot reduce its rigor.'[213]

This statement by Wilkins pinpoints the major difficulties with the clinician's contention of uniqueness, and it reveals the nature of the problems faced by overtures to reconcile the clinical therapeutic and the sociological theoretical roles and perspectives. There is a sanguine note, however, in current writings on these problems, at least in criminology. As Trasler suggests, 'It is surely reasonable to predict that the mutual dependence of clinician and scientist upon the identification of empirical relationships between events will in time give rise to a greater interest in theory among those who are concerned with the practical problems of dealing with offenders. . . . There seem . . . to be strong arguments for the view that competent single-case explanation, and certainly reliable prediction, really demand the adoption of a proper theoretical system.'[214] Intuition, it is generally conceded, is useful because it has heuristic value in science. Many of the notions which psychology and psychiatry have developed in the course of clinical work should not be ignored. But as Marx[215] points out, intuition, whether coming from clinical practice or from the scientist's reflection on data, is restricted in science to the raising of questions and to meaningful suggestions of the direction in which answers may be sought; intuition cannot be used to answer its own questions. Intuitive notions derived from clinical practice must be clearly and explicitly stated (a) so that they may be verifiable by standard scientific methods, and (b) so that their relationship to other psychological and sociological propositions may be properly defined. Trasler's sanguine view of the coming together of clinician and scientist may be justified, if we can judge by the increasing number of clinicians, at least in institutional settings if not in private practice, who appear willing to converse with social scientists. There is some evidence[216] that the process of clinical diagnosis is slowly being subjected to scientific scrutiny and to computer analysis.

The Dangers of Isolation

The present state of affairs tends to create a dangerous split. The clinical and sociological criminologists ignore one another's literature, belong to different professional circles, and rarely work together, while the foundation for progress rests on mutual communication and integration. The gaps between disciplines (sociology, psychology, psychiatry, etc.) are often mentioned but possibly overemphasized and are much less severe than the gap between the clinicians and the general scientists who are working even within the same discipline.

From the viewpoint of mainly sociological criminology, the relation with clinical criminology is essential if a unified and integrated approach is to develop in the scientific study of criminal processes, behavior, and treatment of the offender. A common attitude in the past has been that the sociologist could function in isolation, developing his grand and middle-range theories of the social structure that produced certain social inequities which in turn were criminogenic. With changing phrases and terms, reference has been made to the maldistribution of wealth, social-class differences and pressures towards uniformity or deviancy, the ecological instability of the 'zone in transition', the conflict of values, anomie, differential opportunity structure, culture-conflict, subcultures of delinquency and a lower-class value system, sex-role conflicts, etc. The social disorganization, pathology, or problem of crime has taken on a functional social role in the analysis of general social organization, and interest has been devoted to discussion of crime as a social institution.

Many of the theories, the mental constructs, the logic, the abundant descriptive and empirical studies have been compelling or provocative, if sometimes provincially restricted in terms of calendar or country. It was often the assumed role of the sociologist to examine the macroscopic, to show how the total society manifested dysfunctional characteristics which produced varying probabilities of crime and criminals. It was left to representatives of other disciplines to toy with the individual who, in a deterministic universe, had little chance of being other than he was. It has been argued that comparing criminals with noncriminals is a useless pastime, distracting the intellect and energy from more methodologically sound endeavors, for neither the biology nor the psychology of individuals so dichotomized could explain crime. Most such studies, it has been felt, could do no more than discover traits of personality that might be intrinsically interesting and might even describe differences between the two groups. But without knowledge of the distribution of most of these traits in the general population, or even with that knowledge, not being able to divide into criminal–noncriminal subsets from the trait–nontrait sets, the skeptical sociologist saw no virtue in this methodology typical of medical research. He became bored with the mounting mass of mediocrity which merely counted broken homes, birth order, illness, chest depth, or IQ. He became further isolated and insulated because of the many poor studies by non-sociologists and the difficulties of translating sociological formulations into those employed by the community of social appliers of knowledge. Even with the excellent sociological studies of the prison community, such as those by Clemmer,[217] Sykes,[218] Cressey,[219] Schrag,[220] Wheeler,[221] Ward and Kassebaum,[222] and others,[223] it is not abundantly evident how administrative or treatment personnel might use them. Social workers, from a field that had similar reformistic roots to those of early American sociology, failed to develop sophisticated theory or systematic methodology and have been essentially out of touch with sociology, which increasingly sought not only to distinguish but also to divorce itself from social work and other applied arts of help. Yet it was social workers who could have taken up the tradition, the scientific approach, and the theories and empirical studies of sociology and, as carriers of this knowledge, could have applied it in the diagnostic, classification, and treatment quarters of penology. Social workers could have become the functional liaison between disciplines that need one another.

But there are obvious areas in causation and etiological research that suggest ways of merging sociological and clinical criminology.[224] For example, the ideas of, and derivable operational hypotheses from, the theory of differential association involve learning theory and other psychological and socio-psychological factors. Anomie may be viewed as a state of normlessness or norm-conflict that is incorporated as a facet of personality. The differential response to exogenous stimuli, even to a total or a segmented value system, involves personality variables, some of which lie outside the realm of traditional sociology and outside the competence of sociologists to investigate. Cultures conflict, and crime may occur as a result, but there are also differences between individuals placed in similar environmental circumstances, some of whom are driven into and some of whom escape them. Definitions of subcultures – whether expanded to the parameter of a lower class 'as a generating milieu for delinquency', delimited to juvenile gangs that are negativistic toward middle-class values, or specified in terms of conflict, criminality, or retreatism – are never so holistic that all persons blanketed or all those excluded by the concept are equally committed or equally antipathetic to the subcultural values and norms.

In short, some basic questions often asked have not yet been answered, such as: Why do not all persons exposed to certain assumed criminogenic factors become criminal? Why do many pathological personalities remain noncriminal? More refined questions can easily be raised about equal or unequal intensity of exposure, duration of exposure, etc. The essential issues remain, i.e. so long as the construction of theory and scientific analyses are separated from the work of the clinical observer and these remain as independent functions in the investigation of a phenomenon that requires collaborative efforts, clinical criminology will focus only on the individual, and sociological criminology will be concerned only with pluralities. In one area the clinical science of crime has been principally an application of science directed toward a diagnostic or a therapeutic end. How or why the individual became an offender, relative to other offenders or non-offenders, that is, within the context of a general causation theory, has not been a question of moment to the clinical worker. Progressive elimination of hypotheses, presumably linked to observable symptoms, has been the traditional method of the clinician searching to 'explain' a particular offender's involvement in crime.[225] Knowledge of or concern for the broader questions of causation is usually bypassed in individual diagnosis except for relatively minor therapeutic decisions. This is not to say that the clinician is not using science, but it is especially at this point that integration and cooperation between the general scientist and the clinician would be useful, but has most often been absent in criminology.

Because criminology has been particularly tied to legal, normative structures, and rarely studied empirically from a sociological standpoint, the gap to which we have been referring has become larger and firmer. Many of the crucial decisions concerning the disposition of criminals are taken by legally oriented practitioners who resort either to clinical or to sociological knowledge according to the specific requirements of the case in hand or, unfortunately, according to their personal proclivities.

D

A unifying effort could have come from the legal field, but in spite of important exceptions, its impact has not been felt. It is, after all, for criminologists to put their own house in order, else we continue to be concerned with untransmissible case-material, rarely read and often based on unscientific and unique intuitions, alongside theoretical distinctions, often divorced from reality, or statistical accumulations unpalatable to the decision-maker and unexplained in terms of individual consequences.

It is probably in the area of diagnosis, especially in etiological terms, that the lack of integration has had the most negative effects on progress. But a similar undesirable consequence has also occurred in the two other broad areas of clinical action, prognosis and treatment. Follow-up studies, replications and cross-cultural confirmations, evaluations of programs, assessments of different therapeutic methodologies and techniques have seldom benefited from an integrated research approach. The result has been ignorance of consequences, unwarranted pessimism, or, worse, adoption of catch-all techniques as the only expedient procedure acceptable to all.

So far, we have presented a rather pessimistic, possibly overdrawn picture of a widening gap and a perpetuated isolation. Of course, several efforts have been and can be made toward fostering a unified criminology. We should discuss briefly the major trends along which these efforts might be classified.

Towards a Unified Criminology

Research plans and designs would benefit from constant mutual awareness of the two approaches. The most frequent criticism of clinical studies concerns the lack of sufficient awareness of social variables and of regularities in the general social structure. Conversely, the most frequent criticism of sociological studies concerns the disregard for individuals and their personality variables in the groups under consideration. Mutual understanding and integration should be possible, all the way to combined and integrated research designs.

Another potential area for integration is the strengthening of the feedback from the clinician to the theorist. Too often the clinical impact (or lack of it) which general theories may have is not reported. If constructs such as the differential-association theory or the subcultural hypothesis can be useful to the clinician, the way in which they are transferable from theory to practice should be specified. Moreover, the clinician must become aware of these constructs and be prepared to show that he does or does not function better with them in his clinical role.

A scientific study of the clinician and of his judgement in order to objectify the imponderable elusive qualities which make for a 'good' or a 'bad' clinician would aid the integrative process and reduce the lack of communication between sociological criminologists and clinical criminologists. An example of the need for this kind of study may clarify the reasons for it. One of the areas of greatest irritation and friction between clinicians and sociologists is in the concern with causation. The sociologist looks for cause in a scientific sense, and usually strives for statistical confirmation. The clinician, on the other hand, is satisfied with a partial and pragmatic hypothesis that justifies his action (often, *any* action) and receives confirmation from immediate results but not from statistical manipulations. The consequence for the clinician is the availability of a criterion *ex adjuvantibus*, which the sociologist generally lacks and which reinforces the former's judgement and security in his own diagnostic ability and manipulative power. A clearer definition of their respective roles and a better understanding of their respective limitations in the use of concepts such as causation, prognosis, and treatment should help to develop mutual semantic awareness together with effective practical paths toward combined clinical and social action. Causation, to the clinician, is an almost meaningless term unless it implies an action of some sort, a prognosis and a treatment. To the sociologist it is meaningless unless it fits into a theory or system of theories.

An important way to close the existing gap is training for an integrated criminology. We are aware of no schools of criminology where clinicians and sociologists work side by side in an equally respected position, with equal formative impact. The existing schools are sociological or legal or clinical. Most pay some measure of deference to integration, and a variable degree of awareness of other disciplines is present everywhere. But deference and awareness are insufficient. An integrated training in criminology without exclusive and permanent dominance of any discipline should be tried. The task of creating such a program is difficult, as the failure so far to achieve it demonstrates, but the alternative is continued separation.

NOTES AND REFERENCES

1. See Hermann Mannheim (ed.), *Pioneers in Criminology*, London: Stevens and Sons, 1960.
2. Maurice Parmelee, *Criminology*, New York: The Macmillan Co., 1923.
3. E. H. Sutherland and D. R. Cressey, *Principles of Criminology*, Sixth Edition, Philadelphia: J. B. Lippincott, 1960, p. 3.
4. *Webster's New International Dictionary of the English Language*, Second Edition, Unabridged, Springfield, Mass.: G. & C. Merriam Co., 1959.
5. Thorsten Sellin, *Culture Conflict and Crime*, New York: Social Science Research Council, Bulletin 41, 1938, Chapter I, 'Criminology and the Way of Science', pp. 1-16.
6. Robert C. Hanson, 'Evidence and Procedure Characteristics of "Reliable" Propositions in Social Science', *American Journal of Sociology* (January, 1958) **63**:357-370.
7. Giuliano Vassalli, 'Criminologia e giustizia penale', *Quaderni di Criminologia Clinica* (gennaio-marzo, 1959) **1**:27-87, especially pp. 32-33. Vassalli has recently distinguished criminal anthropology from criminal sociology. He includes in the former, social aspects in the examination of individual cases, and restates an integrated conceptualism of criminology as a fusion of biology, sociology, psychology, and criminal psychopathology.
8. H. Bianchi, *Position and Subject-Matter of Criminology*, Amsterdam: North Holland Publishing Co., 1956. For example, Bianchi says: 'the problems of method and subject-matter are of extreme importance to criminology, particularly because this science is still on the very threshold of becoming an independent science' (*Ibid.*, p. 15). It is our belief that criminology has now passed over this threshold.
9. Roland Grassberger, 'Qu'est-ce que la criminologie?' in *Revue de criminologie et de police technique* (1949), cited by Vassalli, *op. cit.*
10. J. Pinatel, 'La definition criminologique du crime et le caractère scientifique de la criminologie (Chronique de criminologie)', in *Revue de science criminelle et de droit pénal comparé* (1957).
11. Michelangelo Pelaez, *Introduzione allo Studio della Criminologia*, Milano: Giuffrè, 1960.
12. For an excellent sociological analysis of the history of science, see Robert K. Merton, 'Science, Technology and Society in Seventeenth Century England', *Osiris* (1938) **4**:360-632.
13. For a general description of the important differences between 'idiographic' (pertaining to the description of the unique) and 'nomothetic' (pertaining to generalizations and established law), see Howard Becker, 'Culture Case Study and Greek History: Comparison

Viewed Sociologically', *American Sociological Review* (October, 1958) 23:489–504.

14. Lester F. Ward speaks of social evolution generally as having been sympodial. See his *Pure Sociology*, New York: Macmillan, 1903, Second Edition, 1925, pp. 71–79.

15. For discussions of this historical development leading up to Lombroso, see G. Antonini, *I precursori di Lombroso*, Torino, 1950; W. A. Bonger, *An Introduction to Criminology* (trans. by Emil van Loo), London: Methuen, 1936; C. Bernaldo de Quiros, *Modern Theories of Criminality* (trans. by Alfonso da Salvio), Boston: Little, Brown & Co., 1911. See also the discussion and bibliography in Marvin E. Wolfgang, 'Cesare Lombroso', Chapter 9, *Pioneers in Criminology*, London: Stevens & Sons, 1960.

16. Benigno Di Tullio, 'L'opera del medico nella lotta contro la criminalita', *Quaderni di Criminologia Clinica* (1964), No. 2, pp. 135–154.

17. As is reflected in his *Crime: Its Causes and Remedies*, Boston: Little, Brown & Co., 1913.

18. See, for example, de Quiros, *op. cit.*, and Thorsten Sellin, 'En historik aterblick', Chapter I of Ivar Agge *et al.*, *Kriminologi*, Stockholm: Wehlstrom & Widstrand, 1955.

19. Sellin, *ibid.*, p. 19 of the English manuscript.

20. This kind of analysis of institutional patterns is suggested by Talcott Parsons in his discussion of 'integrative institutions', which is part of his structural-functional theoretical system. See Talcott Parsons, *The Social System*, Glencoe, Ill.: The Free Press, 1951; London: Tavistock/Routledge; and *Essays in Sociological Theory*, Glencoe, Ill.: The Free Press, Revised Edition, 1954.

21. Jerome Hall, *Theft, Law, and Society*, Second Edition, Indianapolis: Bobbs-Merrill, 1952.

22. Leon Radzinowicz, *A History of English Criminal Law and Its Administration from 1750*, Vols. 1–3, New York: Macmillan, 1948 and 1957.

23. The works of N. S. Timasheff (*An Introduction to the Sociology of Law*, Cambridge, Mass.: Harvard University Committee on Research in the Social Sciences, 1939) and of G. Gurvitch (*Sociology of Law*, New York: Philosophical Library, 1941) have been standard and well known. For a recent published concern with this topic, see the entire issue of *Social Problems* (Summer, 1959), Vol. 7, 'Symposium on Law and Social Problems'. In Italy, Treves has initiated a revival of interest in this field. See Renato Treves, 'Considerazioni intorno alla sociologia giuridica', *Rivista Trimestrale di Diritto e Procedura Civile* (1960) 1:169–177.

24. Such as the following major works of Sheldon and Eleanor Glueck: *500 Criminal Careers*, New York: Knopf, 1930; *One Thousand Juvenile Delinquents*, Cambridge, Mass.: Harvard University Press, 1934; *Five Hundred Delinquent Women*, New York: Knopf, 1934; *Later Criminal Careers*, New York: The Commonwealth Fund, 1937;

Juvenile Delinquents Grown Up, New York: The Commonwealth Fund, 1940; *Criminal Careers in Retrospect*, New York: The Commonwealth Fund, 1943; *Unraveling Juvenile Delinquency*, New York: The Commonwealth Fund, 1950; *Physique and Delinquency*, New York: Harper, 1956; *Predicting Delinquency and Crime*, Cambridge, Mass.: Harvard University Press, 1959.

25. Marvin E. Wolfgang, '*Uniform Crime Reports*: A Critical Appraisal', *University of Pennsylvania Law Review* (April, 1963) 111:708–738.

26. Thorsten Sellin, *Culture Conflict and Crime*, pp. 57–116.

27. Marshall Clinard, *Sociology of Deviant Behavior*, New York: Rinehart & Co., 1957.

28. E. H. Sutherland, *White Collar Crime*, New York: Dryden, 1949.

29. J. Michael and M. J. Adler, *Crime, Law, and Social Science*, New York: Harcourt, Brace, 1933.

30. Paul W. Tappan, 'Who is the Criminal?' *American Sociological Review* (February, 1947) 12:96–102; and his recent textbook, *Crime, Justice and Correction*, New York: McGraw-Hill, 1960.

31. Clarence R. Jeffery, 'Crime, Law and Social Structure', *Journal of Criminal Law, Criminology and Police Science* (Nov.–Dec., 1956) 47:423–435; and 'Pioneers in Criminology: The Historical Development of Criminology', *Ibid.* (May–June, 1959) 50:3–19.

32. For a discussion of this position in Europe, see Vassalli, *op. cit.*

33. J. L. Gillin, *Criminology and Penology*, New York: D. Appleton-Century Co., Third Edition, 1945, p. 9.

34. In support of this analogy, see Patrick Gardiner (ed.), *Theories of History*, Glencoe, Ill.: The Free Press, 1959.

35. Arnold Hauser, *The Social History of Art*, New York: Vintage Books, Vols. 1–2, 1957, and *The Philosophy of Art History*, New York: Knopf, 1959.

36. E. A. Hoebel, *The Law of Primitive Man: A Study in Comparative Legal Dynamics*, Cambridge, Mass.: Harvard University Press, 1954.

37. See Marshall Clinard, 'The Sociology of Delinquency and Crime', Chapter 14 in Joseph B. Gittler (ed.), *Review of Sociology: Analysis of a Decade*, New York: Wiley, 1957; also, Clinard, 'Criminological Research', Chapter 23 in Robert Merton, Leonard Broom, Leonard Cottrell, Jr., *Sociology Today: Problems and Prospects*, New York: Basic Books, 1959.

38. For recent discussions of the meaning of criminology in the area of penology, or corrections, see the entire issue of *The Prison Journal (Research and Statistics)*, Vol. xxxx, Autumn, 1960.

39. Cf. Bianchi, *Position and Subject-Matter of Criminology*, pp. 19–23.

40. Ernest Greenwood, 'Social Science and Social Work: A Theory of Their Relationship', *The Social Service Review* (March, 1955) 29:20–33.

41. This issue has been discussed in more detail: Marvin E. Wolfgang, 'Research in Corrections', *The Prison Journal* (Autumn, 1960) 40:37–51.

42. Sellin, *Culture Conflict and Crime*, p. 3, where he says, 'The term "criminology" should be used to designate only the body of scientific knowledge and the deliberate pursuit of such knowledge. What the technical use of knowledge in the treatment and prevention of crime might be called, I leave to the imagination of the reader.'

43. The general criteria of the 'professional role' of the criminologist are substantially the same as those used by Parsons in his discussion of the meaning and role of the 'sociologist'. See, Talcott Parsons, 'Some Problems Confronting Sociology as a Profession', *American Sociological Review* (August, 1959) **24**:547–599.

44. E. A. Hooton, *The American Criminal: An Anthropological Study*, Cambridge, Mass.: Harvard University Press, 1939.

45. W. H. Sheldon, *Varieties of Delinquent Youth: An Introduction to Constitutional Psychiatry*, New York: Harpers, 1949.

46. Carl C. Seltzer, 'A Comparative Study of the Morphological Characteristics of Delinquents and Non-Delinquents', Appendix C, in Sheldon and Eleanor Glueck, *Unraveling Juvenile Delinquency*.

47. Cf. Sellin, who says: 'The "criminologist" does not exist who is an expert in all the disciplines which converge in the study of crime' (*Culture Conflict and Crime*, p. 4).

   Concerned with this same problem, Bianchi seems to feel differently: 'Any psychiatrist entering into the field of criminology and reckoning delinquents among his patients, has to be a criminologist into the bargain, from which follows that he should be well acquainted with the entire field and know all the details of the problems of crime and man' (*Position and Subject-Matter in Criminology*, pp. 22–23).

   For a more recent discussion of this same topic, see Denis Szabo, 'Criminology and Criminologists: A New Discipline and a New Profession', *Canadian Journal of Corrections* (January, 1963) **5**:28–39; also, Charles J. Browning, 'Towards a Science of Delinquency Analysis', *Sociology and Social Research* (October, 1961) **46**:61–74.

48. Sellin, *Culture Conflict and Crime*, p. 3.

49. Thorsten Sellin and Leonard Savitz, 'A Bibliographical Manual for the Student of Criminology', *Bulletin*, published by the Societé Internationale de Criminologie (Année 1960) Ier semestre, pp. 81–122. See also, *Selected Documentation on Criminology*, compiled by the International Society of Criminology, Paris: UNESCO, 1961.

50. Two numbers of the 'Criminological Research Bulletin' have been published, one edited by Otto Pollak, *Journal of Criminal Law and Criminology* (March, 1950) **40**:701–728; the other by M. Bressler, *Ibid.* (July, 1953) **44**:185–203.

51. Published annually, with special sections devoted to 'social disorganization' or 'criminology'.

52. Published twice a year under auspices of the Department of Health, Education, and Welfare, Washington, D.C., it contains under the title, 'Juvenile Delinquency', a brief summary of studies in progress, listing under each the title, purpose, subjects, method of

investigation, publication references, duration of project, investigators, and cooperating groups.

53 Several issues have thus far been published. See note 3, Chapter I.

54. For a detailed historical description of clinical criminology, see Jean Pinatel, *Traité de Droit Pénal et de Criminologie*, Vol. III, Paris: Librairie Dalloz, 1963, especially pp. 395–408; Jean Pinatel, 'La Criminologie Clinique', *Quaderni di Criminologia Clinica* (April–June, 1959), pp. 137–164.

A recent analysis of the clinical applied aspects of criminology formulated by Ellenberger, has been discussed by Szabo in 'The Teaching of Criminology in Universities: Contributions to the Sociology of Innovation', *International Review of Criminal Policy* (1964) 22:22.

55. For an analysis of the development of clinical psychological services in criminology, see Leandro Canestrelli, 'Problemi di Psicologia Clinica in campo criminologico', *Corso Internazionale di Criminologia*, Milano: Giuffrè, 1955.

56. Howard B. Gill, 'An Operational View of Criminology', *Archives of Criminal Psychodynamics* (Spring, 1957) 2:278–338.

57. Leon Radzinowicz's recent book, *In Search of Criminology* (London: Heinemann, 1961) has a broad account of the development of criminology in many European countries, which illustrates the different examples of clinical criminological activities in various countries.

58. Olof Kinberg, 'Kriminologie en Empirisk, Klinisk, Vetenskap', (Criminology, An Empirical Clinical Science), from Ivar Agge, et al., *Kriminologi*, XI, Stockholm: Wahlstrom & Widstrand, 1955.

59. Olof Kinberg, *Les Problèmes Fondamentaux de la Criminologie*, Paris: Editions Cujas, 1959.

60. Henrik Sjøbring, *La Personnalité, Structure et Développement*, Paris: Deren & Cie, 1963.

61. Georg K. Stürup, 'Grundsynspunkter for en Klinisk Kriminologi' (Fundamental Viewpoints of a Clinical Criminology), reprinted from *Nordisk Psykologi* (1960) 12:277–289.

62. H. Bianchi, *Position and Subject-Matter of Criminology*, Amsterdam: North Holland Publishing Co., 1956; *Une Nouvelle École de Science Criminelle—L'École d'Utrecht*, Paris: Cujas, 1959.

63. See the proceedings of the Premier Congrès Français de Criminologie, Lyon, les 21–24 Octobre, 1960, published in Marcel Colin, *Examen de Personnalité et Criminologie*, Vol. I, Paris: Masson & Cie., 1961; also *Examen de Personnalité en Criminologie*, Vols. I and II, Premier Congrès Français de Criminologie, Lyon, Octobre, 1960, Paris: Masson & Cie., 1961.

It is also interesting to note that the social defense movement in France has inserted the utilization of psychiatric techniques in its program. See Marc Ancel, 'La Difesa Sociale e il trattamento psichiatrico dei delinquenti', *Quaderni di Criminologia Clinica* (April–June, 1960), pp. 185–198. The psychoanalytic school in

France has consistently shown an awareness of criminological problems. Excellent statements from this school may be found in D. Lagache, 'Contribution à la Psychologie de la Conduite Criminelle', *Revue Française de Psychanalyse* (1948) 4:541 ff.; D. Lagache, 'La Psycho-Criminogenèse', *Revue Française de Psychanalyse* (1951) 1:103 ff.; S. Lebovici, P. Male, and F. Pasche, 'Psychanalyse et Criminologie, Rapport Clinique', *Revue Française de Psychanalyse* (1951) 1:30 ff.

64. See the entire issue of *International Review of Criminal Policy*, No. 3, New York: United Nations, January, 1953.

65. Emanuel Messinger, Benjamin Apfelberg, 'Rapporti esistenti tra comportamento criminale e psicosi, debolezza mentale e tipi di personalità', *Quaderni di Criminologia Clinica* (July–Sept., 1960), pp. 269–316.

66. Bernard Glueck, '608 Admissions to Sing Sing', *Mental Hygiene* (1918) 2:85 ff; 'Psychiatric Aims in the Field of Criminology', *Mental Hygiene* (1918) 2:546 ff.

67. Winfred Overholser, 'The Briggs Law of Massachusetts: A Review and An Appraisal', *Journal of Criminal Law and Criminology* (1935) 35:859 ff; 'Ten Years of Cooperative Effort', *Journal of Criminal Law and Criminology* (May–June, 1938) 29:23 ff.

68. J. G. Wilson and M. J. Pescor, *Problems in Prison Psychiatry*, Caldwell, Idaho: The Caxton Printers, 1939.

69. See, for example, John Lewis Gillin, *Criminology and Penology*, Revised Edition, New York: D. Appleton-Century Company, 1935; Saul D. Alinsky, 'The Philosophical Implications of the Individualistic Approach in Criminology', New York: *Proceedings of the American Prison Association*, 1937.

70. Louis Wirth, 'Clinical Sociology', *American Journal of Sociology* (July, 1931) 37:49–66; Saul D. Alinsky, 'A Sociological Technique in Clinical Criminology', *Proceedings of the American Prison Association* (1934) 64:167–178.

71. A special issue of the *Japanese Journal of Correctional Medicine* (1960), Vol. 9, is devoted to the proceedings of this meeting.

72. The Japanese Criminological Association, directed by S. Yoshimasu, publishes a journal, *Acta Criminologiae et Medicinae Legalis Japonica*, which contains frequent articles on clinical aspects of criminology.

In the field of delinquency, an excellent review has recently been prepared by George A. DeVos and Keiichi Mizushima, 'Research on Delinquency in Japan: An Introductory Review' (mimeographed), n.d. The extensive bibliography covered is a testimony of the variety and interest in clinical criminology in Japan which, regretfully, is not directly available to most Western readers.

73. Benigno Di Tullio, *La costituzione delinquenziale nella etiologia e terapia del delitto*, Rome: Anonima Roma, 1929.

Benigno Di Tullio, 'Il fondamento bio-psicologico ed il Meccanismo di sviluppo delle più comuni manifestazioni di criminalità individuale e collettiva', *Zacchia* (1939) 3:638–667.

Benigno Di Tullio, 'Ancora in difesa dell' Antropologia Criminale', *Criminalia* (1940) 4:1–19.

Benigno Di Tullio, 'Dalla perizia psichiatrica alla perizia criminologica', *Scritti Giuridici in onore di Alfredo De Marsico*, Vol. I, Milano: Giuffrè, 1960, pp. 503–511.

Benigno Di Tullio, *Principi di Criminologia Clinica e Psichiatria Forense*, Roma: Istituto Italiano di Medicina Sociale, 1963; *École de Criminologia Clinique*, Institut d'Anthropologie Criminelle, Rome: Université de Rome, 1956.

74. Cesare Gerin, 'Il metodo di studio medico-legale per l'accertamento della capacità penale dell'individuo antisociale', *Riv. Dif. Soc.*, 1948, No. 3.

Cesare Gerin, Franco Ferracuti, and Aldo Semerari, 'Evaluation Médico-Légale de L'Imputabilité et de la Dangerosité Sociale dans les Anomalies et dans les Maladies Psychiques: Ses Répercussions Criminologiques', *Zacchia* (January–June, 1963), Vol. 26.

Giovanni De Vincentiis, 'Contributo della dottrina e del metodo psicoanalitici allo studio della personalità del delinquente', reprinted from *Archivio Penale* (January–February, 1950), pp. 1–23.

Aldo Franchini and Francesco Introna, *Delinquenza Minorile*, Padova: Cedam, 1961.

Franco Ferracuti and Aldo Semerari, 'Analisi dei motivi nella valutazione della personalità dell'imputato', Atti della Società Romana di Medicina Legale e delle Assicurazioni, *Zacchia*, 1963, 1–2.

W. Lindesay Neustatter, *Psychological Disorder and Crime*, London: Christopher Johnson, 1953.

For the integration of medical sciences and sociology, see Benigno Di Tullio, *Médicine et Sociologie en Etiologie Criminelle*, Paris: Societé Internationale de Criminologie, 1951.

For similar developments in other countries, see Karl Menninger and Joseph Satten, 'The Development of a Psychiatric Criminology', *Bulletin of the Menninger Clinic*, 26:164–172; Leon Radzinowicz, 'Academy Proceedings, 1960, Criminal Law, Criminology and Forensic Science', *Medicine, Science and Law*, 1:7–15.

75. For exceptions, see Aldo Niceforo, *Criminologia*, Rome: Bocca, 1949.

76. Agostino Gemelli, *La personalità del delinquente nei suoi fondamenti biologici e psicologici*, Milano: Giuffrè, 1948.

Luigi Meschieri, 'Contributo metodologico allo studio dell'antisocialità nell'individuo normale', *La Giustizia Penale* (1951) 56:385–408.

Luigi Meschieri, 'Osservazioni critiche sull'applicazione dei metodi psicologici nello studio della personalità del delinquente', Reprinted from *Archivio Penale* (1951), pp. 1–16.

Alberto Marzi, 'Le endocrinopatie come cause di disadattamento sociale, con particolare riguardo alle turbe dello sviluppo puberale', Atti del X Convegno degli Psicologi Italiani, 1954, Firenze: Editrice Universitaria, 1955, pp. 307–309.

Leonardo Ancona, 'Agostino Gemelli e la concezione psicologica della criminologia', *Quaderni di Criminologia Clinica* (October–December, 1959), pp. 402–419.

Tullio Bazzi, 'Psicoterapia e criminologia clinica', *Quaderni di Criminologia Clinica*, Anno I, No. 3 (July–September, 1959), pp. 277–306.

M. Zucchi and L. Stella, 'Lo sviluppo delle tendenze antisociali nel quadro delle anomalie di comportamento di tipo caratteriale del bambino e del ragazzo', *Rivista di Psicologia Sociale* (1960) 4:235–269.

Pasquale Devoto and A. Coppola,' Problemi di criminologia clinica', *Quaderni di Criminologia Clinica* (January–March, 1963), pp. 3–30.

77. For full descriptions of this institution, see:

G. Di Gennaro, Franco Ferracuti, and Mario Fontanesi, 'L'esame della personalità del condannato nell'Istituto di Osservazione di Rebibbia', *Rassegna di Studi Penitenziari* (1955) 3:371–393.

M. Verdun, 'Le Ier Colloque International de Criminologie Clinique et le Nouvel Institut National d'Observation de Rebibbia', *La Presse Médicale* (February 21, 1959), pp. 355–357.

Domingo Teruel Carralero, 'Clinicas criminologicas y jueces de ejecucion de penas', *Boletin de Informacion del Ministerio de Justicia*, Madrid, 1963.

Franco Ferracuti, Mario Fontanesi, and Marvin E. Wolfgang, 'The Diagnostic and Classification Center at Rebibbia, Rome', *Federal Probation* (September, 1963) 27:31–35.

78. *Op. cit.*, pp. 465–499.

79. *Op. cit.*, pp. 509–536.

80. Arthur MacDonald, *Criminology*, New York: Funk & Wagnall, 1893.

81. Maurice Parmelee, *Criminology*, New York: Macmillan, 1923.

82. Maurice Parmelee, *The Principles of Anthropology and Sociology in Their Relations to Criminal Procedure*, New York: Macmillan, 1908.

83. This brief summary of early American criminology is based to some extent upon T. Sellin, 'Les grandes conceptions de la sociologie criminelle américaine', in the volume, *L'examen médico-psychologique et social des délinquents*, Premier Cours International de Criminologie. (Conference published by G. Heuyer and J. Pinatel, Paris, 1953.)

84. See, e.g. Karl Mannheim, 'German Sociology (1918–1933)', *Politica* (February, 1934) 1:12–33, cited by Parsons, 'Some Problems Confronting Sociology as a Profession', *op. cit.*

85. Parsons, *op. cit.*, p. 550.

86. Parsons, *Essays in Sociological Theory*, p. 220.

87. Gillin, *Criminology and Penology*, pp. 247–250.

88. Their work is, of course, the classic American ecological analysis: Clifford Shaw and Henry McKay, *Juvenile Delinquency and Urban Areas*, Chicago: University of Chicago Press, 1942. See also, the excellent summary and critique of the ecological approach in Terence Morris, *The Criminal Area*, London: Routledge and Kegan Paul, 1958.

89. William Healy, *The Individual Delinquent*, Boston: Little, Brown and Co., 1915.

90. For references to Di Tullio, see note 73.

91. Hermann Mannheim, *Juvenile Delinquency in an English Middletown*, London: Kegan Paul, Trench, Trubner and Co., 1943.

92. Bernard Lander, *Towards an Understanding of Juvenile Delinquency*, New York: Columbia University Press, 1954.

93. Morris, *op. cit.*

94. W. I. Thomas, *The Unadjusted Girl*, Boston: Little, Brown & Co., 1923.

95. Alfred R. Lindesmith, *Opiate Addiction*, Bloomington: Principia Press, 1947.

96. Donald R. Cressey, *Other People's Money: A Study of the Social Psychology of Embezzlement*, Glencoe, Ill.: The Free Press, 1953.

97. See note 15.

98. See note 44.

99. See note 45.

100. See note 24.

101. Clifford R. Shaw, *The Jack-Roller*, Chicago: University of Chicago Press, 1930.

102. Clifford R. Shaw, *Brothers in Crime*, Chicago: University of Chicago Press, 1938; also, by the same author, *The Natural History of a Delinquency Career*, Chicago: University of Chicago Press, 1931.

103. E. H. Sutherland, *The Professional Thief*, Chicago: University of Chicago Press, 1937.

104. David W. Maurer, *The Big Con*, Indianapolis: Bobbs-Merrill, 1940.

105. Edwin H. Sutherland, *White Collar Crime*, New York: Dryden, 1949.

106. Marshall Clinard, *The Black Market*, New York: Rinehart, 1952.

107. Cressey, *Other People's Money*, 1953.

108. J. L. Gillin, *The Wisconsin Prisoner*, Madison: University of Wisconsin Press, 1946.

109. Andrew F. Henry and James F. Short, Jr., *Suicide and Homicide*, Glencoe, Ill.: The Free Press, 1954.

110. Marvin E. Wolfgang, *Patterns in Criminal Homicide*, Philadelphia: University of Pennsylvania Press, 1958.

111. Recent additions to the homicide literature include:

Paul Bohannan, *African Homicide and Suicide*, Princeton, New Jersey: Princeton University Press, 1960.

Stuart Palmer, *A Study of Murder*, New York: T. Y. Crowell, 1960.

Manfred Guttmacher, *The Mind of the Murderer*, New York: Farrar, Straus, 1960.

112. Emile Durkheim, *Suicide* (trans. by John A. Spaulding and George Simpson), Glencoe, Ill.: The Free Press, 1951.
113. The development and slight change of Sutherland's thesis of 'differential association' are considered in A. Cohen, A. Lindesmith, and Karl Schuessler, *The Sutherland Papers*, Bloomington: Indiana University Press, 1956, pp. 5–43. Also see note 120.
114. Robert K. Merton, 'Social Structure and Anomie', Chapter 4 in *Social Theory and Social Structure*, Glencoe, Ill.: The Free Press, 1957.
115. Parsons, *The Social System*; see especially his 'Age and Sex in the Social Structure of the United States', *American Sociological Review*, 7:604–616.
116. Albert Cohen, *Delinquent Boys: The Culture of the Gang*, Glencoe, Ill.: The Free Press, 1955.
117. Herbert A. Bloch and Arthur Niederhoffer, *The Gang: A Study in Adolescent Behavior*, New York: Philosophical Library, 1958; also Herbert A. Bloch, 'The Juvenile Gang: A Cultural Reflex', *The Annals of the American Academy of Political and Social Science* (May, 1963) 347:20–29.
118. Walter B. Miller, 'Lower Class Culture as a Generating Milieu of Gang Delinquency', *Journal of Social Issues* (1958) 14:5–19; also, William Kvaraceus, Walter B. Miller, *et al.*, *Delinquent Behavior: Culture and the Individual*, Washington, D.C.: National Education Association, 1959. See also Walter B. Miller, Hildred Geertz, and Henry S. G. Cutter, 'Aggression in a Boys' Street-Corner Group', *Psychiatry* (1961) 24:283–298.
119. Richard A. Cloward and Lloyd E. Ohlin, *Delinquency and Opportunity: A Theory of Delinquent Gangs*, Glencoe: The Free Press, 1960.
120. Donald Cressey, *Delinquency, Crime and Differential Association*, The Hague: Martinus Nijhoff, 1964.
121. Daniel Glaser, 'Criminality Theories and Behavioral Images', *American Journal of Sociology* (March, 1956) 61:433–444.
122. Gresham Sykes and David Matza, 'Techniques of Neutralization: A Theory of Delinquency', *American Sociological Review* (December, 1957) 22:664–670; also, David Matza and Gresham M. Sykes, 'Juvenile Delinquency and Subterranean Values', *American Sociological Review* (October, 1961) 26:712–719. For an expansion of these ideas see David Matza, *Delinquency and Drift*, New York: Wiley, 1964.
123. A. K. Cohen and J. F. Short, Jr., 'Research in Delinquent Subcultures', *Journal of Social Issues* (Summer, 1958) 14:20–37.
124. In addition to Cloward and Ohlin, *Delinquency & Opportunity*, see James F. Short, Jr., 'The Nature of Street Corner Groups: Theory and Research Design' (mimeographed), Youth Studies Program, University of Chicago, 1960.
125. In addition to the studies already mentioned and relative to delinquent forms, see:

Richard Cloward, 'Illegitimate Means, Anomie, and Deviant Behavior', *American Sociological Review* (1959) **24**:164–176.

Robert Dubin, 'Deviant Behavior and Social Structure: Continuities in Social Theory', *American Sociological Review* (1959) **24**:147 164.

Robert K. Merton, 'Social Conformity, Deviation and Opportunity-Structures: A Comment on the Contributions of Dubin and Cloward', *American Sociological Review* (1959) **24**:177–189.

126. Gillin, *Criminology and Penology*.
127. Tappan, *Crime, Justice and Correction*.
128. Robert Caldwell, *Criminology*, New York: Ronald Press, 1956.
129. Walter C. Reckless, *The Crime Problem*, Third Edition, New York: Appleton-Century-Crofts, 1960.
130. Donald R. Taft, *Criminology*, Third Edition, New York: Macmillan, 1956. Also, the Fourth Edition (1964) co-authored by Ralph England.
131. Harry Elmer Barnes and Negley K. Teeters, *New Horizons in Criminology*, Third Edition, New York: Prentice-Hall, 1959.
132. Sheldon Glueck, 'Theory and Fact in Criminology', *British Journal of Delinquency* (October, 1956) **7**:107. Reprinted in Sheldon & Eleanor Glueck, *Ventures in Criminology* London: Tavistock Publications; Cambridge, Mass.: Harvard University Press, 1964.
133. Sutherland and Cressey, *Principles of Criminology*, Sixth Edition, p. 59.
134. Frank E. Hartung, 'A Critique of the Sociological Approach to Crime and Correction', *Crime and Correction*, an issue of *Law and Contemporary Problems* (Autumn, 1958) **23**:703–734.
135. *Ibid.*, p. 711.
136. For references to Weinberg, Tappan, Cavan, and Caldwell, see *ibid.*
137. Ruth Cavan, *Criminology*, Second Edition, New York: T. Y. Crowell, 1955.
138. Sheldon Glueck, 'Theory and Fact in Criminology', *op. cit.*, p. 108.
139. A. K. Cohen, *Juvenile Delinquency and the Social Structure* (Unpublished Ph.D. Dissertation, Harvard University, 1951), pp. 5–13.

Excluding criticisms of the Glueck Social Prediction Table, there are many articles concerned with the kinds of methodological problem raised by the Glueck-type of research in etiology. For examples, see:

D. R. Taft, 'The Glueck Methology for Criminological Research', *Journal of Criminal Law, Criminology, and Police Science* (1951) **42**:300–316; '*Unraveling Juvenile Delinquency*, A Symposium of Reviews', *Journal of Criminal Law and Criminology* (1951) **41**:732–762; 'A Symposium on *Unraveling Juvenile Delinquency*', *The Harvard Law Review*, **64**:1022–1041.
Sol Rubin, '*Unraveling Juvenile Delinquency*: Illusions in a Research Project Using Matched Pairs', *American Journal of Sociology* (Sept., 1951) **57**:107–114.

Albert J. Reiss, Jr., *'Unraveling Juvenile Delinquency*: An Appraisal of the Research Methods', *American Journal of Sociology* (September, 1951) 57:115–120.
Judson T. Shaplin and David V. Tiedeman, 'Comment on the Juvenile Delinquency Prediction Tables in the Gluecks' *Unraveling Juvenile Delinquency*', *American Sociological Review* (August, 1951) 16:544–548.
George B. Vold, 'Some Basic Problems in Criminological Research', *Federal Probation* (March, 1953) 17:37–42.
Martin Gold, 'Assorted Assaults on Delinquency', *Contemporary Psychology* (September, 1963), pp. 357–360.

140. Hartung, 'A Critique of the Sociological Approach to Crime and Correction', *op. cit.*, p. 733.
141. Sutherland and Cressey, *Principles of Criminology*, p. 71.
142. Parsons, *Essays in Sociological Theory*, pp. 223–224.
143. C. Wright Mills, *The Sociological Imagination*, New York: Oxford, 1959.
144. See, e.g., James F. Short, Jr., 'The Nature of Street Corner Groups: Theory and Research Design', *op. cit.*; James F. Short, Jr., 'Differential Association and Delinquency', *Social Problems* (1957) 4:233–239; James F. Short, Jr., 'Differential Association with Delinquent Friends and Delinquent Behavior', *Pacific Sociological Review* (1958), 1220–1225. See also in this relationship:

Donald R. Cressey, 'The Theory of Differential Association', *Social Problems* (Summer, 1960) 8:2–6.
Daniel Glaser, 'Differential Association and Criminological Prediction', *ibid.*, 8:6–14.
James F. Short, Jr., 'Differential Association as a Hypothesis: Problems of Empirical Testing', *ibid.*, 8:14–25.
Henry D. McKay, 'Differential Association and Crime Prevention', *ibid.*, 8:25–37.
Albert J. Reiss, Jr., and A. Lewis Rhodes, 'An Empirical Test of Differential Association Theory', *The Journal of Research in Crime and Delinquency* (January, 1964) 1:5–18.
T. J. Fararo and Morris H. Sunshine, *A Study of a Biased Friendship Net*, New York: Syracuse University Press, 1964.
Harwin L. Voss, 'Differential Association and Delinquent Behavior', *Social Problems* (Summer, 1964) 12:78–85.

Another very useful article dealing with the empirical problem of using a theory is D. R. Cressey, 'Epidemiology and Individual Conduct: A Case from Criminology', *Pacific Sociological Review* (Fall, 1960) 3:47–58. Cressey points out that 'a theory explaining social behavior in general, or any specific kind of social behavior, should have two distinct but consistent aspects. First, there must be a statement that explains the statistical distribution of the behavior in time and space (epidemiology), and from which predictive statements about unknown statistical distributions can be derived. Second, there must be a statement that identifies, at least by implication, the process by which individuals come to exhibit the behavior in question, and from which can be derived predictive statements about the behavior of individuals' (*ibid.*, p. 47).

145. C. H. S. Jayewardene, *Criminal Homicide: A Study in Culture Conflict* (Unpublished Ph.D. Dissertation, University of Pennsylvania, 1960).
146. See the detailed examination of Cohen's book by John I. Kitsuse and David C. Dietrick, 'Delinquent Boys: A Critique', *American Sociological Review* (1959) 24:208–215.
147. For much of this succinct summary of these theories of delinquencies, we are indebted to David J. Bordua, 'Sociological Theories and Their Implications for Juvenile Delinquency', *A Report of a Children's Bureau Conference*, Washington, D.C.: Children's Bureau, 1960.
148. Bloch and Niederhoffer, *The Gang*, 1958.
149. Walter B. Miller, 'Lower Class Culture as a Generating Milieu of Gang Delinquency', *Journal of Social Issues* (1958) 14:5–19.
150. John Barron Mays, *Growing Up in the City: A Study of Juvenile Delinquency*, Liverpool: Liverpool University Press, 1954.
151. Donald R. Cressey, *Delinquency, Crime and Differential Association*, The Hague: Martinus Nijhoff, 1964.
152. Albert J. Reiss, Jr., and A. Lewis Rhodes, 'An Empirical Test of Differential Association Theory', *The Journal of Research in Crime and Delinquency* (January, 1964) 1:5–18.
153. *Ibid.*, p. 18.
154. Ephraim H. Mizruchi, *Success and Opportunity*, New York: The Free Press of Glencoe, 1964.
155. Irving Spergel, *Racketville, Slumtown, Haulburg: An Exploratory Study of Delinquent Subcultures*, Chicago: University of Chicago Press, 1964.
156. Martin Gold, *Status Forces in Delinquent Boys*, Ann Arbor, Michigan: The University of Michigan, 1963.
157. Kurt Lewin, *Field Theory in Social Science*, New York: Harper; London: Tavistock, 1951.
158. Walter C. Reckless, Simon Dinitz, and Barbara Kay, 'The Self Component in Potential Delinquency', *American Sociological Review* (1957) 22:566–570.
Walter C. Reckless, Simon Dinitz, and Ellen Murray, 'Self Concept as an Insulator against Delinquency', *American Sociological Review* (1956) 21:744–746; 'The "Good Boy" in a High Delinquency Area', *Journal of Criminal Law, Criminology and Police Science* (August, 1957) 48:18–26.
Frank R. Scarpitti, Ellen Murray, Simon Dinitz, and Walter C. Reckless, 'The "Good" Boy in a High Delinquency Area: Four Years Later', *American Sociological Review* (August, 1960) 25:555–558.

Walter C. Reckless and Shlomo Shoham, 'Norm Containment Theory as Applied to Delinquency and Crime', *Excerpta Criminologica* (1963) 3:637–645.

Recently, an effort was made to bridge Reckless's ideas of the self concept and other attitudes of children with the Cohen and Cloward–Ohlin subculture theories by using two Likert-type attitude scales. See Judson R. Landis, Simon Dinitz, Walter C. Reckless, 'Implementing Two Theories of Delinquency: Value Orientation and Awareness of Limited Opportunity', *Sociology and Social Research* (July, 1963) 47:408–416.

159. Albert J. Reiss, Jr., 'Delinquency as a Failure of Personal Social Controls', *American Sociological Review* (1951) 16:196–207.
160. Martin Gold, *op. cit.*, p. 35.
161. *Ibid.*, p. 37.
162. *Ibid.*, pp. 182–183.
163. John C. Ball, *Social Deviancy and Adolescent Personality*, University of Kentucky Press, 1962.

Several other suggestions, within a criminological framework, for theoretical development and research in relating personality to the social system appear in the following examples:

Arthur L. Beeley, 'A Social-Psychological Theory of Crime and Delinquency: A Contribution to Etiology', *Journal of Criminal Law, Criminology and Police Science* (1955) 45:391–399.
Frank E. Hartung, 'Methodological Assumption in a Social-Psychological Theory of Criminality', *Journal of Criminal Law, Criminology and Police Science* (1955) 45:652–661.
D. H. Stott, 'Delinquency, Maladjustment and Unfavourable Ecology', *British Journal of Psychology* (1960) 51:157–170.
United Nations Educational, Scientific, and Cultural Organization, *Report on Psychology of the Adolescent and Social Inadaptation: Some Research Trends, Methods and Problems*, Unesco House, June 4–8, 1962, UNESCO/ED/199.
Guy Houchon, 'Le Principe des Niveaux D'Interprétation en Criminologie', *Revue de Droit Pénal et de Criminologie* (December, 1962) 43:185–209.
S. R. Hathaway and E. D. Monachesi, *Adolescent Personality and Behavior*, Minneapolis: University of Minnesota Press, 1963.

164. *Ibid.*, p. 104.
165. David Gottlieb and Jon Reeves, *Adolescent Behavior in Urban Areas*, New York: The Free Press of Glencoe, 1963.
166. Denis Szabo, *La Délinquance Juvénile*, Amsterdam: North-Holland Publishing Co., 1963.
167. David Matza, *Delinquency and Drift*, New York: Wiley, 1964.
168. Leslie T. Wilkins, *Social Deviance*, London: Tavistock Publications; New York: Prentice-Hall, 1964.

169. J. I. Kitsuse and D. C. Dietrick, 'Delinquent Boys: A Critique', *American Sociological Review* (1959) **24**: 208–215
170. Wilkins, *Social Deviance*, pp. 90–91.
171. *Ibid.*, p. 103.
172. T. J. Fararo and Morris H. Sunshine, *A Study of a Biased Friendship Net*, Syracuse, New York: Syracuse University, 1964.
173. Hermann Mannheim and Leslie T. Wilkins, *Probation Methods in Relation to Borstal Training*, London: H. M. Stationery Office, Home Office Research Unit, 1955.
174. Leslie T. Wilkins, *Delinquent Generations*, London: H.M. Stationery Office: Home Office Research Unit, 1960.
175. W. F. Greenhalgh, 'A Town's Rate of Serious Crime against Property and Its Association with Some Broad Social Factors', London: Home Office Scientific Adviser's Branch Police Report, SA/Pol 2, February, 1964; 'Police Correlation Analysis: An Interim Report', London: Home Office Scientific Adviser's Branch Police Report, SA/Pol 5, August, 1964.
176. Georg Karlsson, 'First-Time Legal Deviation as a Stochastic Process', Research Report from the Department of Sociology, Uppsala University, Sweden, n.d.
177. *Ibid.*, p. 1.
178. Isidor Chein, *Some Epidemiological Vectors of Delinquency and Its Control: Outline of a Project*, New York: Research Center for Human Relations, New York University, 1963 (mimeographed).
179. Bernard P. Cohen, *Conflict and Conformity: A Probability Model and Its Application*, Cambridge, Mass.; M.I.T. Press, 1963.
180. Solomon E. Asch, *Social Psychology*, New York: Prentice-Hall, 1952.
181. R. R. Bush and F. Mosteller, *Stochastic Models for Learning*, New York: Wiley, 1955.
182. Thorsten Sellin and Marvin E. Wolfgang, *The Measurement of Delinquency*, New York: Wiley, 1964.
183. From his abundant writings, see for example, S. S. Stevens, 'On the Psychophysical Law', *Psychological Review* (1957) **64**:153–181.
184. For instance, Eugene Galanter, 'The Direct Measurement of Utility and Subjective Probability', *American Journal of Psychology* (1962) **75**:208–220.
185. Bordua, 'Sociological Theories and Their Implications for Juvenile Delinquency', pp. 8–13. Emphasis added.
186. Parsons, *Essays on Sociological Theory*, p. 354.
187. Sutherland and Cressey, *Principles of Criminology*, p. 78.
188. *Ibid.*, p. 79.
189. Sheldon Glueck, 'Theory and Fact in Criminology', *op. cit.*, p. 96.
190. *Ibid.*, p. 103.
191. Sellin, *Culture Conflict and Crime*, p. 45.
192. *Ibid.*, p. 40.
193. *Ibid.*, p. 41.
194. Sutherland and Cressey, *op. cit.*, p. 71.

For similar comments designed to stimulate research and theory in Europe as well as in the United States, see:

Marshall B. Clinard, 'Research Frontiers in Criminology', Reprinted from *The British Journal of Delinquency* (October, 1956) 7:110–122.

Clarence R. Jeffery, 'The Structure of American Criminological Thinking', *Journal of Criminal Law, Criminology and Police Science* (1956) 46:658–672.

H. Bianchi, *Position and Subject-Matter of Criminology*, Amsterdam: North-Holland Publishing Co., 1956.

T. C. N. Gibbens, 'Trends in Juvenile Delinquency', *Public Health Papers*, No. 5, Geneva: World Health Organization, 1961.

Leon Radzinowicz, *In Search of Criminology*, London: Heinemann, 1961.

Nils Christie, 'Scandinavian Criminology', Reprinted from *Sociological Inquiry* (Winter, 1961) 31:93–104.

Armand Mergen (ed.), *Kriminologie-Heute*, Hamburg: Kriminalistik Verlag, 1961. An interesting account of research and theoretical needs for the development of criminology in Germany may be found in Fritz Sack's review of *Kriminologie-Heute* in *Kölner Zeitschrift für Soziologie und Sozialpsychologie* (1964) 2:388–391.

195. J. A. Mack, 'Juvenile Delinquency Research: A Criticism', *Sociological Review* (July, 1955) 3:54–57.

196. The general report on delinquency from various countries and published for the London meeting of the U.N. Congress made abundantly clear the need for integration. The report itself is a review of the problem. See Wolf Middendorff, *New Forms of Juvenile Delinquency: Their Origin, Prevention and Treatment*, New York: Second United Nations Congress on the Prevention of Crime and Treatment of Offenders, 1960.

Relative to many problems of integrating fact with theory, see also:

Clarence R. Jeffery, 'An Integrated Theory of Crime and Criminal Behavior', *Journal of Criminal Law, Criminology and Police Science* (March–April, 1959) 49:533–552.

Ralph H. Turner, 'The Quest for Universals in Sociological Research', *American Sociological Review* (December, 1953) 18:604–611.

George B. Vold, 'Some Basic Problems in Criminological Research', *Federal Probation* (March, 1953) 17:37–42.

197. Robert K. Merton, 'Notes on Problem-Finding in Sociology', *Sociology Today*, New York: Basic Books, 1959, p. xiii.

198. *Ibid.*, p. xiv.

92 · THE SUBCULTURE OF VIOLENCE

199. See especially Talcott Parsons, 'Comment' to L. Gross, 'Preface to a Metatheoretical Framework', *American Journal of Sociology* (September, 1961) **67**:136–140.
200. Clarence Schrag, 'Some Notes on Criminological Theory' in William R. Larson (ed.), *Conference on Research Planning on Crime and Delinquency*, Youth Studies Center, University of Southern California, 1962, p. 2.
201. Gunnar Myrdal, *Value and Social Theory. A Selection of Essays on Methodology*, edited by Paul Streeten, New York: Harper & Brothers, 1958, p. 236.
202. As Llewellyn Gross points out in his 'Preface to a Metatheoretical Framework for Sociology', (*American Journal of Sociology*, September, 1961, **67**:135) the phrase 'analytical theory construction' is used by Don Martindale to identify the body of writings which appeared in Llewellyn Gross (ed.), *Symposium on Sociological Theory*, Evanston, Ill.: Row Peterson, 1959. Don Martindale comments on this new effort in *The Nature and Types of Sociological Theory*, Boston, Mass.: Houghton Mifflin, 1960, pp. x–xi, 537–539. See also Wilbert E. Moore, 'The Whole State of Sociology', *American Sociological Review* (October, 1959) **24**:715–718.
203. Clarence Ray Jeffery, 'An Integrated Theory of Crime and Criminal Behavior', *Journal of Criminal Law, Criminology and Police Science* (April, 1959) **49**:552.
204. William I. Thomas and Florian Znaniecki, *The Polish Peasant in Europe and America*, Vol. I, 2nd Ed., New York: Dover Publications, 1958, p. 44.
205. Alex Inkeles, 'Personality and Social Structure', in Robert Merton, Leonard Broom, Leonard Cottrell (eds.), *Sociology Today*, New York: Basic Books, 1959, p. 254.
206. Gunnar Myrdal, *op. cit.*, pp. 232–233.
207. Melvin H. Marx, 'Sources of Confusion in Attitudes toward Clinical Theory', *Journal of General Psychology* (1956) **55**:19–20; reprinted in Melvin H. Marx (ed.), *Theories in Contemporary Psychology*, New York: Macmillan Co., pp. 311–323.
208. Marx (ed.), *Theories in Contemporary Psychology*, p. 313.
209. W. A. Hunt, 'Clinical Psychology – Science or Superstition', *American Psychology* (1951) **6**:683–687.
210. Gordon Trasler, *The Explanation of Criminality*, London: Routledge & Kegan Paul, 1962.
211. *Ibid.*, p. 23.
212. Paul E. Meehl, *Clinical Versus Statistical Prediction*, Minneapolis, Minn.: University of Minnesota Press, 1954.
213. Leslie T. Wilkins, 'What is Prediction and is it Necessary in Evaluating Treatment?' Report of a Conference on Research and Potential Application of Research in Probation, Parole and Delinquency Prediction, sponsored by the Citizens' Committee for Children of New York, Inc. and the Research Center, New York School of Social Work, Columbia University (mimeographed), quoted from Marvin

E. Wolfgang, Leonard Savitz, Norman Johnston, *The Sociology of Crime and Delinquency*, New York: Wiley, 1962, p. 99.

214. Trasler, *op. cit.*, p. 31. See also Gordon Trasler, 'Strategic Problems in the Study of Criminal Behavior', *British Journal of Criminology* (July, 1964) 4:422–442.

215. M. H. Marx, *op. cit.*, p. 316.

216. For details, see Eugene E. Graziano, *Medical Diagnosis with Electronic Computers: An Annotated Bibliography*, Sunnyvale, California: Lockheed Missiles and Space Company, Special Bibliography SB-63-8, April, 1963. See also, John E. Overall and Clyde M. Williams, 'Models for Medical Diagnosis', *Behavioral Science* (1961) 6:134–141.

For a brief review of experiences in collaborative work, see Leonard S. Cottrell, Jr., and Eleanor B. Shelden, 'Problems of Collaboration between Social Scientists and The Practicing Professions', in *Medicine and Society*, edited by John A. Clausen and Robert Straus, *The Annals of The American Academy of Political and Social Science* (March, 1963) 346:125–137. And in a recent report, David Lavin has both raised some issues of disagreements and provided some interesting suggestions for interdisciplinary reconciliation between sociology and psychiatry. See David Lavin, 'Sociological Aspects of Psychiatric Diagnosis', Paper presented at the annual meeting of the *American Sociological Association*, Montreal, Canada, September 1, 1964.

217. Donald Clemmer, *The Prison Community*, New York: Rinehart, 1940, 1958.

218. Gresham M. Sykes, *The Society of Captives*, Princeton, N.J.: Princeton University Press, 1958.

219. Donald R. Cressey (ed.), *The Prison: Studies in Institutional Organization and Change*, New York: Holt, Rinehart & Winston, 1961.

220. Clarence Schrag, *Crimeville: A Sociometric Study of a Prison Community*, Ph.D. Dissertation, University of Washington, 1950. See also his excellent chapter in Cressey, *The Prison*.

221. Stanton Wheeler, *Social Organization in a Correctional Community*, Ph.D. Dissertation, University of Washington, 1958. See also his insightful chapter in Cressey, *The Prison*.

222. David A. Ward and Gene G. Kassebaum, 'Patterns of Homosexual Behavior among Female Prison Inmates', School of Public Health, University of California, Los Angeles, 1963 (unpublished).

223. Richard A. Cloward, Donald R. Cressey, George H. Grosser, Richard McCleery, Lloyd E. Ohlin, Gresham M. Sykes, Sheldon L. Messinger, *Theoretical Studies in Social Organization of the Prison*, New York: Social Science Research Council Pamphlet No. 15, 1960.

224. For some suggestions, see:

Donald R. Cressey, 'Changing Criminals: The Application of the Theory of Differential Association', *American Journal of Sociology* (September, 1955) 61:116–120.

Mario Ignacio Chichizola, *Objeto y metodo de la sociologia criminal y sus vinculaciones con la criminologia*, No. 8, La Plata, Instituto de Investigaciones y Docencia Criminologicas, 1961. Hermann Mannheim, *Group Problems in Crime and Punishment*, London: Routledge and Kegan Paul, 1955.

225. Kinberg writes: 'In order to study clinically certain forms of human behavior, find their causes, treatment and prophylaxis, the researcher must, however, use methods that belong to a long list of other scientific disciplines, such as morphology, constitutional research, medicine (especially psychiatry), objective psychology, sociology, statistics, forensic psychology, penology, etc. None of these disciplines is, by itself, criminology; their role is only to supply data and work methods that are important for criminology, which is, therefore, in the last analysis, research that always deals with concrete individuals and tries to find the causes of the behavior of such individuals in certain respects.' From Olof Kinberg, 'Kriminologin en empirisk, klinisk vetenskap' (Criminology, an empirical clinical science), Chapter 20 in Ivar Agge *et al.*, *Kriminologi*, Stockholm: Wahlstrom and Widstrand, 1955 (Vol. I of *Kriminologisk Handbok* utgiven av Karl Schlyter), p. 339.

III · Subculture of Violence: An Integrated Conceptualization

THE BASIC MEANING OF SUBCULTURE

Although, or perhaps because, the term 'subculture' has been used by anthropologists and sociologists in a variety of ways and contexts, it contains much ambiguity. There is a reasonable degree of consensus in its use among sociologists, but other social scientists and psychologists may be less familiar with its implications. The prefix 'sub' refers only to a subcategory of culture, a part of the whole; it does not necessarily indicate a derogation unless a particular subculture is viewed as undesirable by the members of the dominant or a contrary value system. For analytical purposes, the sociologist uses the term without a value judgement. In this section we seek to analyze the meaning of 'subculture' and to discuss its definition, with the hope that its conceptual meaning may be made more clear for future theory and research. This task appears particularly necessary in criminology where the subculture concept is being more and more used as both an *a priori* assumption and an *a posteriori* interpretation.

We can only mention some of the many definitions of culture as a clue to the meaning of subculture. E. B. Tylor, in 1871, probably made the first definition in modern anthropological terms, and except for different points of emphasis, his definition has remained the classic one: 'Culture ... taken in its wide ethnographic sense, is that complex whole which includes knowledge, belief, art, morals, law, custom, and any other capabilities and habits acquired by man as a member of society.'[1]

Definitions in the social sciences have proliferated, and by 1962 A. L. Kroeber and Clyde Kluckhohn[2] had analyzed 160 definitions in English by anthropologists, sociologists, psychologists, psychiatrists, and others. Judged by their principal emphasis, the definitions were said to fall into six major groups, labeled as enumeratively descriptive, historical, normative, psychological, structural, or genetic.[3] The definition these authors offer is a synthesis which is intended to embody the elements accepted by most contemporary social scientists. 'Culture consists of patterns, explicit and implicit by symbols, constituting the distinctive achievements of human groups, including their embodiments in artifacts; the essential core of culture consists of traditional (i.e. historically derived and selected) ideas and especially their attached values; culture systems may, on the one hand, be considered as products of action, on the other as conditioning elements of further action.'[4]

In these elements, social scientists usually find the way of life of a society, the prescribed ways of behaving, the norms of conduct, beliefs, values, behavioral patterns and uniformities, as well as the artifacts which these 'non-material' aspects create. The writings of Boas, Linton, Klineberg, Sorokin, MacIver, White are only a few examples among the many important contributions to the embellishment of the meaning of culture.[5] Kroeber and Parsons have drawn a distinction between 'society' and 'culture': 'We suggest that it is useful to define the concept *culture* for most usages more narrowly than has been generally the case in the American anthropological tradition, restricting its reference to transmitted and created content and patterns of values, ideas, and other symbolic-meaningful systems as factors in the shaping of human behavior and the artifacts produced through behavior. On the other hand, we suggest that the term *society* – or more generally, *social system* – be used to designate the specifically relational system of interaction among individuals and collectivities.'[6]

More recently, Jaeger and Selznick[7] emphasize the symbolic aspects of communication in their normative theory of culture: 'Culture consists of everything that is produced by, and is capable of sustaining, shared symbolic experience.'[8] They note that their normative concept of culture entails an appropriate theory of value which requires viewing norms as cultural, not by virtue of being norms, but only in so far as they evoke symbolic responses. Pointing out that not everything that is possessed by a social group has equal status as a cultural value, these authors seem to stress the degree of attachment or intensity of meaning in the 'expressive symbolism' of a culture, a point to which we shall return in more detail later.

The term *subculture*, though not the concept, did not become common in social science literature until after the Second World War. Alfred McClung Lee[9] made use of the term in 1945, and Milton Gordon in 1947 defined subculture as '. . . a subdivision of a national culture, composed of a combination of factorable social situations such as class status, ethnic background, regional and rural or urban residence, and religious affiliation, but *forming in their combination a functional unity which has an integrated* impact on the participating individual'.[10] Although he later comments favorably upon Cohen's use of a 'delinquent subculture', Gordon's definition is also used to refer to a subsociety, and he says that he prefers to reserve the term subculture for 'the cultural patterns of a subsociety which contains both sexes, all ages, and family groups, and which parallels the larger society in that it provides for a network of groups and institutions extending throughout the individual's entire life cycle'.[11] For the cultural patterns of a group more limited and restricted in scope than a subsociety as he would define it, and presumably for Cohen's delinquents, Gordon suggests the term *group culture*.[12] However, without parameters for either term, it is doubtful whether *group culture* adds greater clarity. Moreover, this term does not suggest in its composition, as does subculture, that the group is a subpart of a larger group, a subset of cultural patterns and values subsumed under a set of patterns and values of wider scope. And as Edward Shils[13] has emphasized, the central value system is not the whole of the order of values and beliefs espoused and observed in society. Value systems in any diversified society are distributed along a range; variants from the central value system run from hyper-affirmation of certain of its components to an extreme denial of some of its major elements, which might be coupled with an affirmation of some elements even denied or subordinated in the central value system. It is these variants and their degree of variance that should be of principal concern to those who use the term subculture.

In sociological criminology, Cohen[14] should probably be credited with the first and most fertile theoretical statements about the meaning of subculture. A chapter in *Delinquent Boys* is entitled 'A General Theory of Subcultures', and throughout the book are general descriptions of the elements of a subculture. But as is often true of classic propositions, those of Cohen have become hardened by others into restrictive meanings when they were meant originally as a highly general and schematic presentation leading to a fuller exposition of delinquent subcultures. Cohen describes the term by referring to the cultural patterns of subgroups;[15] the emergence of subcultures 'only by interaction with those [persons] who already share and embody, in their belief and action, the culture pattern';[16] the psychogenic situation of physical limitations and problems requiring solutions;[17] the fact that human problems are not randomly distributed among the roles that make up a social system;[18] reference groups for interaction, for the sharing of values, and as the means of achieving status, recognition, and response.[19]

The mutual sharing of perceived norms makes the emergence of group standards cultural. The *sub*cultural aspect arises 'because the norms are shared only among those actors who stand somehow to profit from them and who find in one another a sympathetic moral climate within which these norms may come to fruition and persist. . . . Once established, such a subcultural system may persist, but not by sheer inertia. It may achieve a life which outlasts that of the individuals who participated in its creation, but only so long as it continues to serve the needs of those who succeed its creators'.[20]

Even before Cloward and Ohlin's *Delinquency and Opportunity*, Milton Yinger[21] noted over one hundred books and articles that made some use, incidental or elaborate, of the idea of subculture. After a comprehensive review of such terms as 'situation', 'anomie', and 'role', which should not, he says, be confused with the meaning of subculture, Yinger introduces the concept of *contraculture*: 'And subculture, I have suggested, is used to designate both the traditional norms of a subsociety and the emergent norms of a group caught in a frustrating and conflict-laden situation. This paper indicates that there are differences in the origin, function, and perpetuation of traditional and emergent norms, and suggests that the use of the concept contraculture for the latter might improve sociological analysis.'[22] He further suggests that hypotheses concerning contraculture can best be derived from social-psychological theories that account for interaction, value confusion, weak social controls, frustration-aggression, and 'value leakage'.

Since Cohen's *Delinquent Boys*, there have been further refinements of delinquent subcultural types in the writings of Cohen and Short, Bloch and Niederhoffer, Cloward and Ohlin, Miller, Kitsuse and Dietrick, Sykes and Matza, Bordua, Yablonsky, Gottlieb and Reeves, Gold, Mays, Mack, Mizruchi, Spergel, Stott, Scott, Wilkins, Bernstein, Bianchi, and others.[23]

These studies are interesting and meritorious contributions in their own right and style; they raise questions about the nature of delinquent subcultural genesis and persistence; they discuss whether the subculture is a negative reaction to, or a positive outgrowth from, the larger culture; they distinguish several types of delinquent subculture; they provide clues to the means for social intervention in order to promote change in these subcultures. But they do not address themselves to the difficult problem of defining the meaning of subculture more precisely. Cohen recognized this need when he said, 'A complete theory of subcultural differentiation would state more precisely the conditions under which subcultures emerge and fail to emerge, and would state operations for predicting the content of subcultural solutions . . . the completion of this theory must await a great deal more of hard thinking and research.'[24] In the sections that follow, we discuss *some* of the thinking we have done on clarifying the general concept and suggest means for researching some of the major components of subcultural differentiation from a central culture. Generally, we build upon the assumption alluded to briefly by Shils and by Jaeger and Selznick, namely, that not all values, beliefs, or norms in a society have equal status, that some priority allocation is made, that the subcultural variants may partially accept, sometimes deny, and even construct antitheses of, elements of the central, wider, or dominant values, yet remain within that cultural system.

SOME FUNDAMENTAL PROPOSITIONS ABOUT THE MEANING OF SUBCULTURES

The Subculture in Relation to the Dominant Culture

A subculture implies that there are value judgements or a social value system which is apart from and a part of a larger or central value system. From the viewpoint of this larger dominant culture, the values of the subculture set the latter apart and prevent total integration, occasionally causing open or covert conflicts. The dominant culture may directly or indirectly promote this apartness, of course, and the degree of reciprocal integration may vary, but whatever the reason for the difference, normative isolation and solidarity of the subculture result. There are shared values that are learned, adopted, and even exhibited by participants in the subculture, and that differ in quantity and quality from those of the dominant culture. Just as man is born into a culture, so he may be born into a subculture. As Sellin has remarked in *Culture Conflict and Crime*, 'He arrives biologically equipped to receive and to adapt knowledge about himself and his relationships to others. His first social contacts begin a life-long process of coordination during which he absorbs and adapts ideas which are transmitted to him formally and informally by instruction or precept. These ideas embody *meanings* attached to customs, beliefs, artifacts, and his own relationships to his fellow men and to social institutions. Looked upon as discrete units, these ideas may be regarded as *cultural elements* which fit into patterns or configurations of ideas, which tend to become fixed into integrated systems of meanings.'[25] There is a culture theme, a sub-ethos, or a cluster of values that is differentiated from those in the total culture. These terms used to describe a subculture have been employed by sociologists in discussing the values of such groups as the Amish, Mormons, delinquents, inmates in prison, ethnic groups, social classes, and others among the heterogeneous groupings in American society. Many of the stereotypes which describe ethnic and geographical groups in Europe reflect and at the same time, perhaps, perpetuate subcultural attributes.

A subculture is only partly different from the parent culture. We use the term 'parent' to refer both to a larger culture from which subcultural elements have stemmed as different offshoots of its own value system and to a larger culture that is willing to adopt a subculture voluntarily grafted to the parent because of a sufficiency in number and type of significant values commonly shared between 'parent' and 'child'. Occasionally this 'adoption' is the almost chance result of political events or of geographical proximity, but still a certain degree, however minimal, of acceptance is necessary. In one sense, the labor union movement that grew up within America was spawned by values inherent but long dormant in the dominant culture and is an example of the first type. The Hasidic Jews in Williamsburg[26] represent a parental cultural adoption. In either case, the subculture by any definition or classification cannot be *totally* different from the culture of which it is a part. The problem of what really defines 'difference' in a culture in today's world of relatively free interchange of opinions and values remains to be solved. Even very different societies from a political and ethnic viewpoint tend to have some common values and behavioral patterns.

Some of the values of a subculture may, however, more than differ from those of the larger culture. They may also be in conflict or at variance with the latter. It may be useful for our analysis to distinguish, as Yinger has done, between subcultures and contracultures. He refers to subcultures as systems which embody values only different from but not antithetical to the broader social system; and to contracultures as those subcultures which have values at variance with the dominant value system. We must again emphasize that no subculture can be totally different from or completely in conflict with the society of which it is a part. ‖The 'conflict' stems from a contrast of two or more normative systems, at least one of which implies strong adherence to a set of moral values that are often codified. To be part of the larger culture implies that some values related to the ends or means of the whole are shared by the part. The subculture that is only different is a tolerated deviation. Values which a culture can tolerate are those that do not cause disruptive conflict or that do not disturb too much the larger normative solidarity. Moreover, tolerated values are not functionally necessary for maintaining allegiance to the core values of the culture. Even a subculture can tolerate values outside its value system so long as they do not disturb allegiance to its own basic values that distinguish it as a subculture, and as long as its own existence, or the existence of its leaders and opinion-makers, is not menaced.

Conduct Norms

The values shared in a subculture are often made evident and can be identified phenomenologically in terms of the conduct that is expected, ranging from the permissible to the required, in certain kinds of life situation. Again, Sellin has noted: 'Some of these life situations, at least, are sufficiently repetitious and socially so defined that they call for definite responses from the type of person who encounters them.‖ There are attached to them, so to speak, norms which define the reaction or response which in a given person is approved or disapproved by the normative group. The social attitude of this group toward the various ways in which a person might act under certain circumstances has thus been crystallized into a rule, the violation of which arouses a group reaction. These rules or norms may be called *conduct norms*.'[27] Conduct of an individual is, then, an external exhibition of sharing in (sub) cultural values, and this form of manifestation of values would surely satisfy Durkheim's emphasis on 'facts' that have the quality of exteriority. The norms that govern conduct will involve varying degrees of expectation of individual conformity to the shared values. The same norms may serve as criteria for defining what is 'normal' or expected conduct and what is not. Abnormal may then be further classified into 'bad' or 'immoral' and 'sick' or 'maladjusted' or psychologically ill, or combinations thereof.

/When we speak of the 'teenage culture', the 'adolescent culture', or even the 'delinquent subculture', we have not yet stated whether we are discussing quantitative variables or qualitative attributes or both. We have not isolated sufficiently the differentiating normative items./The persuasive and provocative arguments about a delinquent subculture that emerge from a working-class ethic are only beginnings toward establishing operational hypotheses, which are needed but which cannot be tested until we have objective and independent measurements of the norms of conduct. Until further clarification is made, Kluckhohn's reference to 'the subculture of anthropologists', Riesman's use of a 'subculture among the faculty', or reference to any other type of 'subculture' cannot easily be rejected as too loose usages of the term.

Social Groups

It is difficult to discuss subcultures and conduct norms without reference to social groups. Values are shared by individuals and individuals sharing values make up groups. In most cases when we refer to subcultures (the Amish, Hutterites, the earlier ghettoes, delinquent conflict gangs) we are thinking of individuals sharing common values and socially interacting in some limited geographical or residential isolation. However, value-sharing does not necessarily require social interaction. Consequently a subculture may exist, widely distributed spatially and without interpersonal contact among individuals or whole groups of individuals. Several delinquent gangs may be spread throughout a city and rarely or never have contacts. Yet they are referred to collectively as the 'delinquent subculture', and properly so, for otherwise each gang would have to be considered a separate subculture. Individual (non-group) behavior can be subcultural so long as it reflects values of an existing subculture./

/ Members of a group use one another as reference points for self-image and for establishing the relationship of self to others. This process implies continuing reinforcement of the subcultural values. A wish to remain an ingroup participant does not necessarily mean, however, a total personal commitment or commitment to the totality of subcultural values. The individual may occasionally be more concerned with maintaining his group association than with sharing the group's values. He may be reluctant to exhibit his group allegiance in a way that is discordant with his own beliefs, but at the same time he may place a higher value on remaining a member of the group than on abrogating the prescriptions of conduct. The juvenile who conforms to the delinquent gang's demands for fighting but who dislikes the resort to violence, and the soldier who goes to combat with deep hatred for war are both unwilling to sever association with their groups but cannot be said to share much in the value of violence. The value these two individuals will share with their groups is that of maintaining the group. Thus, while the manifest representation (conduct) of the subculture may generally be a valid index of normatively induced values, latent and different values may be retained by some individuals who are members of the group that share in this subculture. Several degrees of conflicting situation may occur, and the resulting psychodynamics may find expression in personal psychological disturbances ranging from simple anxiety to more malignant reactions. The need for assessment of the deep personal affiliations and motives decreases reliance on external behavior, or 'facts', for determining cultural and subcultural allegiances in specific individuals.

Because a subculture refers to a normative system of some group or groups smaller than the whole society, it should be possible to examine descriptively the composition of the population that shares the subcultural values. Individuals are, after all, culture-carriers who both reflect and transmit through social learning, the attitudes, ideals, and ideas of their cultures. A subcultural ethos may be shared by all ages. Still, that ethos may be most prominent in a limited, segmental age group. Furthermore, if beyond typical role differentiations there are also normatively induced sex role expectations and social class variations, we may further refine and localize the strongest and most visible group reflecting the subcultural value or values. Although conduct, as we have noted, may not invariably be in accord with the actor's attitude, the social analyst often has little more than forms of conduct to examine and uses them as representations of group values. If a form of conduct is most commonly found among a limited portion of the population, if the conduct is deviant from the dominant culture prescriptions and possesses the other aspects we have considered thus far in our analysis of subcultures, then we should expect to learn something tangible, objective, and empirical about the parameters of the subculture, its etiology, its strength and likelihood of persistence, and how it might be cultivated, modified, or eliminated. To limit ourselves to the external parameters of 'conduct' does not necessarily exclude further 'depth' analysis, but offers a consistent starting-point which can be used to delimit our research 'population'.

Roles

An analytical distinction between role norms and subculture has been suggested by Yinger. But because many role norms are defined within a subcultural complex, the distinction is often empirically unclear. The rights and duties assigned to a specific role in the larger culture may simply be exaggerated, extended, or distorted in the subcultural normative system so that the differences, instead of being sharp, are variable and sometimes situational. For example, the male role may be legally and functionally similar both in the dominant culture and in a particular subculture, but the latter may assign rights to the role that were formerly, but are no longer, aspects of the male role in the dominant culture. Or the different language, drinking habits, sex behavior, leisure pursuits, etc., of males who share subcultural values may be role expectations normatively induced.

Role differentiation exists in all societies, but only heterogeneous societies can have subcultures.[28] And because social interaction in an open society can involve an individual's participation in a considerable diversity of groups, there may be a number of subcultures to which he has commitments so long as these subcultures do not conflict or so long as the individual can withstand the stress of the resulting conflict. The various subcultures in which an individual is involved generally must be complementary or supplementary; otherwise his personality might become unintegrated or disintegrated. Occasionally, life situations will cause psychological disintegration through enforced participation in conflicting sets of values, as can often be the case in migrating groups. If these assumptions are correct, we can assume the presence of common subcultural themes, or normative aspects, that appear in some or all of the subcultures in which the individual shares values. With the same thread he weaves his way through and ties together more than one set of values. He can do this because each set has some common link with every other set. Specific value elements will not appear in all sets because of their limitation to only one set. But we have already said that a subculture must have some major values in common with the dominant culture in order to be designated a *sub*culture, otherwise the prefix indicating connective values should be dropped. Therefore, some minimal similarity must also exist between (or among) subcultures in which an individual is immersed.

Situational and Subcultural Norms

Some ideas, attitudes, means, goals, or conduct may be 'situationally induced, not simply normatively induced'.[29] If the situation changes, in these circumstances, presumably values and behavior change, thus indicating no real and enduring normative allegiance. This is not an entirely satisfactory distinction. If it were, the issue would then be how permanent the situation has been or might be, or, particularly, whether attitude or behavior is unisituational, i.e. whether there is only a single situation that induces a typically common response. The statistical rather than the subcultural norm is more likely to be used in analysis of behavioral reactions to a specific situation. For a response to be normatively induced, it seems that we must resort to such a phrase as 'style of life' in order to indicate the pervasiveness involved in the normative character of action. But again, what this means quantitatively and empirically is that the action at least must be multisituational. If we were to use permanence of a social response as a criterion of normativeness, any modification of the norm would require our classifying it ex post facto as situational. But if values change when situations change, it is also likely that situations change when values change, or that varied adherence to the values causes a differential choice of situations on the part of the individual.

We are suggesting, then, that a given conduct norm or a set of values must function to govern the conduct in a variety of situations in order to classify that norm or value-set as a (sub)culturally expected or required response and not merely as a statistical modal reaction. This suggestion means that we must examine many different kinds of personal and social interaction to establish a firm empirical basis for the classification. The resulting categories will be meaningful from a psychological standpoint as well as from a pure sociological perspective. Moreover, the presence, even in a latent sense, of potential employment of a normatively induced and supported response calls attention to the pervasive, penetrating, and diffusive character of the response. An individual carrier of a norm may be consciously or subconsciously prepared to react in the same way in various social situations, or does in fact react similarly in diverse circumstances. The reaction may differ phenotypically, but the choice of the 'problem-relieving' mechanism may be the same. The degree of the individual's assimilation of the norm may in part be measured by the number and kinds of situations in which he uses the norm as supportive explanation for his behavior. When he

E

shares this tendency to act ('attitude' in Thomas and Znaniecki) with others, and especially when there are residential, age, ethnic, and sex similarities between him and the others who are sharing the attitude with him, we may be approaching still another dimension in the meaningful understanding of subculture: i.e. the differential distribution of the presence and exhibition of the norm.

Sanctions

Every norm seems to have its counter-norm and sanction to support its continuance. However we may ultimately define the parameters of a subculture, it seems safe to assert that any group will have formal and informal sets of sanctions to apply to members who violate the major subcultural themes. If some form of punitive action were not taken the group would soon lose its separate identity. Sellin adds:

'A conduct norm may, for instance, be regarded as a rule supported by sanctions which reflect the value attached to the norm by the normative group. The sanction which is an integral part of the norm – since no conduct norm without a sanction can be imagined – raises a barrier against violation. The strength of this barrier depends on the attitude of the normative group toward the conduct in question. If the barrier is weak it can be due only to the fact that the group does not offer much resistance to the violation of the norm. If the rule has powerful sanctions the group resistance must be great.

'We may in a sense regard this group resistance as crystallized in the norm, giving it an intrinsic quality of strength or weakness, a power which may be measured in degrees of what the group regards as the severity of the sanction. It is not the external means or the form of the sanction which is important here, but the deterrent value which the group attaches to it. . . . A conduct norm then becomes a rule which governs a specific type of life situation and is authoritative to the extent of the group's resistance to violation.

'The inherent energy or power of the norm, as just described, may be called its *resistance potential.*'[30]

If membership in any group may in part be gained by adopting those values peculiar to the group that distinguish it from other groups, then it would seem that violation of those values would function to sever membership. This severance is generally viewed by the group as a punitive action imposed on the violator, although, of course, there may be other sanctions applied that are less severe and are designed to retain the violator within the group. From the violator's viewpoint, severance may actually resolve his conflicts of identification with the subculture. Capital punishment as a sanction of severance is the most extreme used by the larger society and by such groups as organized criminals and the occasional delinquent gang. But usually the subculture, which is territorially limited by the residential isolation of its representatives, does not or cannot resort to such extreme measures. By excluding, sending away, ostracizing, 'kicking out' the norm violator, the subcultural group is using sanctions similar to exile, banishment, deportation. The very adherence and involvement of the individual in the subculture make enforcement of these sanctions relatively easy, occasionally easier and more effective than law enforcement in larger societies.

Transmission of Values

The transmission of subcultural values obviously involves analysis of the personality factors of individual participants. The 'sharing of values' means that there has been a learning process that established a dynamic lasting linkage between the values and the individuals. It is at this point of analysis that the psychological theory of personality and the sociological theories of subcultures can best be integrated both with one another and with empirical data. Whether or not a subculture is principally the product of interaction with the dominant culture, whether or not the primary element of a subculture is a contradiction of, or is in conflict with, the larger culture, personality variables are involved in the acceptance or rejection of the whole or a part of the subcultural values. Allowing for individual variations, the learning process must have generated common 'motives', common reaction patterns, and differential perceptual habits. Occasional evidence of the differential psychology of members of a subculture is available, but it has seldom been linked to a general subcultural frame of reference.

The Problem of Quantification

Perhaps the major difficulty in trying to define the elusive meaning of subculture has been the lack of parameters that suggest some form of quantification. Although the concept may be qualitative and absolute, there seems every reason to believe that subcultural variations are mostly quantitative and relative and thus may be viewed as appearing on a continuum of differentiation from the larger culture. Often, of course, quantitative and qualitative differences can only be made *a posteriori* and may be conceptually meaningless. Theoretical analyses thus far have usually tended to view cultural elements as discrete units. But the analyst must enter the real world with the kind of mental constructs that permit him to cope with degrees of variation of norms, and he must try to determine how and where the line denoting a subculture should be drawn on a continuum or continua. Recently, Leslie Wilkins[31] and Ruth Cavan[32] have graphically depicted culture norms and deviations from them as a continuum of actions representing norm-abiding and norm-violating conduct. 'It is convenient', says Wilkins, 'to envisage human acts as a continuum from the most saintly to the most depraved. . . . There are few extremely saintly acts, and few extremely depraved; the majority of our actions are "normal".'[33] The figure below crudely represents this hypothesis.

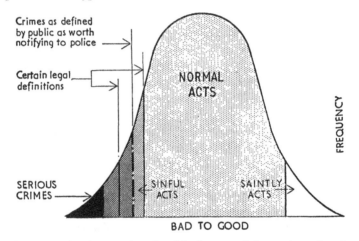

Figure 1   *Continuum of good and bad acts, and the cutting points for various types of definition*

Source: Leslie T. Wilkins, *Social Deviance*, p. 46.

Cavan's statement also is represented by a bell-shaped curve; the extremes of behavior are suggested as being criminal and idealized, with the idealism being tolerated within conventional society but the dark area to the left being untolerated contracultural conduct. It is not entirely clear from the descriptions of these two authors whether they are referring to subcultures on the extreme ends of the continuum. Probably they are not, nor does the hypothesis of a continuum of actions require a corollary hypothesis of subcultural elements. Cavan, for example, suggests that the idealized behavior, or what Wilkins calls 'saintly acts', may be performed by a single individual. The inference is strong on the part of both authors that these types of act need not be collectively performed or performed by reason of values shared in concert. The same may, perhaps, be said of delinquent and criminal acts. Thus, if this figure is applied to subcultures, the following additional propositions should be contained in the hypothesis: (a) groups of individuals exist throughout the continuum; (b) sharing and exchanging values and value orientations; (c) groups identified on the continuum have a tradition of transmission of values; (d) a socialization process shall be observable; and (e) sanctions may be noted when members of the groups deviate within the boundaries of their own subcultural areas on the continuum.

It should be noted that the continuum approach automatically creates a particular problem in criminology, for to identify criminal behavior with the subcultural end of the continuum means to deny, at least in principle, the existence of qualitatively differentiating aspects for the criminal-subculture behavior. The continuum suggests an opportunity for movement from one part of the culture to another, and may at first glance imply only a quantitative change. But it must be emphasized that both ends of the continuum are statistically abnormal, although only the contraculture end contains culturally pathological or criminal aspects. Thus there is a normative dimension to the continuum such that cultural definitions of 'good' and 'bad', 'criminal' and 'noncriminal', become labels attached to any locus on the abscissa. Moreover, the point where subculture norms begin to function and to be accepted as prevalent values is not necessarily congruent with the point where codified prohibitions begin. Both are relative over time and space, and to determine greater precision in the identification of these two subuniverses requires more research than has yet been done on the meaning of social values, the strength of normative prescriptions throughout the continuum, and the degree of introspection by the individuals who can be identified within subcultures. These items could also constitute a very interesting research area for the field of experimental jurisprudence. Although some limited efforts have been made by this new integrating field, emerging from an interchange between the social sciences and the law, we are not aware of any legal studies in this area. In the field of psychopathology, the continuity of behavior from normal to abnormal has been, of course, an important focus of interest. The identification of the 'pathological' is a baffling enterprise and often a matter of conventional agreement. 'Normal' is equally difficult to define, and various criteria, such as the behavior's being functional or consistent with the previous life history, have sometimes been introduced in psychiatry and strongly defended.

Our study of subcultures implies moving from references to the social universe, from the sociological perspective, to the idioverse, or individual's perceptual world, from the psychological viewpoint. In one sense, the collection of like idioverses, relative to important items of values and norms, defines the universe of a subculture. The individual absorbs culturally transmitted values, but, passing them through the prism of his own psychophysiology, he possesses a specific perception and response. That the idioverse is unique does not preclude the scientific classification of individuals, nor does recognition of the idioverse imply acceptance of the existential-phenomenological stance. For taken to its extreme position, as in existentialism, we would lose all or most points of reference in social and/or legal norms, and would be reduced, not to a cultural relativity that is willing to take into account the individual, but to individual relativity. Furthermore, in existentialism, to engage in violative thought could be interpreted as dynamically equivalent to actual criminal behavior.

But what criteria can be used to provide findings that would enable us to designate a set of values as subcultural, particularly in the field of criminology? First, if a subculture is denoted by values that are different from those of the dominant culture, we should determine whether the values are (a) tolerated differences that are not disruptive, that do not cause injury or possess potential threat of social injury to the dominant culture; or are (b) conflicting differences that are disruptive, that do cause injury or possess potential threat of social injury to the dominant culture. The Amish in Pennsylvania share values that by and large are tolerated deviations from American culture; however, there are a few values that the Amish possess that are much at variance and in conflict with the larger culture.[34] The 'delinquent subculture' is characterized principally by conduct that reflects values antithetical to the surrounding culture; but a variety of their activities are acceptable juvenile and not delinquent behavior. The different but tolerated values are concordant with the broader culture themes, for the two flow together without discord and the one is but an exaggeration of or an addendum to the other. The conflicting values are discordant and negative because of their disrupting effect upon the broader culture themes.[35] We are, therefore, suggesting at this point that there are two major types of subcultural values: (a) *tolerated concordant values*; and (b) *untolerated discordant values*.

This suggested dichotomy is commonly recognized, but has not been made explicit or described value by value in sufficient detail. It calls, first, for a classification of norms assumed to be different in *kind*. But before this division can be empirically performed, we need clear ideas of the values that constitute the dominant value system so that we have a base line from which to determine the category of values that presumably are different. The process of classifying values becomes the first and necessary task leading toward measurement of value differentiation. As has been suggested, 'Any classification . . . serves no more purpose than the catalog of events in chemistry, but without such a catalog, the study of combination of norms, their relationship to other cultural phenomena, etc., cannot be placed on a high scientific plane and thus aid in the scientific description of the phenomena of social life.'[36]

Second, the *number* of values that a subculture possesses that are different from those of the dominant culture is important, but only as each is considered in relation to its similar or antithetical value in the dominant culture. Thus a prerequisite of establishing the parameters of a subculture would appear to be the construction of a scale of values in the dominant culture. This scaling seems necessary if we are to weigh the importance of particular variant values or of their interacting patterns. For instance, two values that conflict with the larger culture may be of supreme evaluative importance to the latter; the apposition, therefore, could be sufficient to constitute a subculture. On the other hand, ten untolerated and discordant values may be of little importance and should consequently be viewed relative to the position of the previous two. This may be an individual, temporary phenomenon which calls for analysis of another area; i.e. the *stability* of a subculture. Relating a subcultural value element by the position of its directly opposite value in the hierarchy of the scale of values of the dominant culture might be part of the measurement process. If the subcultural element is a tolerated concordant value, relating it to the distance from the position of the parent value from which it is an offshoot would be one aid in measurement.

We should be able to measure the degree of value variance in terms of the reactions of agents of the dominant culture, according to whether they view a subcultural difference with tolerance or see variance as an actual or potential threat to the value of the dominant culture. An attitude scale could be used to obtain data on the direction (tolerated concordant vs. untolerated discordant) and on the extent to which subcultural values or conduct norms are thought to differ from the larger culture values. The perspective of a group representative of the dominant value system could help to determine the degree of variance.

(Temporal, situational variations in the group perspectives would have to be taken into account.)

The intensity or strength of a value is conceived as a mensurable item. We are here referring to the extent to which the value is internalized, absorbed, and consequently shared by agents of the subculture. An attitude scale could be constructed to register the degree of allegiance owed by members of a subculture to subcultural values. This could be done with the help of attitude-measuring through questionnaires, as has been attempted by Reckless, or, at a deeper level of personality assessment, through analysis of values and social motives derived from projective instruments.

Sellin has suggested that the intrinsic quality of a norm might be measurable in degrees. We have noted that he refers to this inherent energy or power of the norm as its resistance potential. He adds: 'This quality could perhaps be utilized as one basis for a preliminary and experimental classification of norms. Its utility would, of course, depend on the development of some technique of measurement, whereby conduct norms, regardless of the group evolving them, could be fitted into divisions on a scale.'[37] We have earlier referred to deviations within each subculture. The sanctions applied to these deviations can provide some measurement of the strength of the conduct norm based entirely upon the degree of severity of the penalty assigned to the violations. Deviations within a subcultural value system that have the same penalty would be grouped together and would carry the same weight, regardless of any other characteristics of these offenses.

It could be argued that we might establish a scale of values for the dominant culture in much the same way; i.e. by measuring the severity of the penalty ('resistance potential') for deviations from conduct norms. Although this position might be valid for legal norms generally, sanctions assigned for deviations from non-legal norms reflecting non-legal values would probably be extremely difficult to designate, and might have entirely different strengths and connotations in similar but geographically separated subcultures. A dominant culture that can exist with a variety of satellite subcultures will itself be heterogeneous and characterized by mobile degrees of support or mild rebuke within the range of acceptable conduct. Conformity generally is less required and demanded by the dominant culture than by any subculture, and the number, range, and variety of alternative forms of conduct are probably greater in the larger culture. Likewise, in the larger culture there is range and variety to the informal modes of control (sanctions) assigned to deviations that do not themselves amount to subcultural variations. To maintain its distinctive form of value differentiation, to preserve its identity, a subculture must generally attach stronger demands for conformity to those very value elements that are different from those of the larger culture. Because these different values are but a part of a subcultural system that mostly shares the values of the dominant culture (else, as we have said, it could not be a part of the whole), they are relatively few and the sanctions assigned to deviations from them should be more obvious and measurable. Thus we are suggesting that either a scaling analysis of individual attitudes of allegiance to subcultural values, or a scaling analysis of penalties for deviations from subcultural norms, could be used to provide a measure of the intensity or strength of subcultural values.

THE CONCEPTION
AND CLASSIFICATION OF VALUES

To develop more fully an operational definition of subcultures it is necessary to examine classification schemes and the methods for measuring norms and values. There is also the unresolved problem of whether classification and measurement should be made of norms or of values.

The Distinction Between Norms and Values

Kluckhohn and others have provided a distinction that should be kept in mind.[38] Values may be viewed as virtually synonymous with individual beliefs, which, of course, may nevertheless be held in concert and shared. They may connote what is or is believed (existential), what people want (desire), or what people ought to want (desirable).[39] Values do not necessarily have sanctions designed to support related norms. Norms, however, are always group-held prescriptions for or prohibitions against certain conduct. Because a belief may be idiosyncratic, a theory involving analysis of a subculture, such as the subculture of violence, requires a delimitation to those values that are shared by a substantial proportion of a population, even if there is cognitive unawareness by that population of the extent of the sharing. To determine the extent to which certain values are shared and to determine whether there is a normative system developed around a cluster of values, i.e. sanction-supported values, it is necessary to catalogue, classify, and measure commitment and sanction. We take our cue from and agree with Dewey, who believed that values are a proper subject for scientific study, when he said: 'Valuations exist in fact and are capable of empirical observation so that propositions about them are empirically verifiable. What individuals and groups hold dear or prize and the grounds upon which they prize them are capable, in principle, of ascertainment, no matter how great the practical difficulties in the way.'[40]

Thus, for operational theory we are inclined to view values as normative standards that are part of the repertoire of response which an individual may use as alternatives for action.[41] Biological impulses that are not a function of learned behavior would be excluded. With the exception of his willingness to include personal, individual beliefs, one of Kluckhohn's definitions presents this same view: 'A value is a conception, explicit or implicit, distinctive of an individual or characteristic of a group, of the desirable which influences the selection of available modes, means and ends of action.'[42] Aberle defined a value as 'an effectively charged idea or attitude in terms of which objects, events, actions, individuals, etc., are judged on a scale of approval–disapproval, whether the approval and disapproval are moral, aesthetic, hedonic, or in terms of some other dimension'.[43]

We have used in our own definition the term 'normative', referring to desirable, instead of 'norm', referring to a standard to which a social group generally conforms or which the group manifests in conduct. The distinction may be theoretically crucial for purposes of classification and measurement. In the real world, we are convinced, norms are created and emerge from a normative or value system that, properly measured, can reveal how norms are dictated. Moreover, as we have argued, the values to which we refer in subcultural theory are part of a group standard and are not responses merely to a specific or immediate situation. A specific situation may provoke a subcultural response, of course, but in Thomas and Znaniecki's sense, a cultural or subcultural response exists prior to the situation, new as it may be, and is, in short, a prepotent tendency to act that has been internalized by the individual as a commanding choice.

There may be a question about the difference which MacIver[44] raised with respect to 'interest', that is, between *like* and *common* values. In one sense, we avoid this issue of communication among individuals, an issue which MacIver's dichotomy raises. If persons have like values which determine the repertoire of response, and if we assume that these values create the normative standards governing conduct, many individuals with like values, knowing that the values are shared by others, function in ways indistinguishable from persons who commonly communicate their values by direct social interaction. That some communication is necessary to produce a subcultural response seems evident, but *Gemeinschaft* living is not a requisite. Thus individuals who are spatially remote from one another may constitute a plurality who hold a value or values in common, hence have shared values. Moreover, these same individuals may be involved in an institutional complex which requires subscription to the same value system. If 'like' were to mean similar but without any felt sense of sharing, then reference would again be made to individual beliefs, not to values as part of normative standards or group prescriptions or proscriptions. A subculture is composed of a group or groups but is not restricted by spatial proximity, although the kind of deviant subcultures with which criminology is mostly concerned are also often characterized by propinquity of group members.

Some Criteria of Values

In general, and to some extent following ideas summarized by Jacob and link,[45] we may say that the values lying behind the norms represented in a subculture have the following properties:

externality – they arise outside the individual, are the products of group living, and make us captives of conformity.

internalization – they are absorbed by the individual as part of his personality structure and self-inhibiting or self-fulfilling content.

selectivity – a limited range of alternatives with some functional consistency is available to the individual.

order – the options are arrayed in some kind of priority allocation of significance.

variability – even within a small and restricted subculture there is probably no social situation in which there is one and only one type of response dictated by the normative standards, although a generalized value of 'proper' conduct may offer only a few specific alternative courses of action in specific situations.

social obligation – they are part of the functioning and fulfillment of role requirements in a subsociety.

personal imperative – they are part of the ego demands in an evaluation of self.

We should stress that we are not contending that values *cause* norms or that values are necessarily *motives* of action. Both causes and motivations are complex phenomena, and neither the sociological nor the psychological literature has yet escaped the circularity expressed in explanations that infer that values derive from specific norms and then use the values to explain the norms. Values may be viewed as the subjective linkages between actors and action, between the individual and social norms, but using values in this way does not impose a causal nexus.[46] We have suggested or assumed that some norms exemplify some values, that some values may be reflected in norms that prescribe and prohibit certain conduct. If a set of norms can logically be said to cluster around a value concept, a normative system develops, and if values can be arrayed in hierarchical order, a value system may be described. If value systems are empirically derivable, then variances, divergencies, contranormative, and contra-value systems – in short, subcultures – can also be measured.

Some Criteria of Norms

There has been no shortage of efforts to classify norms. Our purpose is not to add to this effort but to suggest a method for deriving a classification. A brief summary list of some of the major aspects of norms, the ways in which they vary and may be classified, has been provided by Blake and Davis:[47]

‘1. *Content*
  (a) Societal requirement involved. (Norms ordinarily concern some functional requirement such as reproduction, division of labor, allocation of power. Norms clustered around a given functional requirement are often collectively designated as ‘institutions’.)
  (b) Whether the norm relates to a goal or to the means.
  (c) How the norm is stated – whether put negatively (should not) or positively (should).

‘2. *Types of Sanction*
  (a) Maximum or minimum.
  (b) Reward or punishment.
    Repressive or restitutive (in the case of punishment).

‘3. *Acceptance of the Norm*
  (a) Extent of acceptance (accepted as obligatory by virtually everyone or accepted as obligatory by only certain groups, such as certain ethnic groups).
  (b) Degree of acceptance (felt to be mildly obligatory or felt to be mandatory).

'4. *Mode of Transmission*

(*a*) Primary socialization.
(*b*) Secondary socialization.

'5. *Source of Imputed Authority for the Norm*

(*a*) Tradition.
(*b*) Law.
(*c*) A nonempirical or supernatural agency ('natural law', God, some member of a pantheon, ghosts, etc.).
(*d*) Public opinion.

'6. *Extent of Application of the Norm*

(*a*) To which statuses does the norm apply? (The reader will note that the extent of application of a norm is different from the extent of its acceptance. A norm which applies only to the occupant of a particular status may nonetheless be accepted by everyone as the proper conduct for that status. Example: Everyone thinks a judge should be fair and impartial.)
(*b*) To what groups does the norm apply?

'7. *Mode of Origination*

(*a*) Formal enactment.
(*b*) Informal, traditional accretion.

'8. *Formal Properties of the Statement of the Norm*

(*a*) Explicit (a body of law, regulations, codes).
(*b*) Implicit ('gentlemen's agreements', rarely verbalized but understood ways of behaving and thinking).
(*c*) Vague, diffuse statement.
(*d*) Specific, detailed statement.
(*e*) Rigid (requires exact conformity).
(*f*) Flexible (latitude in the precision with which the normative demand must be met).'

Some of the main features suggested by Barton,[48] Linton,[49] Morris,[50] and Williams[51] are included in this listing. There have been many other schemes for classifying norms, depending on the purpose and type of analysis, from the time Sumner[52] introduced his classification of norms into folkways and mores. Linton's[53] categories included universals, specialities, and alternatives. Sorokin[54] spoke of law-norms, technical norms, norms of fashion, and etiquette. Williams[55] built upon these efforts and suggested technical, conventional, aesthetic, moral, and institutional norms. G. H. von Wright[56] developed a scheme of normative concepts within 'denotic' logic, or the logic of the modes of obligation, and included as modal categories obligatory, permitted, indifferent, and forbidden. These were elaborated and presented in formal, symbolic notation by Anderson and Moore.[57] More recently, Mizruchi and Perrucci,[58] building upon a two-dimensional pro-scriptive/prescriptive basis, have set up a typology designed to specify the nature of these dimensions and to place them in a content of social system analysis. After reviewing several studies on alcoholism, these authors aver that norms may be classified ideal-typically in terms of the degree of elasticity, elaboration, pervasiveness, and functional inter-relatedness.

Recently Jack Gibbs[59] has pointed out the lack of agreement in generic definitions of norms, the absence of what he believes is an adequate classificatory scheme for distinguishing types of norm, and the lack of consistent distinction between attributes of norms. He takes the position that the degree of conformity to norms is a contingent[60] but not a definitional attribute, and emphasizes, as we have, that if we identify norms in terms of behavior, it is tautological to refer to the former as influencing or controlling the latter. Gibbs provides a typology of nineteen norms based primarily upon his distinctions between norms that include (1) a collective evaluation of behavior in terms of what *ought* to be; (2) a collective expectation as to what behavior *will* be, in a predictive sense; and (3) particular reactions to behavior, including attempts to apply sanction or otherwise induce a particular kind of conduct. Our own definition of values and emphasis for classi-fication and measurement purposes embraces Gibbs's first criterion, e.g. collective evaluation, or a shared belief that persons ought or ought not to act in a certain way. Gibbs announces that his typology 'is not concerned with the obvious fact that norms are relative'.[61] Our interest in value measurement and the significance of establishing parameters of a subculture are directly concerned with this very relativity that, though obvious, has not been adequately described or analytically interpreted.

Modes of Value-orientations

Finally, the 'modes of value-orientations' distinguished by Parsons and Shils *et al.* are well known and involve commitments to different types of selective standard of evaluation. The modes are the cognitive, the appreciative, and the moral, and are briefly defined as follows:

> 'The *cognitive* mode of value-orientation involves the various commit-ments to standards by which the validity of cognitive judgments is established. These standards include those concerning the relevance of data and those concerning the importance of various problems. They

also include those categories (often implicit in the structure of a language) by which observations and problems are, often unconsciously, assessed as valid.

'The *appreciative* mode of value-orientation involves the various commitments to standards by which the appropriateness or consistency of the cathexis of an object or class of objects is assessed. These standards sometimes lay down a pattern for a particular kind of gratification; for example standards of taste in music. The criterion in formulating such appreciative standards is not what consequences the pursuit of these patterns will have upon a system of action. Rather, these standards purport to give us rules for judging whether or not a given object sequence or pattern will have immediate gratificatory significance.

'The *moral* mode of value-orientation involves the various commitments to standards by which certain consequences of particular actions and types of action may be assessed with respect to their effects upon systems of action. These standards define the actor's choices with a view to how the consequences of these choices will affect (a) the integration of his own personality system and (b) the social system in which he is a participant.'[62]

Talcott Parsons's concern with ideas or systems of belief that are cognitive and evaluative has a direct bearing on our interest in defining, classifying, and measuring values. In *The Structure of Social Action*, reference is made to 'ultimate value attitudes', and, in *The Social System*, the phrase 'value-orientation patterns' is common. Elsewhere in his writings, Parsons speaks of 'moral norms', 'evaluative standards', or 'role expectations'. These are surely closely related items and are contrasted, as Charles Madge clearly points out, with cognitive ideas and beliefs.[63] Yet the contrast is not sustained in Parsons's writings, for he also stresses that 'man is a cognizing animal, and so his values do not exist apart from beliefs which give them cognitive meaning'.[64] Using Durkheim's concept of a common value system as a required condition for a society to maintain a system in equilibrium, Weber's concept of ultimate ends, the notion of patterned consistency in role expectations, and expanding on Freud's original concept of internalization to include internalization in the personality of the common value system that is also externally present as a shared system of symbols,[65] Parsons gives almost equal importance to cognition while stressing the evaluative mode. In *The Social System* he writes: 'The primary emphasis of this volume has been on the integration of social systems at the level of patterns of value-orientation as institutionalized in role-expectations. These patterns of value-orientations are elements of the cultural tradition, but are only part of it. Man is a cognizing animal, and so his values do not exist apart from beliefs which give them cognitive meaning. The dimension of cognitive orientation to the situation is just as essential to a total system of cultural orientation as is that of value-orientation to the choice-alternatives of action. . . . Since there must be *relative consistency* in the value-orientation patterns of a collectivity – though perfect consistency is not possible – this consistency must extend to the system of beliefs which give cognitive meaning to these value-orientations, again imperfectly to be sure. . . . Hence, there must be a set of beliefs, subscription to which is in some sense an obligation of collectivity membership roles, where the cognitive conviction of truth and the "moral" conviction of rightness are merged. . . . Value-orientation patterns, it will be remembered, always constitute definitions of the situation in terms of directions of solution of action-dilemmas.'[66]

These comments by Parsons about 'value-orientation patterns' and their cognitive meaning express notions with which we not only agree but wish to emphasize, for, as we shall contend, values can be captured on the cognitive level by socio-psychological investigation, they can be operationally defined and measured for intensity of subscription by individuals and groups, and they can be clustered in a way that denotes relative consistency, thereby promoting and producing a social system and subsystem.

Commitment and Conformity

In the literature on values and norms, much emphasis is placed on the assumption that commitment and conformity are correlated closely with role-status obligations. Values are held by individuals and are expressed through conduct conforming to group norms. But as William Goode[67] observes, while there is no concrete norm to be observed, there are many concrete role models. 'The norm,' he says, 'has no independent, original source of power other than persons, and their spontaneous censure usually focuses on the role relationship.'[68] He goes on to suggest that to understand better how norms, values, and roles are inter-related, research should be concerned with measuring the intensity of commitment to values, the degree of group consensus, and the degree of emotional and behavioral conformity to various role obligations. Moreover, as Ralph Turner,[69] Kelley and Shapiro,[70] and, more recently, as many studies in the tradition of sociometry and small-group analyses have indicated, the acceptance of the individual by his group members, the existence of conflicting role situations, or a conflict between the individual's relation to his friends and to authority, and the size of the group (dyad, triad, etc.) are a few of the variables affecting conformity to and deviance from normative standards. How the individual perceives his role; how his group perceives his role; how, in a Cooley looking-glass sense, he perceives the group's conception of his role; and how, in Matza's conceptualization, the group members wander and drift in a state of 'pluralistic ignorance' of one another's perception – are all dimensions of importance in determining the genesis and development of values and norms. But these are dynamic qualities helpful in explaining the child and adult socialization processes, the ways in which we adjust and readjust to changes in our roles or changes in the composition of groups around us. These variables are important in understanding why individuals possess certain values. However, if we are to produce parameters of significance in defining and delimiting subcultures, the primary focus should be on efforts to capture the values, to classify and to measure the values and the intensity of commitment to them.

THE MEASUREMENT OF VALUES

The abundant researches on perception, attitudes, social distance, prejudice, and discrimination, etc., provide examples of value measurement on a limited scale and with narrowly defined situations. Much less common has been research designed to classify, order, and measure a variety of culture values. In sociology, the writings of Stuart C. Dodd and of William R. Catton, Jr., probably represent the most detailed and methodologically refined thinking directly aimed at the measurement of values on a large scale that would help us to distinguish a subculture from its central culture.

Dodd's Classification

Dodd[71] was involved in a project on 'specifications for a national values scale' and limited the study 'to verbalized values as a first approximation to all values'. Using operational units, Dodd defined 'value' as a desideratum, i.e. anything desired or chosen by someone sometime. Values could be positive or negative, means or ends, minute or magnificent. Intensity of holding a value ('valuing') was based on a subject's claim of how strongly he felt about the value or what he would give or do to get or retain the physical manifestations of the value. 'Valuation' or 'tension ratio' became the ratio of an index of intensity of desiring to an index of the amount of the desideratum. 'Valuers' referred to the actors or respondents to questionnaires or interviews. As he describes 'valuation' or 'tension ratio':

> 'Thus, "I'll give $10 for two tickets" states a valuation of $5 per ticket; while "I'll give an evening a month for this committee job" states a valuation or tension ratio in time units for a unitary value, "the committee job." Tension may be measured either by a ratio or by an arithmetic product. The product of indices of desiring and of a desideratum defines a "tension product." This measures how much of a value one wants *and* how intensely one wants it. Thus a population's tension or victory depends both on the magnitude of the victory they want *and* how strongly they want it.'
>
> 'A valuation may be thought of in various terms, such as a "give/get" ratio, or as the "exchange ratio," or as the "price," or "worth per unit," or "unit cost" of any value.'[72]

Aberle also referred to the necessity to consider kind, intensity, and *role systems* in measuring values. He added: 'They [values] must be related to the analysis of the amount of latitude for apathy, expediency, and conflict which can exist with a tolerable degree of integration.' And among the pertinent questions to be asked in an empirical situation, he suggested, was 'the relative weight of two value-commitments when there is conflict, with the possibility that one commitment may be greatly attenuated'.[73]

Finally, Dodd suggested that time and space dimensions may be important in measuring values, but that these variables would have to be worked out as research progressed. Value systems, he believed, would have to consist of frequencing values or ordering them along a time dimension. An algebraic formula would become a *dimensional formula* (as physicists use the term), defined as 'a sum of products of powers of basic factors'. Representative samples of people in different cultures (and, presumably, subcultures) could be used to obtain a classifying system. Dodd suggested a dozen institutional subclasses of culture, namely: (1) domestic; (2) scholastic; (3) economic; (4) political; (5) religious; (6) philanthropic; (7) hygienic; (8) recreational; (9) artistic; (10) scientific; (11) linguistic; (12) military. If alternative classifying systems were explored, the one that yielded the smallest percentage of responses classified differently by different classifiers, working independently, would be the most reliable; and the one that yielded variables most highly correlated with later relevant behavior to be predicted would be the most predictive.

The essence of these suggestions is that values are not absolute, but relative. Moreover, it should be possible to produce a single scale of valuing, to borrow Dodd's phrasing, such that measurement could lead to more valid prediction of behavior. As indicated below, we accept Dodd's suggestion of reaching these research goals via psychophysical techniques and regression equations.

Catton's Concept of 'Value-space'

Following the lead of Stuart Dodd, William R. Catton, Jr.,[74] has sought to refine some of the dimensions useful for research on values. After defining value as 'a conception of the desirable which is implied by a set of preferential responses to symbolic desiderata',[75] he asserts that, in part, the value of an object is a function of its spatial proximity. Both social space and psychological time become important, and his general thesis suggests that a goal is perceived as less valuable when the relevant social distance is increased. Thus Catton introduces the element of desire or motivation for an object into the general discussion of values and formally states his position as follows: 'When values are held constant, desiring (or "motivation") varies inversely with the "distance" (in an *n*-dimensional psychological space, or value-space) between the values and the desideratum.'[76] Although he introduces the notion of 'value-space' and discusses some of its coordinates, he does not specify the procedures necessary for determining them experimentally. If 'value-space' exists, as for example when perceptions of time vary by age or when immediately attainable goals are selected over postponed and doubtfully attained goals, etc., it is clear that it is a socio-psychological and cultural product. 'It may appear', says Catton, 'to have different subsets of dimensions in different cultures and subcultures.'[77]

In one small experiment, this same author produced a 'hierarchy index' based on five simple items, using a paired-comparison questionnaire.[78] But of more importance to our concern, he attacked the problem of 'infinite' values, that is, those items which E. L. Thorndike had referred to earlier as 'utterly desirable or intolerable' to which he applied the term 'obsessional behavior'.[79] Seeking to determine whether there are values thought to be of infinite worth to human beings ('human life itself', 'worship of God and acceptance of God's will', etc.), Catton obtained several samples of clergymen to respond to questionnaires. Using six abstract values, he asked several sets of ministers to compare them in paired comparisons, another set to rank the six values, and a third set to indicate which were, in their opinion, of 'infinite worth'.

Because the ministers' responses on the paired-comparison questionnaire were not random, it was concluded that the respondents were able to discriminate between the relative worths of the different items and that values are not 'infinite' in the literal mathematical sense, for they can be measured according to established scaling techniques. As Catton said:

'... human values, including those which are regarded by certain authorities as being of infinite worth, become *measurable relative to each other* in exactly the same manner as other verbal stimuli. ...

'The measurability of any class of values, "infinite" or otherwise, may thus be regarded as a function of the ingenuity of the experimenter in devising techniques for obtaining discriminal responses to those values, of the sort described by the law of comparative judgment. The mere fact that the stimuli in question are labelled "values" does not make them non-measurable, nor does the fact that responses to such stimuli are called "value judgments" prevent them from displaying empirical regularities which may enable social scientists to make predictions.'[80]

The Measurement of Values in Different Populations

There have been several other experiments in, or suggestions for, measuring values. Briefly, Roy E. Carter, Jr., used the paired-comparison technique to measure 'the relative importance and/or acceptability of certain value concepts to three groups of subjects: 42 Indian nationals, 79 Filipinos, and 60 upper-division Stanford University students'.[81] The focal purpose of the study was to develop a procedure to be used for measuring responses of representative samples drawn from clearly defined populations. The author himself did not use a random sample. Using seven value items concerned with racial equality, population control, ownership of land, religion, central government, family stability, and education, Carter carefully examined the issue of 'circular trials', or non-rational preference rankings. (Thus, if A was preferred to B, and B to C, but C to A, the choices represented a non-rational preference.)[82] The so-called 'Koloman' procedure was used in which a group of 'explorers' discussed national goals and priorities for these goals in 'Koloman', a mythical new country. A single value concept was introduced in each paragraph of the dialogue, and subjects were asked to place a plus or minus mark (or double marks to indicate intensity) beside every argument with which they felt they could agree or disagree.

William Scott[83] has reported another interesting sociological effort to assess values and designate cultural ideologies. Defining 'personal value' or 'moral ideal' as 'a particular individual's concept of an ideal state of affairs or relations among people, which he uses to assess the "goodness" or "badness", the "rightness" or "wrongness" of actual relations which he observes',[84] the author selected samples from three different midwestern United States populations and analyzed by content analysis answers to open questions concerning traits which the subjects claimed they admired or disliked in other people. Traits such as honesty, integrity, genuineness, intelligence, dependability, fairness, love of people, generosity, friendliness, humility, up to twenty-one items were included. A particular moral ideal was judged dominant, and hence a cultural value, to the extent that it was widely shared within the group. Cultural ideologies were inferred from intercorrelations between moral ideals within the group of respondents. Chi-square analyses were used, and the author concluded that these admittedly crude items none the less did cluster, albeit with some inconsistencies, to produce observable cultural ideologies of an upper-middle-class suburban community, of university students, and of a minority Fundamentalist religious sect. Scott considers that when a sample is selected from a larger population that constitutes a society or subsociety, the procedure he used is appropriate for determining the values and ideologies of the entire culture, provided that each individual's moral ideals are given equal weight in the total. He suggests, however, that if the group culture is defined, not by the shared psychological attributes of its members, but as an external system of ideas and cultural products, some other method of determining values should be used. He infers that individuals responding to questionnaires, whether structured or open-ended, produce results that measure values principally from a psychosocial definitional perspective. What he refers to as the 'external system' and 'direct assessment of relevant cultural products' for assessing values and culture ideologies are language, art forms, mass communication, etc. Scott seems aware of the difficulty of using these 'external' attributes of a culture as indices of culture values. However, we would suggest using, whenever possible, the available phenomenologically perceived culture items, first, as exterior indices of culture values, and, second, as independent criteria for comparison with the group's cognitive expression of their value-orientations.

Analysis of Moral Values

Role conflicts and moral decisions are research areas explored by many authors. We can only cite as examples, without description, the works of Stouffer[85] on role conflicts, of William McCord and Joan McCord[86] on measuring conscience by using a moral-decision test, and of Patrick Suppes[97] in using mathematical statistics and game theory in developing formal models for justice involving a two-person non-cooperative game situation. Studies such as these provide clues to the variables in subjects' responses, to the procedures best fitted to measure values in a given population, to the means for making *a priori* selections of subpopulation units designed to provide carriers of subcultures, and to the methods for symbolically formalizing the results mathematically.

Some mention should be made of the literature concerned with the development of moral values in children and adults. Most of this work, as, for instance, the early empirical studies of Hartshorne and May,[88] has been devoted to intelligence, social class, and other personality and social factors related to behavioral manifestations of morality. Others, like the classic work of Piaget[89] on the child's moral judgement, discuss the developmental processes of acquiring an assessment of moral obligations and prohibitions. More recently, the thorough and sophisticated summary analyses by Kohlberg[90] on the development of moral character and the experiments by Aronfreed[91] on moral responses to transgression characterize the work being done in this socio-psychological area of values. Excellent as they are as contributions to our understanding of the socialization and learning processes, they stand just on the periphery of our interest in classifying and measuring cultural values to obtain the parameters of subcultures. Attempts at measuring 'moral judgements' psychometrically have rarely been successful, although they have enjoyed a limited popularity in Europe with tests like 'Tsedek'.[92]

Factor analysis of moral values, conducted by Rettig and Pasamanick, constitutes an example of a method of ranking and weighing the strength of about fifty moral values. These authors have conducted several studies on moral values among Koreans, Israelis, and Americans, including differences between generations.[93] In a factor analysis, six orthogonal moral values factors were extracted from each group studied. The clusters obtained were identified as: Factor A – general morality, which loaded on almost all items used; Factor B – religious morality, which loaded primarily on religious issues; Factor C – family morality, which loaded on those items which represented primary as well as more general functions of the family; Factor D – puritanical morality, which loaded on items considered 'conventionally' rather than 'intrinsically' wrong; Factor E – exploitative-manipulative morality, which included various morally prohibited activities that are considered wrong but that are likely to be risked for exploitative gain; and Factor F – economic morality, which loaded on items involving a financial motive. These studies by Rettig and Pasamanick represent carefully designed and statistically analyzed efforts to classify and to measure the strength of certain values. The method is complex, the values are limited to moral ones, and the results of factor analysis are not always easy for producers or consumers to interpret.

Cross-cultural Studies

In political science and international relations there has been an increasing interest in national values and efforts to measure values cross-culturally. Philip Jacob, at the University of Pennsylvania, has initiated a large-scale research on the interaction of social values and political leadership, as part of a program of international cooperative research on social values and political behavior.[94] Building upon many of the references to values and value measurement already cited in this chapter, upon such recent behavioral research on political integration and the influence of social values on political leadership as discussed by Jacob, Deutsch, *et al.*, in *The Integration of Political Communities*,[95] upon the work of Charles Morris and of Allen Barton who have, respectively, suggested a cross-cultural scale for measuring values and an operational definition of values,[96] Jacob and his associates are endeavoring to obtain an empirical assessment of social values from critically positioned local, regional, and national leaders in order to determine, among other things, how these values affect decisions and affect lower-status persons with whom the leaders interact. This elaborately planned study expects to collect data on values and value differentiations in India, Poland, Yugoslavia, and perhaps several other cooperating countries. Values are viewed as 'the norms which guide and influence persons in making decisions; the yardsticks by which they judge whether conduct is legitimate or not; the standards by which they feel obligated to do something or refrain from doing it'.[97] The study design announces that 'the main focus of the study is on the identification, comparison and measurement of the influence of the normative values held by leaders, which act as a major determinant of their policy decisions. These leadership values are considered a principal intervening variable in the process of political integration'.[98]

This study is of interest to us in our concern about measuring subcultures, and especially in measuring a subculture of violence, because the status leaders in a delinquent gang or a broader subculture of violence might be the principal carriers of the pervasive values of delinquency or violence. Moreover, we concur with a major notion of Jacob's proposed study, i.e.: 'Values . . . are empirically demonstrable through the manner in which given persons experience, perceive and interpret the concrete situations which they confront in life.'[99]

Indirectly related to this ambitious study of Jacob and his associates, and similarly concerned with national (political) or cross-cultural values, was the earlier work of Ruesch, Jacobsen, and Loeb.[100] In 1948 these authors developed a crude scale for measuring the degree of conformity to the 'American core culture', defined as 'general attitudes and assertions which are shared by the majority of Americans'. Their scale consisted of twenty-four items and a four-point scale for degree of conformity to a given aspect of the core culture. A scale point 4 indicated complete conformity, and a scale point 1, the greatest deviation from the core. The study was limited in many respects but represents an insightful beginning to research on values.

More recently and in this same cross-cultural vein, Leonard Doob reports a study of values using the paired-comparison technique.[101] Subjects included German-speaking South and North Tyrolean and Italian secondary-school students and Ladin children in primary school. Sixty pairs of words or phrases, each separated by the word 'or' were used, and subjects were requested to draw a line under the word which better represented their point of view. Four groups of pairs included notions of 'pleasantness, importance, friendliness and health'. This study is basically on the topic of patriotism among geographically close yet ethnically distinct groups. There were twenty-three statistically significant differences noted, including such things as the fact that South Tyroleans, compared with Italians, felt that soup was more healthful than spaghetti and preferred Goethe to Dante. To some extent, the study fails to avoid the pitfall to which Jacob, in the previously mentioned study, draws attention; i.e. confusing the meaning of values with preferences, goals, and wants. Nonetheless, we draw the reader's attention to the Doob reference because once again an effort has successfully been made to designate, empirically, value clusters. The well-known work of Charles Osgood and his associates[102] in the field of psycholinguistics emphasizes the importance of this approach and its interdisciplinary relevance. By a 'semantic differential' technique, different dimensions of values, expressed in verbal communications in different languages and cultural environments, become a refined tool of assessment which can be, and has been, used in a variety of research and experimental situations.

The relevance of the above-quoted literature obviously lies in the fact that it is an hypothesis of value-clustering capable of measurement that underlies any meaningful theory of subcultures.

The Measurement of Values in Criminological Studies

Except for our previous reliance upon Sellin's *Culture Conflict and Crime*, our discussion of value measurement has generally been devoid of references from criminological literature. Solomon Kobrin's[103] lucid statements about constructing a typology of delinquency areas based on degrees of integration of opposing value schemes should not be overlooked; nor should the hypotheses of distinguishing delinquent from the broader American values, by Milton Barron.[104] These articles concur with our general discussion about subcultures and the need to measure values. Relative to our axiomatic statement that subcultural value systems are a part of, not apart from, the parent culture, Kobrin says, for example: 'Competing value systems tend to accommodate to one another by mutual incorporation of elements common to or compatible with each other.'[105] His general conclusions are that a delinquent subculture originates from cross-group hostility, that such a subculture is a group elaboration of individual adaptations serving ego-defense needs, and that the conflict of cultures has a social psychological reflection in the dual value-orientation introjected by the delinquent individual. There are implicit but clear requests in these observations for measurement of the value items that are in conflict and that overlap.

Perhaps more explicit are the questions raised by Barron nearly fifteen years ago: How do social values differ from other cultural constructs such as standards, ideals, goals, morals, mores, and norms? What are the values of our society? Do social values include social processes as well as social objectives or goals?[106] He spoke of 'official' values, 'private or unofficial' values, and the need for discovering differences or correlations between delinquent values and delinquent behavior. He strongly asserted, '. . . it is our contention that Sellin deserves more credit for the revitalization of the values approach to delinquency and crime'.[107] And, finally, he referred to the need to develop more versatile utilization of methodological techniques for measuring delinquent and nondelinquent values.

Under the direction of Denis Szabo in Montreal, a pilot study is being conducted in an effort to describe the moral value system of delinquents.[108] Analytically, three value systems have been assumed, each with its own *région morale*. The first is designated 'conventional morality', or that of the dominant culture, and researchers hope to capture elements of this system by examining the personal morality of officials of the social and legal institutions. The second is referred to as 'marginal morality', loosely indicating several social-class, adolescent, and ethnic subcultures that have, in their own adaptation processes, somewhat modified the more 'global moral value system'. Finally, the third system is the 'contracultural morality' associated with the development of norms and values of delinquents. The four hypotheses governing this pilot study are common assumptions to current sociological theory: (1) there exists among delinquents an arrangement of moral values particular to their group; (2) delinquents share certain values with the conventional global culture; (3) the moral system of delinquents contains a set of values peculiar to their adaptation patterns and proper to their socioeconomic and adolescent subculture; and (4) the moral system of delinquents includes some values appropriate to their contraculture.

Methodologically, there appear to be gross limitations and problems in this study as now conceived, and the responses to questionnaires given to each of the three groups fail to provide consistent patterns of values. This failure seems to lie less in the error of the hypotheses of value-system differentiation than in the lack of precision in defining units of investigation, inadequate classification of values, premature efforts to apply statistical manipulation to sketchy data that probably could not yield discriminal points of variance, and other similar weaknesses. But pilot studies are expected to highlight problems of this kind, and it is hoped that this research will be improved and pursued further, for it is one of the few studies in criminology seeking to describe empirically values and value systems.

The Use of Psychophysical Methods: Magnitude Estimation

As we have seen, there are many types of scale and statistical manipulation that might be employed to measure the degree of acceptance or rejection of specific values. After a typology and classification system have been established, we are inclined to believe that one of the most efficient and successful types of scale for measurement purposes is the magnitude estimation scale described most fully by S. S. Stevens, of Harvard University, in the development of psychophysical measurements. Sellin and Wolfgang[109] have introduced the use of this ratio scale in the field of criminology to obtain from several sets of subjects responses regarding the seriousness of specific types of crimes, and the experience of these authors suggests that this same scaling procedure might effectively be used to obtain information about the relative degrees of allegiance to, or unacceptability of, a set of values. Once having established a value set, and after hypothesizing a cluster of characteristics as denoting certain groups in society which share certain values in degrees significantly different from other groups, magnitude estimation scale scores, once properly handled statistically, could provide tests for the major and sub-hypotheses. This effort would at least be a beginning of the task of determining where the central culture starts to merge with a subcultural component, i.e. the parameters of a subcultural entity of whatever form or phenomenology.

The history of psychophysics is relatively short, dating in modern terms from Fechner[110] in 1860, but the literature on this topic in psychology is extensive. Initially emphasis was on the relation between physical objects and psychological, i.e. subjective, responses to them. The development of the underlying mathematical ideas in measurement and of the psychology of perception converged to produce the scales of modern psychophysics. Fechner's early interests were concerned with the mind–body problem and the nature of the function that connected physical measures of energy, to which people were sensible, to their mental effect. Thus a 'heavy' weight weighed more than a 'light' weight. But how many more grams had to be added to a weight of 10 grams to make it appear twice as 'heavy'? The answer was not 10 grams if 'heavy' and 'light' referred to the psychological effect of the weights. To find this psychophysical rule, Fechner had to have a measure of 'heaviness', which was not available. But he developed a theory of psychological measure and used this theory to establish the psychological scale, after which he derived the psychophysical rule about the relation between mental and physical measures. Much later, in the 1920s, L. L. Thurstone,[111] developing the law of comparative judgement, brought to the attention of scholars the fact that psychological events with no intrinsic physical counterpart could also be given quantitative values. Thurstone's scaling techniques were widely adopted, and psychological measures became common currency in much of social psychology.

In the middle and late 1930s, S. S. Stevens developed a number of techniques for the assessment of psychological magnitudes of physically measurable events and, along with his collaborators, has shown that the current methods in psychophysics can be applied to many non-physical dimensions.

Scales measuring attitudes and values are not new, as any current book on scaling analysis will readily show. In sociology, for example, the work of Likert, Guttman, Stouffer, and the use of factor analysis in moral values by Rettig and Pasamanik are well known. But of the four types of scales – nominal, ordinal, interval, and ratio – the first three have been predominant in sociological research, while the ratio scale, developed most intensively in psychophysics, has almost entirely been neglected by sociologists. It is a ratio scale in the form of the magnitude estimation, which we are suggesting without our present context as the best means for measuring the strength of social values both in the dominant or central culture and in subcultural segments.

'Scales are possible in the first place', says Stevens, 'only because there exists an isomorphism between the properties of the numeral scales and the empirical operations that we can perform with the aspects of objects.'[112] But he further warns us:

'Not *all* the properties of numbers and not *all* the properties of objects can be paired off in a systematic correspondence. But *some* properties of objects can be related by semantical rules to *some* properties of the numerical series. In particular, in dealing with the aspects of objects we can invoke empirical operations for determining equality (the basis for classifying things), for rank ordering and for determining when differences and when ratios between the aspects of objects are equal. The conventional series of n numerals – the series in which by definition each member has a successor – yields to analogous operations: We can identify the members of the series and classify them. We know their order as given by convention. We can determine equal differences, as $7-5 - 4-2$, and equal ratios, as $\frac{10}{5} = \frac{6}{3}$. This isomorphism between the formal system and the empirical operations performable with material things justifies the use of the formal system as a *model* to stand for aspects of the empirical world.

'The type of scale achieved when we deputize the numerals to serve as representatives for a state of affairs in nature depends upon the character of the basic empirical operations performed on nature. These operations are limited ordinarily by the peculiarities of the thing being scaled and by our choice of concrete procedures, but, once selected, the procedures determine that there will eventuate one or another of four types of scale: *nominal, ordinal, interval,* or *ratio.* Each of these four classes of scales is best characterized by its range of invariance – by the kinds of transformations that leave the "structure" of the scale undistorted.'[113]

As we have indicated, the method called magnitude estimation has come to be the most widely used in psychophysics, probably because it is simple, straightforward, and gives results that seem to stand up under efforts at validation. Magnitude estimation refers to a procedure in which the observer makes direct numerical estimations of a series of subjective impressions. The experimenter typically presents a stimulus of medium intensity and tells the subject to call it 10. (Any number could, of course, be used.) The subject is then told that a series of intensities will be given and that to each of them he should assign a number proportional to the apparent magnitude as he perceives it. The subject is permitted to use any numbers that seem appropriate, i.e. whole numbers, decimals, or fractions. If a stimulus seems to the subject to be twice as great as the original modulus or standard, he should call it 20, if five times as great, 50, if only a twentieth as great, 0·5, etc. It is best if a different ordering of stimuli is used for each subject, and the results, usually for at least ten subjects, are averaged by taking a mean or median value.[114]

Although many methodological problems of measurement theory are involved in research techniques that use the magnitude estimation scale, and although most of the previous research has used prototethic continua such as apparent duration, apparent thickness, vibration on the finger tip, loudness, there have been interesting efforts to apply the magnitude estimation scale to metathetic non-physical continua, as in a study of the subjective utility of money, and the previously mentioned study of seriousness of delinquency. Our suggestion now is to apply these efforts to the study of values, value priorities, intensity, strength, degree of allegiance, or similar terms that can be operationalized through quantitative measurement.

Because our immediate concern is with criminal conduct, and particularly with violence, the rather ambitious task of scaling major values of the central culture and a variety of subcultures would be reduced for the present purposes by limiting the scaling to those values concerned with the use of violence.

In the Sellin–Wolfgang study, measurement of the seriousness of delinquency was limited to 141 versions of offense descriptions that avoided the use of traditional legal labels. The phrasing was such that cross-cultural replications could be made with little difficulty, and the resulting numerical weights for criminal acts were theoretically defended and empirically treated as a ratio scale. Both the more traditional category scale and the magnitude estimation scale were used, compared, and found to correlate highly with one another. Moreover, several sets of raters (judges, police officers, university students) and different ages of offenders (27 years old, 17, 13, unidentified age) were used; and no statistically significant differences were found between rating groups or for offenders of different ages. For illustrative purposes here, the instructions to respondents on the magnitude estimation scale are presented below:[115]

'This booklet describes a series of violations of the law, each violation is different. Your task is to show how serious *you* think each violation is, *not* what the law says or how the courts might act.

'You do this by writing down in a score box on each page a number which shows how serious each violation seems to you. The first violation has been done as an example. It shows a violation which is given a seriousness score of 10. Use this violation as a standard. Every other violation should be scored in relation to this standard violation. For example, if any violation seems ten times as serious as the standard violation, write in a score of 100. If a violation seems half as serious as the standard, write in a score of 5. If a violation seems only a twentieth as serious as the standard, write in a score of ½ or ·50. You may use *any* whole or fractional numbers that are greater than zero, no matter how small or large they are just so long as they represent how serious the violation is compared to the standard violation.

'Take your time. Every page should have a number in the score box. Do not turn back once you have finished a page. Remember, this is not a test. The important thing is how *you* feel about each violation. Do not write your name on any of the sheets for you will not be identified.'

Approximately one thousand subjects were asked to give numerical scores of relative seriousness; the raw scores were converted to means; standard deviations and z-scores were obtained; and, by the use of a constant divisor and rounding, a set of mathematical weights was developed for computing meaningful weighted rates of crime and delinquency based on seriousness. These score values benefit from the attributes of additivity and of being ratio scales; thus a seriousness score of 14 is twice as serious as a score of 7.[116] The process for deriving the scores was statistically complicated but not complex, and the results were presented and can be used in simple and efficient forms.

As a brief example from this study, some of the final seriousness scores for personal injuries were: 26 for criminal homicide, 10 for forcible rape, 7 for a physical injury causing hospitalization, 4 for an injury requiring medical treatment and discharge without hospitalization, and 1 for minor injury without medical treatment. It should be kept in mind that all of these injuries resulted from criminal acts and could occur as separate discrete assaults or as components of a single but complex criminal event like rape or robbery. A criminal event may have more than one victim, and each victim of an assaulting crime was separately scored. In forcible rape, the kind of physical injury is added to the score of 10 for the rape itself. There are, of course, many intricate problems in this kind of measurement, of counting events, victims, and scores; but, once clearly described, the operational aspects appear to be relatively simple. In this study, Sellin and Wolfgang were able to reduce crimes against the person and against property to a unidimensional base, i.e. the judged seriousness of the offenses. While the authors did not explicitly suggest that physical injuries could thereby be plotted with money values and that money could be used as a scale of seriousness, the suggestion is not unreasonable.[117] In the scaling analysis of the delinquency, the judged pain of loss of money was capable of being isolated from certain components of the law violation. That is, from a burglary or a robbery, the authors were able to extract the score value for the breaking and entering alone, or for the intimidation alone, etc., and thus obtain the score value for the money loss due to the theft. The loss of money through a theft was represented in a mathematical formula that expressed a power function. Thus losing two hundred dollars was not twice as serious as losing one hundred dollars; the amount lost had to exceed $250 and could go as high as $2,000 in order to be perceived as twice as serious. The magnitude scale scores and money values were plotted on arithmetic coordinate and then on log-log paper as shown in the following figures (pp. 136, 137).

The computed relation between the scores and the selected reference points of money value is described as a power function. As the authors claim:

'These results fit closely previous research on the subjective utility of money. Although this is not surprising, they are an important addition to this literature because the present study is the first to show the power function of money in an experimental situation for which different assigned amounts described as stolen constitute loss instead of gain. It should be emphasized that the raters did not scale amounts of money but, rather, their own subjective reaction, along an implicit continuum of seriousness, to the loss of different amounts of money. The data show that the form of the function relating the seriousness of the offense to the amount of money stolen is similar to ratio scales for many other analogous perceptual continua.'[118]

There are many other aspects of this study that are relevant to the present discussion, but enough has been said to reveal the general aspects of the methodology. As indicated, this kind of scaling of values has the benefit of a ratio scale and of additivity, thus capturing discriminal points of reference that would permit analysis of subcultural values according to priority assignment, intensity of commitment, clusters of

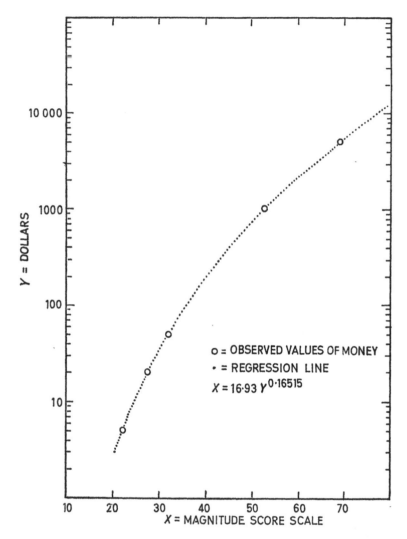

Figure 2   *The power function of money. The relation between magnitude scale scores of University of Pennsylvania raters (N = 105) and points of the value of money thefts.*

Source: Sellin and Wolfgang, *The Measurement of Delinquency*, p. 285.

values added together as components of a value system, and the relational strength of values in one subculture compared to another subculture or to the central culture.

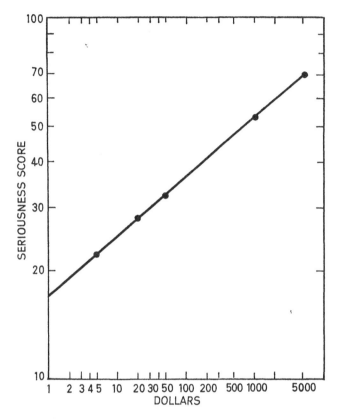

Figure 3   *The power function of money. The relation between magnitude scale scores of University of Pennsylvania raters (N = 105) and points of the value of money thefts (log-log plot).*

Source: Sellin and Wolfgang, *The Measurement of Delinquency*, p. 286.

We are suggesting, therefore, that research on values in general should be pursued by means of a psychophysical method, such as the magnitude estimation scale of Stevens, used effectively in the Sellin–Wolfgang study of crime. It would be necessary to establish through a base-line survey sets of values to be scaled. Then, representative samples of population could be used as subjects selected on the basis of sociological variables,

F

hypothesized (or empirically derived) as meaningful for delineating the carriers of central culture or subcultural value themes.

This suggestion is made with some awareness of the limitations of such scaling techniques. As a measurement of subjective allegiances to specific values, these scales could be extremely useful. That the techniques measure subjective responses at a point in time that may not correspond to some other point in time is admitted. There may be temporary, fleeting, or enduring attitudes expressed; but testing and retesting can determine the temporal character of the values. We wish to emphasize, however, that the psychophysical scale may not tell us all we wish to know about overt behavior responses to real-life situations or about projections of the subjects outside themselves. Thus no brief is made here that psychophysical scaling serves all the necessary requirements of diagnosis.

It may be argued that asking people to rate the relative importance of some set of values, and to give ratings to the degree of individual support they offer to these values, measures only the expressed opinion and not the actual behavior or the unconscious or latent attitudes, feelings, or thoughts. To interpret from the manifest content of subjective responses to questions of the magnitude of allegiance and significance of values to the individual to *latent* attitudes, and to extrapolate from one situation to another that presumably carries the same value-orientation, may be highly suspect forms of analysis from such responses. Rosenzweig,[119] particularly, has made us aware of the three major levels of behavior in the typical methods of personality assessment. He says: 'It is possible conveniently to classify these methods as subjective, objective, or projective according to whether the subject takes himself as a direct object of observation, whether the observer takes the subject as a direct object of observation, or whether the subject in cooperation with the observer "looks the other way" at some ego-neutral object. The subjective methods include the questionnaire or inventory and the autobiography, in both of which the individual expresses from his standpoint opinions or judgments about himself or about other objects and situations. The objective methods comprise such direct observations of gross behavior as can be made through one-way screens and such more covert methods as become possible by employing physiological indicators, e.g. the psychogalvanometer. The projective methods embrace, among other instruments, the Rorschach technique, the Thematic Apperception Test, word association, play technique, and motor-expressive types of performance like handwriting gait, and voice.'[120] Although noting in ideal form the existence of these three different levels in psychodiagnosis, Rosenzweig admits that the levels are apt to mingle and merge in everyday life and in test situations to such a degree that analysis is often difficult. None the less, the heuristic value of the classification is self-evident.

Moreover, the old question cannot be entirely ignored of whether the responses of individuals, albeit anonymously, to a set of questions regarding their priority allocation of a predetermined set of values and their intensity of allegiance to them, may not be different from (a) the latent content of the response, or (b) how the individual may in fact conduct himself in specific social situations. None the less, experimental research and logic suggest that the testing situation does not produce reponses alien to the subjects' personality and cultural orientations. In a quite different context, Galanter's comments on his analysis of the utility function of money are relevant:

'. . . we have asked people about hypothetical increments of money and we do not have any information about what would happen if they *actually* got the money. This is often stated as an argument against techniques of this kind, but the fact of the matter is that prior to a decision one always considers the alternatives as hypothetical and, presumably, bases his action on these considerations. To argue that we use in hypothetical situations a scale of values and, therefore, that the scale does not represent what people do, is to prejudge the usefulness of the scale as a characterization of the hypotheses that antedate the decision.'[121]

We believe that despite the plethora of acts, tendencies to act, feelings, thoughts, attitudes, despite the multitudinous values, norms, prescriptions and proscriptions of conduct, and despite the variability of personality and behavior, an effort to locate dominant values in a culture and in its subcultural components, to classify and to measure them, should and can be made. While the individual may be unique as a composite, he and his values can be clustered with other individuals and values. One of the functions of science is to distinguish regularities, patterns, configurations, and classifications. And this function serves the additional one of prediction. If individuals may be grouped on the basis of certain likenesses, so may value-orientations and value-laden and norm-demanding situations. It is in the pursuit of this goal that the parameters of a subculture and, concomitantly, the collection of individuals constituting a subculture, may be located. It is doubtful whether a subculture requires formal social organization or even highly structured roles; therefore the absence of formal means of communication may be noted without damage to the thesis of the existence of a specified subculture. But values shared in similar rank order and with similar intensity would seem to be the critical elements in the definition and precision of the meaning of subcultures.[122]

THE THESIS
OF A SUBCULTURE OF VIOLENCE

This section examines the proposition that there is a subculture of violence. Since results of the kinds of scaling analysis suggested in the last section are not available, it is necessary to build upon previous related research and theory in order to extend a theoretical formulation regarding the existence of subcultures in general if we are to hypothesize a particular subculture of violence. It would be difficult to support an argument that a subculture exists in relation to a single cultural interest, and the thesis of a subculture of violence does not suggest a monolithic character. It should be remembered that the term itself – subculture – presupposes an already existing complex of norms, values, attitudes, material traits, etc. What the subculture-of-violence formulation further suggests is simply that there is a potent theme of violence current in the cluster of values that make up the life-style, the socialization process, the interpersonal relationships of individuals living in similar conditions.

The analysis of violent aggressive behavior has been the focus of interest of many social and biological researches, and psychology has attempted to build several theories to explain its phenomenology, ranging from the death-aggression instinct of the psychoanalytic school to the frustration-aggression hypothesis. The present discussion is the result of joint explorations in theory and research in psychology and in sociology, using the concept of subculture as a learning environment. Our major area of study has been assaultive behavior, with special attention to criminal homicide. The following chapter will present a more detailed analysis of the pertinent literature, but some of the main trends in criminological thinking related to this topic must now be anticipated for the proper focus of the present discussion.

Isolated sectional studies of homicide behavior are extremely numerous, and it is not our intention to examine them in this chapter. There are basically two kinds of criminal homicide: (1) premeditated, felonious, intentional murder; (2) slaying in the heat of passion, or killing as a result of intent to do harm but without intent to kill. A slaying committed by one recognized as psychotic or legally insane, or by a psychiatrically designated abnormal subject involves clinical deviates who are generally not held responsible for their behavior, and who, therefore, are not considered culpable. We are eliminating these cases from our present discussion, although subcultural elements are not irrelevant to the analysis of their psychopathological phenomenology.

Probably fewer than five per cent of all known homicides are premeditated, planned intentional killings, and the individuals who commit them are most likely to be episodic offenders who have never had prior contact with the criminal law. Because they are rare crimes often planned by rationally functioning individuals, perhaps they are more likely to remain undetected. We believe that a type of analysis different from that presented here might be applicable to these cases. [123]

Our major concern is with the bulk of homicides – the passion crimes, the violent slayings – that are not premeditated and are not psychotic manifestations. Like Cohen, who was concerned principally with most delinquency that arises from the 'working-class' ethic, so we are focusing on the preponderant kind of homicide, although our analysis, particularly in the next chapter, will include much of the available data on homicide in general.

Psychoanalytic Theories of Aggression

One of the most popularized theoretical approaches to the explanation of violence is that presented by the psychoanalytic school. Aggression is conceived as the actualization of a so-called 'death instinct', a general aggressive instinctual drive. Freud maintained that a somatically based instinct toward aggression exists, 'an active instinct for hatred and destruction'. This basic drive, for which Freud provided a fascinating, if unproven, theoretical foundation, could, of course, be modified through its interaction with the opposed 'life instinct' and through education, sublimation, and socialization of its objectives. However, its basic teleological nature and the tension-reducing characteristics of the behavior which it elicited remained unvaried. Basic to this formulation is the innate aspect and the universality of the existence of this drive.

Since Freud's original formulation, psychoanalysts have taken divergent positions. Sometimes, like K. Menninger[124] or Waelder,[125] they have accepted entirely the original formulation of a death instinct. At other times, like Alexander[126] and Hartmann, Kris, and Loewenstein,[127] they have accepted the instinctual aspects, although rejecting the general concept, of a 'death instinct.' Other psychoanalysts, like

Saul,[128] reject the 'innate' aspects of the aggression instinct. Although, as usual, many different kinds of criticism could be adduced against the 'instinct' theory of aggression, the most basic rebuttal of the 'innate', 'inborn' aspects is that we lack any biologically acceptable explanation for the concept of the innate 'aggression' drive, and that we find no confirmation of its existence in the many carefully controlled and executed studies of animal behavior. We do find evidence of physiological mechanisms that control fighting behavior, but their stimulation must come from the external environment. The psychoanalytic hypothesis, so far, lacks confirmation, but does constitute an interesting research approach, which unfortunately has not been subjected to any large-scale investigation and has received only scarce and somewhat tautological clinical confirmation.

Medical and Biological Studies

Medical and biological studies have contributed only partial and incomplete data to the problem of violence. Several medical investigations have been conducted, particularly in the field of criminology, on homicidal groups, without, however, any general value. Leptosomes, or mesomorphs, appear to predominate in the homicide populations, and a variety of biological disturbances, from hyperthyroidism to hypoglycemia, may cause aggressive reactions. Although some endocrinological abnormalities and neuropsychiatric syndromes may occasionally be provocative of aggression and violence in normal subjects, this behavior seems to be unrelated to systematic and/or unique biological differences. The Gluecks' study on juvenile offenders has found that hostility, although highly associated with delinquency, does not differ significantly among the four types of delinquents and nondelinquents, classified according to Sheldonian somatotyping.[129] Electroencephalographic studies elicit a greater proportion of abnormalities, often of an aspecific type, in violent offenders, particularly in those showing motiveless violence. Again, no consistent biological disturbances can be isolated, and this lack of consistency reflects the uncertainty of our knowledge about the underlying neural mechanisms of emotion in general, and specifically of anger.

We cannot adequately or clearly differentiate between fear and anger at a physiological level. We find no physiological evidence for any spontaneous stimuli for fighting arising within the body in a normal organism. This lack of evidence leads to an important consideration – the chain of causation of aggression traces back to outside the organism, and although there may be individual differences in the reactivity to external stimuli evoking aggression, these inner characteristics do not, by themselves, explain aggressive behavior. We are led back to the external social environment as the area where the causative key to aggression must at present be found.

Psychometric Techniques

One particular approach to research on violence, which should be briefly mentioned, is that which utilizes psychological tests for the study of groups of violent subjects. Many investigations have been published, particularly in the field of criminology, which make use of modern psychometric tools, projective or questionnaire type, in an attempt to define and describe a 'differential' psychology of the violent offender. Many of the psychometric researches are on homicides. Often, these studies have been poorly planned and poorly executed, with fundamental faults in design, sampling, and administration. However, from an analysis of their results, we obtain the general picture of a personality characterized by egocentrism and lack of emotional control. The murderer can be described as an explosive, immature, hyperthymic person who is unable to establish social contact. He displays a deficit of conscious control and a strong need for the immediate gratification of impulses.

No attempts, however, have so far been made to link meaningfully the psychometric evaluation of aggressive traits to a theory of aggression, and these studies remain descriptive and isolated. They are undoubtedly relevant to the diagnosis and prediction of proneness to aggressive behavior, and they are useful tools in a variety of clinical situations, but their general interest and theoretical value are limited, as we shall observe more fully in the next chapter.

The Frustration–Aggression Hypothesis

The frustration–aggression hypothesis has been readily accepted by many sociologists and psychologists as a useful research tool. It is a 'classic' approach to the problem of violence, and its heuristic value has probably not been matched by any other theory. However, few psychologists would today assert that the presence of frustration inevitably leads to some form of aggression. Less criticism is met by the statement that aggressive behavior always presupposes a frustrating situation. Scientific research on the frustration–aggression hypothesis is not easy, since it is difficult to avoid a circular logic. As McNeil has observed, 'If the experimenter predicts that an increase in aggressive behavior will result from an increase in frustration, he cannot then use the aggressive behavior as proof that he has increased the frustration.'[130] Also, the different forms of frustration vary very much, and the same applies to the phenomenology of the aggressive reaction to the frustration, as Rosenzweig[131] pointed out. A recent report of the studies on this hypothesis, conducted by Berkowitz,[132] provides a redefinition of the basic terms. His work has been particularly useful in considering instrumental aggression – a construct that Dollard and his collaborators did not include in their analysis – as separate from reactive aggression. In Berkowitz's definition, '*frustration* produces an emotional state, *anger*, which heightens the probability of occurrence of drive-specific behaviors, namely *aggression*'.[133] The probability that aggression will actually take place depends, however, on the presence or absence of restrainers against aggressive, hostile actions. The strength (and, we should like to add, the quality and phenomenology) of the aggressive responses arising from a frustration should be 'a joint function of anger intensity and of the degree of association between the instigator and the releasing cue'.[134] This new formulation, with its awareness of the importance of outside stimuli, which, in most instances can be equated to social determinants of the learning process and of the differential reactions to frustration, constitutes a welcome improvement of the rigid mechanistic process originally presented in the work of Dollard and his collaborators.[135] The non-applicability of the general hypothesis and the importance of the arbitrariness or non-arbitrariness of frustration (as perceived by the subject) have been firmly stated by Pastore, Cohen, and others.[136] The status of the hypothesis is far from settled, but quite recently the predictive capacity of the thesis has been reaffirmed.[137] On the other hand, Masserman[138] has denied its validity and claims that animal behavior resulting from external frustration is adaptive, initiative behavior and needs no new rubric of 'aggressivity' to account for its dynamics or economics. Extensions of the hypothesis to include the concepts of conflict and hostility have generated a widened range of theoretical and experimental studies.[139]

In making one of the most comprehensive analyses of the concept of frustration, Berkowitz has modified the hypothesis in order to enlarge its basis of support and includes recent experimental research findings and theoretical formulations.[140] His inclusion of instrumental aggression, consequent to non-aggressive motivations, and his eclectic awareness of stimulus-response and cognitive theory enhance the value of the original frustration–aggression formulation. These modifications still do not account for divergent experimental results and insert many more conditions and prerequisites in the hypothesis. Important to our subcultural approach, however, is the fact that the perceptual process is introduced into the frustration–aggression formula. This perceptual process directly affects the definition of the situation as frustrating and determines the type of reaction. When frustration includes a perceptual, quasi-existential element, the way is open for integration with the subcultural hypothesis, which, after all, involves the important ingredient of the differential perceptual characteristics of the subculture members.

The heuristic value of the frustration-aggression hypothesis is unquestionable in the area of general and clinical psychology. In criminology, however, it has been little used. The hypothesis has been employed in two studies on homicides, one by Henry and Short[141] and the other by Palmer.[142] However, the causal nexus between frustration and overt aggression that ends in homicide has not been specified in these studies, nor have the different reactions of human subjects to frustration been adequately accounted for. As we suggest elsewhere, some of the Henry and Short data could be better explained through the use of Reckless's containment theory, in terms of external restraint.[143] Objective studies conducted by McCary[144] with the Rosenzweig Picture-Frustration Test have failed to confirm some of the interpretations of the differential homicide rates of the Southern Negro groups studied by Henry and Short. In fact, some of the data yielded contradictory results. Southern Negroes appeared to be less extra-punitively aggressive toward others than were Southern whites or other Negro groups. Thus, the Southern Negroes may be more frustrated and do commit more homicide, but no causal link has been established between the frustration and homicide, even when using diagnostic tools theoretically derived from the frustration–aggression hypothesis. In the New Hampshire study, on the other hand, Palmer defined frustration in such a general way that items like epilepsy, severe measles, head trauma, etc., were taken as 'frustrating' factors, and no concern was indicated for the fact that these items can by themselves, exclusive of any 'frustration' hypothesis, cause ixothymic or aggressive personality deformations.

It is virtually axiomatic that frustration is inevitable and necessary in the socialization process. The frustration–aggression thesis has been one of the most challenging in social psychology and is not likely to be abandoned.[145] But its present value for empirical research purposes is indeed limited. Especially is the thesis of limited utility with regard to large subcultural groups known for their recorded high rates of aggressive violent crime. There are no comparable data on 'rates of frustration', the 'factors causing frustration', or whether these factors and the degrees of frustration are related to aggressive crime. The empirical gap left by applying the frustration–aggression thesis to large social groups renders the thesis relatively inoperable in criminology.

Containment Theory

The internal and external containment theory proposed by Reckless[146] has been used by its author as an alternative to the Henry and Short hypothesis. Containment theory represents a 'middle-of-the-road' approach which has received confirmation, notes Reckless, from studies on the social-psychiatric aspects of the Hutterites, Reiss's personal and social control theory, and Nye's social control theory. One of its advantages is that some of its postulates can be formulated in psychological terms amenable to objective research. An example of this point can be seen in the case of the ego and superego functions included in Redl's 22-item list of the 'behavior control system'.[147] Employing questionnaire-type tools, Reckless and his collaborators have carried out studies which appear to support his theory.[148] However, the central position of the theory and Reckless's attempts to realize a broad conceptual eclecticism do not make containment fully satisfactory as an etiological theory. There is the common and implicit danger of exposing the researcher to ex-post-facto interpretations. For example, the absence of crime among the Hutterites can readily be redefined as allegiance to a *non*violent subculture, and psychological traits which result from subcultural allegiance can enter into the 'behavior control system' of the individual.

The Concept of Catharsis

Another group of the Berkowitz investigations concerned with the concept of catharsis[149] has considerable practical interest and is an important aspect of the researches on aggression and violence. From the original Aristotelian formulation to the more recent Freudian hypotheses and to the present concern with the effect of filmed or televised violence on children, the view has been maintained that the observation of portrayed violence not only does not lead to actual violence on the part of the observer, but, instead, can exert a positive effect through a mechanism which purges the observer of his aggressive impulses. Opinions on these issues are divided and the matter is of vital importance to preventive programs, affecting such basic issues as the need for control and regulation of mass media, the effect on predisposed subjects, and the general policy of educational programs.

In several studies on the catharsis hypothesis, it seems that portrayed violence is not as innocuous or even beneficial as several authors have maintained. The reinforcing effect of observed violence is of interest to the subcultural approach, for one of the mechanisms of the subcultural transmission of values and attitudes is undoubtedly direct behavioral observation, something which, in the case of violence and aggression, the catharsis hypothesis appears to contradict.

The proneness to aggression and violence decreases with age, as Rosenzweig and Rosenzweig have demonstrated with the P-F study on children.[150] External controls diminish the extra-punitive reactivity of normal subjects. Other relevant factors are the development of internal controls and of adequate ego-strength, particularly if this is viewed in terms of frustration-tolerance, ability to cope with anxiety-producing factors and situations, and flexibility in delaying gratification.

Child-rearing Practices and Aggression

Of great interest is the relationship between aggression-proneness and child-rearing. Adequate knowledge on this point is essential in view of the importance of parent–child relationships in the general development of the personality and in the transmission of cultural and subcultural themes and values, as well as in consideration of the possibility of constructive preventive and treatment efforts through the modification of parental attitudes or the establishment of positive alternate parental figures. A number of significant investigations have been conducted on this topic by Bandura and his associates,[151] by Sears,[152] by Lovaas,[153] and by many others.[154] The consensus of opinion appears to be that parental, particularly father, identification plays a major role in the learning of aggressive behavioral patterns. It has been maintained by A. Freud,[155] and confirmed by Bandura and Huston,[156] that identification is unnecessary, imitation being sufficient and adequate to explain the transmission of the behavior from the meaningful adult to the child. The quality of the child–adult relationship seems to be another non-essential characteristic, for both nurturant and non-nurturant adults appear to be imitated. However, the importance of the dependency relationship and of its adequate handling in the parent–child interaction has been underlined by Saul[157] and reconfirmed by the Bandura–Walters[158] study of aggressive antisocial adolescents. Parental rejection appears to be a meaningful factor in the etiology of aggressive behavior and, apparently, rejection does not prevent imitation. As Bandura and Walters state, the social environment (cultural or subcultural) makes available the 'content' of the value system to be transmitted from the adult to the child, but the conditions necessary for the introjection and internalization of values must be found in the personality development of the individual child. This 'personality' qualification of the adult–child value and cultural transmission process is also essential in explaining the cases which are spared from the cultural or subcultural criminal transmission in high-delinquency ecological areas and in delinquent families. At the same time, the selectivity and the highly individualized quality of the identification–imitation process explain the internalization of antisocial aspects of parents and meaningful adults in predominantly nondelinquency areas and from nondelinquent families.

Social Learning and Conditioning

Studies of child-rearing practices in relation to the development of aggressive traits lead us to consider briefly one important theoretical development from the field of general and social psychology which, in our opinion, provides the theoretical bridge between an individual's violent behavior and his subcultural value allegiance. We are referring to what is generally included under the heading of 'social learning'.[159] Issues which arise in any analysis of the structure and phenomenology of subcultures are the process of transmitting the subculture values, the extent of individual differences in the strength of allegiance to those values, and the fact that not all the individuals with ecological propinquity share value and motive identity with the surrounding culture. The process of social learning, through a number of mechanisms ranging from repetitive contacts to the subtler forms of imitation and identification, involves the acquisition of value systems in early childhood and their integration in the complex personality trait–value–motive system, which makes up the adult global individuality.

A recent paper by Jeffery[160] summarizes a number of theoretical statements accepting the general principle that criminal behavior can be explained as learned behavior if conceptualized as operant behavior and reinforced through reward and immediate gratification. However, the complexity of learning theory and the serious uncertainties that still plague its core concepts have thus far produced an heuristic deficiency in transferring from theory and experimental laboratory research to field applications. The same may be said about transferring to diagnostically oriented studies of the differential psychology of violent offenders. Admittedly, the transposition from laboratory and animal experimentation to the street corner and the prison is not easy, is somewhat speculative, and may prove impossible until the social-learning approach can produce measurable, economical, and valid diagnostic instruments.

An interesting beginning towards such a development in criminology has been made by Eysenck[161] and his collaborators[162] A general restatement of the thoery can be found in Trasler,[163] and earlier statements appear in Mowrer,[164] for example. Bandura's rich production follows a social-learning approach, and his recent books with Walters provide a detailed discussion of mechanisms, patterns, and implications for the application of a behavioristic learning approach to analysis of personality development.[165]

Indoctrination into a subculture can take place through early-infancy learning processes. However, not only does this indoctrination prove difficult to reconstruct in an individual diagnostic process, or impossible to demonstrate in the laboratory, but it is confused with individual differences. These differentials in the imitation and identification processes beg the central question of why equally exposed individuals terminally behave differently and exhibit values and norms that resist attempts to classify them into discrete, yet uniform categories.

Eysenck has approached this problem through introduction of the concept of individual differences in conditioning, including, by extension, social conditioning. This approach assumes that, whereas introverts are easier to condition and therefore more readily absorb socialized values, extroverts are resistant to conditioning and dominated by antisocial impulsive reactions. The conceptualization can be extended to include social learning of whole antisocial value systems.[166] These notions, if logically followed, would postulate two types of violent offender: (1) the introversive, who are socialized into a subculture of violence through conditioning, and are frequent in specific ecological settings; (2) the extroversive, impulsive, unsocialized types, who cut across social, cultural, and subcultural strata. Both types can exhibit violent behavior, but the etiology and the probability of such behavior vary along with basic psychological make-up, i.e. a set of inherited characteristics which, in Eysenck's terms, dichotomize individuals according to biological determinants that place them in a given position on the introversion–extroversion continuum. Only modest confirmation is so far available for this far-reaching conceptualization.

An extension of the behavioristic learning theory into therapy has been proposed by Bandura and Walters and analyzed by several others.[167] The advisability of granting scientific status to an approach which is still highly experimental has been seriously questioned.

Although the social-learning approach still awaits confirmation, it does provide a conceptually useful bridge between the sociological, the psychological, and clinical constructs which we have discussed in the preceding pages. It also furnishes us with the possibility of utilizing two other personality theories which have a definite place in the transposition of the concept of subculture from sociology to psychology. Dissonance theory,[168] as one of these, constitutes an elegant, if yet unproved, link between the cognitive aspects of subcultural allegiance, the psychoanalytic mechanism of projection, and the internal consistency (with consequent reduction of the anxiety level) which constitutes the differential characteristics of members of the subculture. No dissonance is experienced so long as the value system of the individual is not confronted by different or certainly conflicting values. The treatment implications of the concept of cognitive dissonance in relation to subculture allegiance are obvious, and point to the need to fragment and rearrange antisocial group alliances. The utilization of cognitive dissonance in this way in the prevention of international conflict has been advocated, for example, by Stagner[169] and Osgood.[170] Stagner has, however, carefully analyzed the importance of perceptual personality theory to individual and group aggression. A subculture allegiance entails an organization or reorganization of the process of personality formation as a process of learning to perceive objects, persons, and situations as attractive or threatening,[171] in accordance with subcultural positive and negative valences.

The general psychological contributions from conditioning, learning theory, cognitive dissonance, perceptual personality theory, are indeed far from providing a total theoretical system as a counterpart to the sociological notions about subcultures. However, we are convinced that these behavioral constructs of social learning not only are the most directly related to subculture theory but also are capable of generating an integrated theory in criminology.

The Cultural Context

Like all human behavior, homicide and other violent assaultive crimes must be viewed in terms of the cultural context from which they spring. De Champneuf, Guerry, Quetelet early in the nineteenth century, and Durkheim later, led the way toward emphasizing the necessity to examine the *physique sociale*, or social phenomena characterized by 'externality', if the scientist is to understand or interpret crime, suicide, prostitution, and other deviant behavior. Without promulgating a sociological fatalism, analysis of broad macroscopic correlates in this way may obscure the dynamic elements of the phenomenon and result in the empirical hiatus and fallacious association to which Selvin refers.[172] Yet, because of wide individual variations, the clinical, idiosyncratic approach does not necessarily aid in arriving at Weber's *Verstehen*, or meaningful adequate understanding of regularities, uniformities, or patterns of interaction. And it is this kind of understanding we seek when we examine either deviation from, or conformity to, a normative social system.

Sociological contributions have made almost commonplace, since Durkheim, the fact that deviant conduct is not evenly distributed throughout the social structure. There is much empirical evidence that class position, ethnicity, occupational status, and other social variables are effective indicators for predicting rates of different kinds of deviance. Studies in ecology perform a valuable service for examining the phenomenology and distribution of aggression, but only inferentially point to the importance of the system of norms. Anomie, whether defined as the absence of norms (which is a doubtful conceptualization) or the conflict of norms (either normative goals or means),[173] or whether redefined by Powell[174] as 'meaninglessness', does not coincide with most empirical evidence on homicide. Acceptance of the concept of anomie would imply that marginal individuals who harbor psychic anomie that reflects (or causes) social anomie have the highest rates of homicides. Available data seem to reject this contention.

Anomie as culture conflict, or conflict of norms, suggests, as we have in the last section, that there is one segment (the prevailing middle-class value system) of a given culture whose value system is the antithesis of, or in conflict with, another, smaller, segment of the same culture. This conceptualism of anomie is a useful tool for referring to subcultures as ideal types, or mental constructs. But to transfer this norm-conflict approach from the social to the individual level, theoretically making the individual a repository of culture conflict, again does not conform to the patterns of known psychological and sociological data. This latter approach would be forced to hypothesize that socially mobile individuals and families would be most frequently involved in homicide, or that persons moving from a formerly embraced subvalue system to the predominant communal value system would commit this form of violent deviation in the greatest numbers. There are no homicide data that show high rates of homicides among persons manifesting higher social aspirations in terms of mobility. It should also be mentioned that anomie, as a concept, does not easily lend itself to psychological study.[175]

That there is a conflict of value systems, we agree. That is, there is a conflict between a prevailing culture value and some subcultural entity. But commission of homicide by actors from the subculture at variance with the prevailing culture cannot be adequately explained in terms of frustration due to failure to attain normative-goals of the latter, in terms of inability to succeed with normative-procedures (means) for attaining those goals, nor in terms of an individual psychological condition of anomie. Homicide is most prevalent, or the highest rates of homicide occur, among a relatively homogeneous subcultural group in any large urban community. Similar prevalent rates can be found in some rural areas. The value system of this group, we are contending, constitutes a subculture of violence. From a psychological viewpoint, we might hypothesize that the greater the degree of integration of the individual into this subculture, the higher the probability that his behavior will be violent in a variety of situations. From the sociological side, there should be a direct relationship between rates of homicide and the extent to which the subculture of violence represents a cluster of values around the theme of violence.

Except for war, probably the most highly reportable, socially visible, and serious form of violence is expressed in criminal homicide. Data show that in the United States rates are highest among males, non-whites, and the young adult ages. Rates for most serious crimes, particularly against the person, are highest in these same groups. In a Philadelphia study of 588 criminal homicides,[176] for example, non-white males aged 20–24 had a rate of 92 per 100,000 compared with 3·4 for white males of the same ages. Females consistently had lower rates than males in their respective race groups (non-white females, 9·3; white females, 0·4, in the same study), although it should be noted, as we shall discuss later, that non-white females have higher rates than white males.

It is possible to multiply these specific findings in any variety of ways; and although a subcultural affinity to violence appears to be principally present in large urban communities and increasingly in the adolescent population, some typical evidence of this phenomenon can be found, for example, in rural areas and among other adult groups. For example, a particular, very structured, subculture of this kind can be found in Sardinia, in the central mountain area of the island. Pigliaru has conducted a brilliant analysis of the people from this area and of their criminal behavior, commonly known as the *vendetta barbaricina*.[177]

In Colombia, the well known *violencia* has been raging for the last 15 years, causing deaths of a total estimated between 200,000 and 300,000.[178] The homicide rate in several areas has been among the highest in the world, and homicide has been the leading cause of death for Colombian males aged between 15 and 45. Several causes, some political, initially associated with the rise of this phenomenon continue to exist, and, among them, a subcultural transmission of violence is believed to play an important role. More will be said later about the subcultural traditions of violence in Sardinia, Colombia, and elsewhere.

We suggest that, by identifying the groups with the highest rates of homicide, we should find in the most intense degree a subculture of violence; and, having focused on these groups, we should subsequently examine the value system of their subculture, the importance of human life in the scale of values, the kinds of expected reaction to certain types of stimulus, perceptual differences in the evaluation of stimuli, and the general personality structure of the subcultural actors. In the Philadelphia study it was pointed out that:

'. . . the significance of a jostle, a slightly derogatory remark, or the appearance of a weapon in the hands of an adversary are stimuli differentially perceived and interpreted by Negroes and whites, males and females. Social expectations of response in particular types of social interaction result in differential "definitions of the situation." A male is usually expected to defend the name and honor of his mother, the virtue of womanhood . . . and to accept no derogation about his race (even from a member of his own race), his age, or his masculinity. Quick resort to physical combat as a measure of daring, courage, or defense of status appears to be a cultural expression, especially for lower socioeconomic class males of both races. When such a culture norm response is elicited from an individual engaged in social interplay with others who harbor the same response mechanism, physical assaults, altercations, and violent domestic quarrels that result in homicide are likely to be common. The upper-middle and upper social class value system defines subcultural mores, and considers many of the social and personal stimuli that evoke a combative reaction in the lower classes as "trivial." Thus, there exists a cultural antipathy between many folk rationalizations of the lower class, and of males of both races, on the one hand, and the middle-class legal norms under which they live, on the other.[179]

This kind of analysis, combined with other data about delinquency, the lower-class social structure, its value system, and its emphasis on aggression, suggest the thesis of a violent subculture, or, by pushing the normative aspects a little further, a *subculture of violence*. Among many juvenile gangs, as has repeatedly been pointed out, there are violent feuds, meetings, territorial fights, and the use of violence to prove 'heart', to maintain or to acquire 'rep'.[180]

Physical aggression is often seen as a demonstration of masculinity and toughness. We might argue that this emphasis on showing masculinity through aggression is not always supported by data. If homicide is any index at all of physical aggression, we must remember that in the Philadelphia data non-white females have rates often two to four times higher than the rates of white males. Violent behavior appears more dependent on cultural differences than on sex differences, traditionally considered of paramount importance in the expression of aggression. It could be argued, of course, that in a more matriarchal role than that of her white counterpart, the Negro female both enjoys and suffers more of the male role as head of the household, as parental authority and supervisor; that this imposed role makes her more aggressive, more male-like, more willing and more likely to respond violently. Because most of the victims of Negro female homicide offenders are Negro males, the Negro female may be striking out aggressively against the inadequate male protector whom she desperately wants but often cannot find or hold.[181]

It appears valid to suggest that there are, in a heterogeneous population, differences in ideas and attitudes toward the use of violence and that these differences can be observed through variables related to social class and possibly through psychological correlates. There is evidence that modes of control of expressions of aggression in children vary among the social classes.[182] Lower-class boys, for example, appear more likely to be oriented toward direct expression of aggression than are middle-class boys. The type of punishment meted out by parents to misbehaving children is related to this class orientation toward aggression. Lower-class mothers report that they or their husbands are likely to strike their children or threaten to strike them, whereas middle-class mothers report that their type of punishment is psychological rather than physical; and boys who are punished physically express aggression more directly than those who are punished psychologically. As Martin Gold[183] has suggested, the middle-class child is more likely to turn his aggression inward; in the extreme and as an adult he will commit suicide. But the lower-class child is more accustomed to a parent–child relationship which during punishment is for the moment that of attacker and attacked. The target for aggression, then, is external; aggression is directed toward others.[184]

The existence of a subculture of violence is partly demonstrated by examination of the social groups and individuals who experience the highest rates of manifest violence. This examination need not be confined to the study of one national or ethnic group. On the contrary, the existence of a subculture of violence could perhaps receive even cross-cultural confirmation. Criminal homicide is the most acute and highly reportable example of this type of violence, but some circularity of thought is obvious in the effort to specify the dependent variable (homicide), and also to infer the independent variable (the existence of a subculture of violence). The highest rates of rape, aggravated assaults, persistency in arrests for assaults (recidivism) among these groups with high rates of homicide are, however, empirical addenda to the postulation of a subculture of violence. Residential propinquity of these same groups reinforces the socio-psychological impact which the integration of this subculture engenders. Sutherland's thesis of 'differential association', or a psychological reformulation of the same theory in terms of learning process, could effectively be employed to describe more fully this impact in its intensity, duration, repetition, and frequency. The more thoroughly integrated the individual is into this subculture, the more intensely he embraces its prescriptions of behavior, its conduct norms, and integrates them into his personality structure. The degree of integration may be measured partly and crudely by public records of contact with the law, so high arrest rates, particularly high rates of assault crimes and high rates of recidivism for assault crimes among groups that form the subculture of violence, may indicate allegiance to the values of violence.

We have said that overt physical violence often becomes a common subculturally expected response to certain stimuli. However, it is not merely rigid conformity to the demands and expectations of other persons, as Henry and Short[185] seem to suggest, that results in the high probability of homicide. Excessive, compulsive, or apathetic conformity of middle-class individuals to the value system of their social group is a widely recognized cultural malady. Our concern is with the value elements of violence as an integral component of the subculture which experiences high rates of homicide. It is conformity to *this* set of values, and not rigid conformity *per se*, that gives important meaning to the subculture of violence.

If violence is a common subcultural response to certain stimuli, penalties should exist for deviation from *this* norm. The comparatively nonviolent individual may be ostracized,[186] but if social interaction must occur because of residential propinquity to others sharing in a subculture of violence, he is most likely to be treated with disdain or indifference. One who previously was considered a member of the ingroup, but who has rebelled or retreated from the subculture, is now an outgroup member, a possible threat, and one for the group to avoid. Alienation or avoidance takes him out of the normal reach of most homicide attacks, which are highly personal offenses occurring with greatest frequency among friends, relatives, and associates. If social interaction continues, however, the deviant from the subculture of violence who fails to respond to a potentially violent situation, may find himself a victim of an adversary who continues to confrom to the violence values.

It is not far-fetched to suggest that a whole culture may accept a value set dependent upon violence, demand or encourage adherence to violence, and penalize deviation. During periods of war the whole nation accepts the principle of violence against the enemy. The nonviolent citizen drafted into military service may adopt values associated with violence as an intimately internalized re-enforcement for his newly acquired rationalization to kill. War involves selective killing of an outgroup enemy, and in this respect may be viewed as different from most forms of homicide. Criminal homicide may be either 'selective' or nondiscriminate slaying, although the literature on homicide consistently reveals its intragroup nature. However, as in wartime combat between opposing individuals when an 'it-was-either-him-or-me' situation arises, similar attitudes and reactions occur among participants in homicide. It may be relevant to point out that in the Philadelphia study of criminal homicide, 65 per cent of the offenders and 47 per cent of the victims had previous arrest records. Homicide, it appears, is often a situation not unlike that of confrontations in wartime combat, in which two individuals committed to the value of violence came together, and in which chance, prowess, or possession of a particular weapon dictates the identity of the slayer and of the slain. The peaceful non-combatant in both sets of circumstances is penalized, because of the allelomimetic behavior of the group supporting violence, by his being ostracized as an outgroup member, and he is thereby segregated (imprisoned, in wartime, as a conscientious objector) from his original group. If he is not segregated, but continues to interact with his original group in the public street or on the front line that represents the culture of violence, he may fall victim to the shot or stab from one of the group who still embraces the value of violence.

An internal need for aggression and a readiness to use violence by the individual who belongs to a subculture of violence should find their psychological foundation in personality traits and in attitudes which can, through careful studies, be assessed in such a way as to lead to a differential psychology of these subjects. Psychological tests have been repeatedly employed to study the differential characteristics of criminals; and if a theoretical frame of reference involving a subculture of violence is used, it should be possible to sharpen the discriminatory power of these tests. The fact that a subject belongs to a specific subculture (in our case, a deviant one), defined by the ready use of violence, should, among other consequences, cause the subject to adopt a differential perception of his environment and its stimuli. Variations in the surrounding world, the continuous challenges and daily frustrations which are faced and solved by the adaptive mechanism of the individual, have a greater chance of being perceived and reacted upon, in a subculture of violence, as menacing, aggressive stimuli which call for immediate defense and counter-aggression. This hypothesis lends itself to objective study through appropriate psychological methodologies. The word of Stagner[187] on industrial conflict exemplifies a similar approach in a different field. This perceptual approach is of great importance in view of studies on the physiology of aggression, which seem to show the need of outside stimulation in order to elicit aggressive behavior.[188] This point will be discussed in more detail in the next chapter.

Confronted with many descriptive and test statistics, with some validated hypotheses and some confirmed replications of propositions regarding aggressive crime in psychological and sociological studies, interpretative analysis leading to the building of a theory is a normal functional aspect of the scientific method.

But there are two common and inherent dangers of an interpretative analysis that yields a thesis in an early stage of formulation, such as our thesis of a subculture of violence. These are: (a) the danger of going beyond the confines of empirical data which have been collected in response to some stated hypothesis; and (b) the danger of interpretation that produces generalizations emerging inductively from the data and that results in tautologous reasoning. Relative to the first type of danger, the social scientist incurs the risk of 'impressionistic', 'speculative' thinking, or of using previous peripheral research and trying to link it to his own data by theoretical ties that often result in knotted confusion typically calling for further research, the *caveat* of both 'good' and 'poor' analyses. Relative to the second danger, the limitations and problems of tautologies are too well known to be elaborated here. We hope that these two approaches to interpretation are herein combined in degrees that avoid compounding the fallacies of both, but that unite the benefits of each. We have made an effort to stay within the limits imposed by known empirical facts and not to become lost in speculative reasoning that combines accumulated, but unrelated, facts for which there is no empirically supportive link.

We have said that overt use of force or violence, either in interpersonal relationships or in group interaction, is generally viewed as a reflection of basic values that stand apart from the dominant, the central, or the parent culture. Our hypothesis is that this overt (and often illicit) expression of violence (of which homicide is only the most extreme) is part of a subcultural normative system, and that this system is reflected in the psychological traits of the subculture participants. In the light of our discussion of the caution to be exercised in interpretative analysis, in order to tighten the logic of this analysis, and to support the thesis of a subculture of violence, we offer the following corollary propositions:

1. *No subculture can be totally different from or totally in conflict with the society of which it is a part.* A subculture of violence is not entirely an expression of violence, for there must be interlocking value elements shared with the dominant culture. It should not be necessary to contend that violent aggression is the predominant mode of expression in order to show that the value system is set apart as subcultural. When violence occurs in the dominant culture, it is usually legitimized, but most often is vicarious and a part of phantasy. Moreover, subcultural variations, we have earlier suggested, may be viewed as quantitative and relative. The extent of difference from the larger culture and the degree of intensity, which violence as a subcultural theme may possess, are variables that could and should be measured by known socio-psychological techniques.[189] At present, we are required to rely almost entirely upon expressions of violence in conduct of various forms – parent–child relationships, parental discipline, domestic quarrels, street fights, delinquent conflict gangs, criminal records of assaultive behavior, criminal homicides, etc. – but the number of psychometrically oriented studies in criminology is steadily increasing in both quantity and sophistication, and from them a reliable differential psychology of homicides should emerge to match current sociological research.

2. *To establish the existence of a subculture of violence does not require that the actors sharing in these basic value elements should express violence*

in all situations. The normative system designates that in some types of social interaction a violent and physically aggressive response is either expected or required of all members sharing in that system of values. That the actors' behavior expectations occur in more than one situation is obvious. There is a variety of circumstances in which homicide occurs, and the history of past aggressive crimes in high proportions, both in the victims and in the offenders, attests to the multisituational character of the use of violence and to its interpersonal characteristics.[190] But, obviously, persons living in a subcultural milieu designated as a subculture of violence cannot and do not engage in violence continuously, otherwise normal social functioning would be virtually impossible We are merely suggesting, for example, that ready access to weapons in this milieu may become essential for protection against others who respond in similarly violent ways in certain situations, and that the carrying of knives or other protective devices becomes a common symbol of willingness to participate in violence, to expect violence, and to be ready for its retaliation.[191]

3. *The potential resort or willingness to resort to violence in a variety of situations emphasizes the penetrating and diffusive character of this culture theme.* The number and kinds of situations in which an individual uses violence may be viewed as an index of the extent to which he has assimilated the values associated with violence. This index should also be reflected by quantitative differences in a variety of psychological dimensions, from differential perception of violent stimuli to different value expressions in questionnaire-type instruments. The range of violence from minor assault to fatal injury, or certainly the maximum of violence expected, is rarely made explicit for all situations to which an individual may be exposed. Overt violence may even occasionally be a chance result of events. But clearly this range and variability of behavioral expressions of aggression suggest the importance of psychological dimensions in measuring adherence to a subculture of violence.

4. *The subcultural ethos of violence may be shared by all ages in a subsociety, but this ethos is most prominent in a limited age group, ranging from late adolescence to middle age.* We are not suggesting that a particular ethnic, sex, or age group all share in common the use of potential threats of violence. We are contending merely that the known empirical distribution of conduct, which expresses the sharing of this violence theme, shows greatest localization, incidence, and frequency in limited subgroups and reflects differences in learning about violence as a problem-solving mechanism.

5. *The counter-norm is nonviolence.* Violation of expected and required violence is most likely to result in ostracism from the group. Alienation of some kind, depending on the range of violence expectations that are unmet, seems to be a form of punitive action most feasible to this subculture. The juvenile who fails to live up to the conflict gang's requirements is pushed outside the group. The adult male who does not defend his honor or his female companion will be socially emasculated. The 'coward' is forced to move out of the territory, to find new friends and make new alliances. Membership is lost in the subsociety sharing the cluster of attitudes positively associated with violence. If forced withdrawal or voluntary retreat are not acceptable modes of response to engaging in the counter-norm, then execution, as is reputed to occur in organized crime, may be the extreme punitive measure.

6. *The development of favorable attitudes toward, and the use of, violence in a subculture usually involve learned behavior and a process of differential learning,*[192] *association,*[193] *or identification.*[194] Not all persons exposed – even equally exposed – to the presence of a subculture of violence absorb and share in the values in equal portions. Differential personality variables must be considered in an integrated social-psychological approach to an understanding of the subcultural aspects of violence. We have taken the position that aggression is a learned response, socially facilitated and integrated, as a habit, in more or less permanent form, among the personality characteristics of the aggressor. Aggression, from a psychological standpoint, has been defined by Buss as 'the delivery of noxious stimuli in an interpersonal context'.[195] Aggression seems to possess two major classes of reinforcers: the pain and injury inflicted upon the victim and its extrinsic rewards.[196] Both are present in a subculture of violence, and their mechanism of action is facilitated by the social support that the aggressor receives in his group. The relationship between aggression, anger, and hostility is complicated by the habit characteristics of the first, the drive state of the second, and the attitudinal interpretative nature of the third. Obviously, the immediacy and the short temporal sequence of anger with its autonomic components make it difficult to study a criminal population that is some distance removed from the anger-provoked event. Hostility, although amenable to easier assessment, does not give a clear indication or measure of physical attack because of its predominantly verbal aspects. However, it may dispose to or prepare for aggression.[197]

Aggression, in its physical manifest form, remains the most criminologically relevant aspect in a study of violent assaultive behavior. If violent aggression is a habit and possesses permanent or quasi-permanent personality trait characteristics, it should be amenable to psychological assessment through appropriate diagnostic techniques. Among the several alternative diagnostic methodologies, those based on a perceptual approach seem to be able, according to the existing literature,[198] to elicit signs and symptoms of behavioral aggression, demonstrating the existence of this 'habit' and/or trait in the personality of the subject being tested. Obviously, the same set of techniques being used to diagnose the trait of aggression can be used to assess the presence of major psychopathology, which might, in a restricted number of cases, have caused 'aggressive behavior' outside, or in spite of, any cultural or subcultural allegiance.

7. *The use of violence in a subculture is not necessarily viewed as illicit conduct and the users therefore do not have to deal with feelings of guilt about their aggression.* Violence can become a part of the life style, the theme of solving difficult problems or problem situations. It should be stressed that the problems and situations to which we refer arise mostly within the subculture, for violence is used mostly between persons and groups who themselves rely upon the same supportive values and norms. A carrier and user of violence will not be burdened by conscious guilt, then, because generally he is not attacking the representatives of the non-violent culture, and because the recipient of this violence may be described by similar class status, occupational, residential, age, and other attribute categories which characterize the subuniverse of the collectivity sharing in the subculture of violence. Even law-abiding members of the local subculture area may not view various illegal expressions of violence as menacing or immoral. Furthermore, when the attacked see their assaulters as agents of the same kind of aggression they themselves represent, violent retaliation is readily legitimized by a situationally specific rationale, as well as by the generally normative supports for violence.

Probably no single theory will ever explain the variety of observable violent behavior. However, the subculture-of-violence approach offers, we believe, the advantage of bringing together psychological and sociological constructs to aid in the explanation of the concentration of violence in specific socio-economic groups and ecological areas.

Some questions may arise about the genesis of an assumed subculture of violence. The theoretical formulation describes what is believed to be a condition that may exist in varying manifestations from organized crime, delinquent gangs, political subdivisions, and subsets of a lower-class culture. How these variations arise and from what base, are issues that have not been raised and that would require research to describe Moreover, the literature on the sociology of conflict, derived principally from Simmel,[199] on the social psychology of conflict,[200] and on the more specific topic of the sociology of violence[201] would have to be carefully examined. That there may be some universal derivatives is neither asserted nor denied. One could argue (1) that there is a biological base for aggressive behavior which may, unless conditioned against it, manifest itself in physical violence; (2) that, in Hegelian terms, each culture thesis contains its contraculture antithesis, that to develop into a central culture, nonviolence within must be a dominant theme, and that therefore a subtheme of violence in some form is an invariable consequence. We do not find either of these propositions tenable, and there is considerable evidence to contradict both.

Even without returning philosophically to a discussion of man's pre-political or pre-societal state, a more temporally localized question of genesis may be raised. The descriptions current in subcultural theorizing in general sociology or sociological criminology are limited principally to a modern urban setting, although applications of these theories could conceivably be made to the criminal machinations in such culture periods as Renaissance Florence. At present, we create no new statement of the genesis of a subculture of violence, nor do we find it necessary to adopt a single position. The beginning could be a Cohen-like negative reaction that turned into regularized, institutionalized patterns of prescription. Sufficient communication of dominant culture values, norms, goals, and means is, of course, implicitly assumed if some subset of the population is to react negatively. The existence of violent (illegitimate) means also requires that some of the goals (or symbols of goals) of the dominant culture shall have been communicated to subcultural groups in sufficient strength for them to introject and to desire them and, if thwarted in their pursuit of them, to seek them by whatever illegal means are available. The Cloward–Ohlin formulation is, in this context, an equally useful hypothesis for the genesis of a subculture of violence. Miller's idea of a 'generating milieu' does not assume – or perhaps even̄denies – the communication of most middle-class values to the lower class. Especially relevant to our present interest would be communication of attitudes toward the use of violence. Communication should, perhaps, be distinguished from absorption or introjection of culture values. Communication seems to imply transmission cognitively, to suggest that the recipients have conscious awareness of the existence of things. Absorption, or introjection, refers to conative aspects and goes beyond communication in its power to affect personalities. A value becomes part of the individual's attitudinal set or predisposition to act, and must be more than communicated to be an integral element in a prepotent tendency to respond to stimuli. It might be said that, both in Cohen's and in Cloward–Ohlin's conceptualizations, middle-class values are communicated but not absorbed as part of the personality or idioverse of those individuals who deviate. In Miller's schema, communication from middle to lower class is not required. A considerable degree of isolation of the latter class is even inferred, suggesting that the lower-class ethic had a developmental history and continuity of its own.

We are not prepared to assert how a subculture of violence arises. Perhaps there are several ways in different cultural settings. It may be that even within the same culture a collective conscience and allegiance to the use of violence develop into a subculture from the combination of more than one birth process, i.e. as a negative reaction to the communication of goals from the parent culture, as a positive reaction to this communication coupled with a willingness to use negative means, and as a positive absorption of an indigenous set of subcultural values that, as a system of interlocking values, are the antithesis of the main culture themes.

Whatever may be the circumstances creating any subculture at variance, the problems before us at present are those requiring more precision in defining a subculture, fuller descriptions and measurements of normative systems, and research designed to test hypotheses about subcultures through psychological, sociological, and other disciplinary methods. In the present chapter we have tried to provide an outline of how some of these problems might be resolved. We have used the conceptualization of a subculture of violence as a point of theoretical departure for an integrated sociological and psychological approach to definition, description, and measurement. It now seems appropriate to examine in more detail some of the relevant theory and data on homicide and other assaultive offenses in order to show how these formulations and empirical facts may lead into and be embraced or rejected by the thesis of a subculture of violence.

NOTES AND REFERENCES

1. E. B. Tylor, *Primitive Culture*, London: John Murray, 1871, p. 1.
2. A. L. Kroeber and Clyde Kluckhohn, *A Critical Review of Concepts and Definitions, Papers of the Peabody Museum of American Archeology and Ethnology*, Vol. 47, No. 1, 1952.
3. For a brief review of these groups, with illustrations, see Clyde Kluckhohn, 'Culture' in Julius Gould and William L. Kolb, *A Dictionary of the Social Sciences*, Compiled under the auspices of UNESCO, London: Tavistock Publications; New York: The Free Press of Glencoe, 1964, pp. 165–168.
4. *Ibid.*, p. 165.
5. Typical statements of these authors may be found in:

   Franz Boas, 'Anthropology', in E. R. A. Seligman (ed.), *Encyclopedia of the Social Sciences*, New York: The Macmillan Co., 1930, Vol. 2, p. 79.
   Ralph Linton, *The Study of Man*, New York: D. Appleton-Century, 1936, p. 78.
   Otto Klineberg, *Race Differences*, New York: Harper & Brothers, 1935, p. 255.
   Pitirim Sorokin, *Society, Culture and Personality*, New York: Harper & Brothers, 1947, p. 133.
   Robert M. MacIver, *Social Causation*, Boston: Ginn and Company, 1942, pp. 269–290.
   Robert M. MacIver and Charles H. Page, *Society: An Introductory Analysis*, New York: Rinehart, 1949, pp. 498 ff.
   Leslie White, *The Science of Culture*, New York: Farrar & Strauss, 1949, p. 25.

   For a detailed effort to analyze culture groups, see Alan P. Merriam *et al.*, 'The Concept of Culture Clusters Applied to the Belgian Congo', *Southwestern Journal of Anthropology* (1959) **15**:373–395.
6. A. L. Kroeber and Talcott Parsons, 'The Concepts of Culture and of Social Systems', *American Sociological Review* (October, 1958) **23**:582–583.
7. Gertrude Jaeger and Philip Selznick, 'A Normative Theory of Culture', *American Sociological Review* (October, 1964) **29**:653–669.
8. *Ibid.*, p. 663.
9. Alfred McClung Lee, 'Levels of Culture as Levels of Social Generalization', *American Sociological Review* (August, 1945) **10**:485–495; 'Social Determinants of Public Opinion', *International Journal of Opinion and Attitudes Research* (March, 1947) **1**:12–29; 'A Sociological Discussion of Consistency and Inconsistency in Intergroup Relations', *Journal of Social Issues* (1949) **5**:12–18.

10. Milton M. Gordon, 'The Concept of the Sub-Culture and Its Application', *Social Forces* (October, 1947) **26**:40 (italics in original). For additional discussions by Gordon using the term *subculture*, see also 'A System of Social Class Analysis', Drew University Studies, No. 2 (August 1951), pp. 15–18; *Social Class in American Sociology*, Durham, North Carolina: Duke University Press, 1958, pp. 252–256; 'Social Structure and Goals in Group Relations', in Morroe Berger, Theodore Abel, and Charles H. Page (eds.), *Freedom and Control in Modern Society*, New York: D. Van Nostrand, 1954. In these references, Gordon uses the term to refer to subsociety as well.

For another early reference to subcultures, see Mirra Komarovsky, S. S. Sargent, and M. W. Smith (eds.), *Culture and Personality*, New York: The Viking Fund, 1949, p. 143.

For more recent usage of the term subculture in general, see:

Murray Straus, 'Subcultural Variations in Ceylonese Mental Ability: A Study in National Character', *Journal of Social Psychology* (1954) **39**:129–141.

Charles Wagley and Marvin Harris, 'A Typology of Latin American Subcultures', *American Anthropologist* (1955) **57**:428–451.

Evon Z. Vogt, 'American Subcultural *Continua* as Exemplified by the Mormons and Texans', *American Anthropologist* (1955) **57**:1163–1172.

B. Bernstein, 'Some Sociological Determinants of Perception: An Enquiry into Sub-cultural Differences', *British Journal of Sociology* (1958) **9**:159–174.

Bernice M. Moore and Wayne H. Holtzman, 'Subcultural Variations in Youth Attitudes and Concerns', paper presented at the annual meeting of the American Sociological Association, Washington, D.C., August 29, 1962.

Burton R. Clark, *Educating the Expert Society*, San Francisco: Chandler Publishing Co., 1962, Chapter 7, 'Student Culture in High School', pp. 244–270.

11. Milton M. Gordon, *Assimilation in American Life*, New York: Oxford University Press, 1964, p. 39.

12. Gordon goes further and proposes a new term, *ethclass*, to refer to 'the subsociety created by the intersection of the vertical stratifications of ethnicity with the horizontal stratifications of social class. . . .' (*ibid.*, p. 51).

13. Edward A. Shils in Donald P. Ray (ed.), *Trends in Social Science*, New York: Philosophical Library, 1961, pp. 63–64.

14. Albert K. Cohen, *Delinquent Boys*, Glencoe, Ill.: Free Press, 1955.

15. *Ibid.*, p. 12.

16. *Ibid.*, p. 13.

17. *Ibid.*, pp. 51–54.

18. *Ibid.*, p. 54.

19. *Ibid.*, pp. 56–59.

20. *Ibid.*, p. 65.

21. Milton Yinger, 'Contraculture and Subculture', *American Sociological Review* (October, 1960) 25:625–635.

22. *Ibid.*, p. 635.

23. We have previously documented most of these sources in Chapter II. For the latter two, see B. Bernstein, 'Some Sociological Determinants of Perception: An Enquiry into Sub-cultural Differences', *British Journal of Sociology* (1958) 9:159–174; H. Bianchi, 'Delinquentie en subcultuur', *Nederlands Tijdschrift voor Criminologie* (February, 1962) 4:20–25.

Other recent useful references to delinquency and subcultures include Robert E. Forman, 'Delinquency Rates and Opportunities for Subculture Transmission', *Journal of Criminal Law, Criminology and Police Science* (1963) 54:317–321; Brahm Baittle and Solomon Kobrin, 'On The Relationship of a Characterological Type of Delinquent to the Milieu', *Psychiatry* (1964) 27:6–16; C. H. S. Jayewardene, 'Criminal Cultures and Subcultures', *The Probation and Child Care Journal* (Ceylon) (1963) 2:1–9.

24. Cohen, *Delinquent Boys*, p. 72.

25. Thorsten Sellin, *Culture Conflict and Crime*, New York: Social Science Research Council, Bulletin 41, 1938, p. 25.

For some interesting examples, mostly from recent literature, of discussions of the ways in which culture elements become 'integrated systems of meanings', see:

William Torrence and Paul Meadows, 'American Culture Themes: An Analysis of Foreign Observer Literature', *Sociology and Social Research* (1958) 43:3–7.

Lucy K. Ackernecht, *'Life Meanings' of Future Teachers: A Value Study*, New York: Philosophical Library, 1964.

T. E. H. Reid (ed.), *Values in Conflict, 32nd Couchiching Conference of the Canadian Institute on Public Affairs*, Toronto, Canada: University of Toronto Press, 1963.

Freemont Shull and André Del Beque, 'Norms, A Feature of Symbolic Culture: A Major Linkage Between the Individual, Small Group, and Administrative Organization', in William J. Gore and J. W. Dyson (eds.), *The Making of Decisions*, New York: The Free Press of Glencoe, 1964, pp. 242–275.

C. L. Shartle, G. B. Brumback, and J. R. Rizzo, 'An Approach to Dimensions of Value', *Journal of Psychology* (1964) 57:101–111.

Morris S. Viteles, ' "Human Relations" and the "Humanities" in the Education of Business Leaders: Evaluation of a Program of Humanistic Studies for Executives', *Personnel Psychology* (1959) 12:1–28.

Melvin Tumin, 'Business as a Social System', *Behavioral Science* (1964) 9:120–130.

Herman Turk, 'Social Cohesion Through Variant Values: Evidence from Medical Role Relations', *American Sociological Review* (1963) 28:28–37.

Cyril S. Belshaw, 'The Identification of Values in Anthropology', *American Journal of Sociology* (1959) **64**:555–562.
Robert J. Smith, 'The Japanese World Community: Norms, Sanctions, and Ostracism', *American Anthropologist* (1961) **63**:522–533.

26. Solomon Poll, *The Hasidic Community of Williamsburg*, New York: The Free Press of Glencoe, 1962.
27. Sellin, *Culture Conflict and Crime*, p. 28.
28. Yinger, 'Contraculture and Subculture', *op. cit.*, p. 627.
29. *Ibid.*, p. 634.
30. Sellin, *Culture Conflict and Crime*, pp. 33–34. For an interesting sociological discussion, with some data, of social (meaning formal and informal) as distinguished from societal (meaning formal culture system) reactions to deviations, see Alexander L. Clark and Jack P. Gibbs, 'Social Control: A Reformulation', *Social Problems* (Spring, 1965) **12**:398–415.
31. Leslie T. Wilkins, 'Criminology: An Operational Research Approach', in A. T. Welford, M. Argyle, D. V. Glass, and J. N. Morris (eds.), *Society: Problems and Methods of Study*, London: Routledge and Kegan Paul, 1962, p. 307; also, Leslie T. Wilkins, *Social Deviance*, London: Tavistock Publications; Englewood Cliffs, N.J.: Prentice-Hall, 1964, pp. 46–48.
32. Ruth S. Cavan, *Criminology*, New York: Thomas Crowell, 3rd Edition, 1962, Chapter 3.
33. Wilkins, 'Criminology: An Operational Research Approach', p. 307. For an earlier discussion of the notion of a culture continuum, see Evon Z. Vogt, 'American Subcultural *Continua* as Exemplified by the Mormons and Texans', *American Anthropologist* (1955) **57**:1163–1172.
34. See for example, John A. Hostetler, *Amish Society*, Baltimore: Johns Hopkins Press, 1963.
35. The analyst is not necessarily required to determine whether description may have ultimately good or bad effects if these effects should change the larger culture. Such a determination would obviously involve an ethical judgement.
36. Sellin, *Culture Conflict and Crime*, p. 35.
37. *Ibid.*, p. 34.
38. See the bibliographic notes in Clyde Kluckhohn and others, 'Values and Value-Orientations in the Theory of Action', in Talcott Parsons and Edward A. Shils (eds.), *Toward A General Theory of Action*, Cambridge, Mass.: Harvard University Press, 1951, pp. 388–533.
39. *Ibid.*, p. 394. See also Morris Opler, 'Themes as Dynamic Forces in Culture', *American Journal of Sociology* (1945) **51**:198–206; Talcott Parsons, 'The Place of Ultimate Values in Sociological Theory', *International Journal of Ethics* (1935) **45**:282–316.
40. John Dewey, 'Theory of Valuation', *International Encyclopedia of*

Unified Science, Vol. 2, No. 4, Chicago, Ill.: University of Chicago Press, 1939.

41. Cf. the definition by Philip E. Jacob and James J. Flink in 'Values and Their Function in Decision-Making', a supplementary issue of The American Behavioral Scientist (May, 1962) Vol. 5, No. 9, p. 10.

42. Kluckhohn in Parsons and Shils, Toward a General Theory of Action, p. 395. For an interesting discussion of Clyde Kluckhohn and philosophers, see Cornelius Golightly, 'Value as a Scientific Concept', Journal of Philosophy (March, 1956) 53:7:233 ff.

43. David F. Aberle, 'Shared Values in Complex Societies', American Sociological Review (1950) 15:495–502, p. 495 cited.

44. Robert M. MacIver, Society.

45. See supra, note 41.

46. For a recent and critical discussion of sociological references to this kind of nexus, see Judith Blake and Kingsley Davis, 'Norms, Values, and Sanctions', in Robert E. L. Faris (ed.), Handbook of Modern Sociology, Chicago: Rand McNally, 1964, Chapter 13, pp. 456–484.

47. Ibid., pp. 464–465.

48. Allen Barton, 'The Concept of Property-Space in Social Research', in P. Lazarsfeld and M. Rosenberg (eds.), The Language of Social Research, Glencoe, Ill.: The Free Press, 1955, pp. 40–52; also Allen Barton, Measuring the Values of Individuals, New York: Bureau of Applied Social Research, (A354), 1962.

49. Ralph Linton, The Study of Man, New York: Appleton-Century, 1936, Chapter 10.

50. Richard T. Morris, 'A Typology of Norms', American Sociological Review (1956) 21:610–613.

51. Robin M. Williams, Jr., American Society, New York: Alfred Knopf, 1960, Chapter 3.

52. William Graham Sumner, Folkways, Boston: Ginn & Co., 1906.

53. Linton, op. cit.

54. Pitirim A. Sorokin, Society, Culture and Personality, New York: Harper & Brothers, 1947, p. 87.

55. Williams, op. cit.

56. G. H. von Wright, An Essay in Modal Logic, Amsterdam: North-Holland, 1951.

57. Alan Ross Anderson and Omar Khayyam Moore, 'The Formal Analysis of Normative Concepts', American Sociological Review (1957) 22:9–17.

58. Ephraim H. Mizruchi and Robert Perrucci, 'Norm Qualities and Differential Effects of Deviant Behavior: An Exploratory Analysis', American Sociological Review (June, 1962) 27:391–399.

59. Jack Gibbs, 'Norms: The Problem of Definition and Classification', American Journal of Sociology (1965) 70:586–594.

60. By 'contingent', the author means 'attributes which vary from one norm to the next and therefore are not relevant for a generic definition of norms' (ibid., p. 586).

61. *Ibid.*, p. 592.

In a recent article that recognizes this relativity, and which is devoted mainly to justifying a fivefold classification of values in order to provide a basis for empirically studying values, Harold Fallding defines value as 'a generalized end that guides behavior toward uniformity in a variety of situations, with the object of repeating a particular self-sufficient satisfaction' (Harold Fallding, 'A Proposal for the Empirical Study of Values', *American Sociological Review* (1965) **30**:223–234, p. 224 cited). With reference to a small-scale study in Australia, Fallding seeks to distinguish between values, pleasures, interests, compulsions, and benefits. He approaches value mainly in terms of an end achievement or satisfaction, not from the normative, 'bright', viewpoint. He is cognizant of differential perspective; he alludes to, but does not call for, a scaling analysis when he criticizes the forced choice in the paired-comparison method; and he distinguishes five values based on Parsons's bifurcation of his fifth pattern variable, self-collectivity. The five Fallding values are: (1) membership values, (2) partisanship values, (3) ownership values, (4) interest values, (5) face values.

62. Talcott Parsons and Edward A. Shils (eds.), *Toward a General Theory of Action*, p. 60. See also Talcott Parsons, *The Structure of Social Action*, Glencoe, Ill.: The Free Press, 1949; *The Social System*, Glencoe, Ill.: The Free Press, 1951; London: Tavistock/Routledge.

63. Charles Madge, *Society in the Mind: Elements of Social Eidos*, New York: The Free Press of Glencoe, 1964, p. 97.

64. Talcott Parsons, *The Social System*, p. 350.

65. We are indebted to Madge, *op. cit.*, p. 102, for this succinct summary.

66. Parsons, *The Social System*, pp. 350–351. Emphasis added.

67. William J. Goode, 'Norm Commitment and Conformity to Role-Status Obligations', *American Journal of Sociology* (1960) **66**:246–258.

68. *Ibid.*, p. 252.

69. Ralph Turner, 'Moral Judgment: A Study in Roles', *American Sociological Review* (1952) **17**:70–77.

70. Harold H. Kelley and Martin M. Shapiro, 'Conformity to Group Norms', *American Sociological Review* (1954) **19**:667–677.

71. Stuart C. Dodd, 'On Classifying Human Values: A Step in the Prediction of Human Valuing', *American Sociological Review* (1951) **16**:645–653, p. 645 cited. The author reported that this article was a pilot research on 'The Classification, Measurement and Theory of Human Values'. See also, Stuart C. Dodd, 'How to Measure Values', *Proceedings of the Pacific Sociological Society*, 1950, cited in *ibid.*

72. Stuart C. Dodd, 'On Classifying Human Values: A Step in the Prediction of Human Valuing', *op. cit.*, p. 646.

73. David Aberle, 'Shared Values in Complex Societies', *op. cit.*, p. 501.

74. William R. Catton, Jr., 'Exploring Techniques for Measuring Human Values', *American Sociological Review* (1954) **19**:49–55; 'A Retest of

G

the Measurability of Certain Human Values', *American Sociological Review* (1956) **21**:357–359; 'A Theory of Value', *American Sociological Review* (1959) **24**:310–317.

75. William R. Catton, Jr., 'A Theory of Value', *op. cit.*, p. 312.
76. *Ibid.*, p. 314. For a recent report on perception of time by age differentials, see John Cohen, 'Psychological Time', *Scientific American* (1964) **211**:116–124.
77. *Ibid.*, p. 317.
78. William R. Catton, Jr., 'Exploring Techniques for Measuring Values', *op. cit.*
79. E. L. Thorndike, 'Valuations of Certain Pains, Deprivations, and Frustrations', *Journal of Genetic Psychology* (1937) **51**:235–236; cited by *ibid.*, p. 52.
80. William R. Catton, Jr., 'Exploring Techniques for Measuring Values', *op. cit.*, p. 55 (emphasis added). See also, William R. Catton, Jr., 'A Retest of the Measurability of Certain Human Values', *American Sociological Review* (1956) **21**:357–359.
81. Roy E. Carter, Jr., 'An Experiment in Value Measurement', *American Sociological Review* (1956) **21**:156–163.
82. *Ibid.*, p. 162. See also:

    Kenneth Arrow, 'Alternative Approaches to the Theory of Choice in Risk-Taking Situations', *Econometrica* (1951) **19**:404–437.
    Donald Davidson, J. C. C. McKinsey, and Patrick Suppes, *Outlines of a Formal Theory of Value*, I, Stanford University: Stanford Value Theory Project, Report No. 1, February, 1954.
    Patrick Suppes, 'The Role of Subjective Probability and Utility in Decision-Making', *Proceedings of the Third Berkeley Symposium on Mathematics, Statistics and Probability* (1956) **5**:61–73.

83. William A. Scott, 'Empirical Assessment of Values and Ideologies', *American Sociological Review* (1959) **24**:299–310. This research is reported as being the first phase of a long-term study of personal values supported initially by the Foundation for Research on Human Behavior at Ann Arbor, Michigan.
84. *Ibid.*, p. 301.
85. Samuel Stouffer, 'An Analysis of Conflicting Social Norms', *American Sociological Review*, (1949) **14**:707–717.
86. William McCord and Joan McCord, 'A Tentative Theory of the Structure of Conscience', in Dorothy Willner (ed.), *Decisions, Values and Groups*, New York: Pergamon Press, 1960, pp. 108–134.
87. Patrick Suppes, 'Two Formal Models for Moral Principles', *Technical Report No. 15*, Stanford, California: Applied Mathematics and Statistics Laboratory, Stanford University, November 1, 1957.
88. H. Hartshorne and M. A. May, *Studies in the Nature of Character*: Vol. I, *Studies in Deceit*; Vol. II, *Studies in Self-Control*; Vol. III, *Studies in the Organization of Character*, New York, Macmillan, 1928–1930.
89. Jean Piaget, *The Moral Judgment of the Child*, London: Routledge &

Kegan Paul; Glencoe, Ill.: The Free Press, 1948 (originally published 1932).

90. Laurence Kohlberg, 'The Development of Children's Orientations Toward A Moral Order: I, Sequence in the Development of Moral Thought', *Vita Humana* (1963) **6**:11–33; 'Development of Moral Character and Moral Ideology', in *Review of Child Development Research*, Volume One, New York: Russell Sage Foundation, 1964.

91. Justin Aronfreed, 'The Nature, Variety, and Social Patterning of Moral Responses to Transgression', *Journal of Abnormal and Social Psychology* (1961) **63**:223–241; 'The Effect of Experimental Socialization Paradigm Upon Two Moral Responses to Transgression', *Journal of Abnormal and Social Psychology* (1963) **66**:437–448.

92. H. Baruk and M. Buchet, *Le test 'Tsedek' – Le jugement moral et la délinquance*, Paris: Presses Universitaires de France, 1950.

93. The following are some of these types of studies by Salomon Rettig and Benjamin Pasamanick: 'Moral Codes of American and Korean College Students', *Journal of Social Psychology* (Spring, 1959) **50**:65–73; 'Changes in Moral Values Among College Students: A Factorial Study', *American Sociological Review* (1959) **24**:856–863; 'Differences in the Structure of Moral Values of Students and Alumni', *American Sociological Review* (1960) **25**:550–555; 'Moral Value Structure and Social Class', *Sociometry* (1961) **24**:21–35; 'Invariance in Factor Structure of Moral Value Judgments from American and Korean College Students', *Sociometry* (1962) **25**:73–84. See also, Peter G. Grasso, 'Valori morali-sociali in transizione', *Orientamenti pedagogici* (1961) **8**:233–268.

94. See, for example, 'The Interaction of Social Values and Political Responsibility: A Pilot Cross-Cultural Study of the Integration of Political Communities' (mimeographed), Philadelphia: University of Pennsylvania, April and May 15, 1964; and the previously cited supplement to the *American Behavioral Scientist*, May, 1962, by Philip E. Jacob and James Flink, *Values and Their Function in Decision-Making*.

95. Philip E. Jacob, Karl W. Deutsch, William L. C. Wheaton, Henry Teune, and James Toscano, *The Integration of Political Communities*, Philadelphia: J. B. Lippincott, 1964.

96. Charles Morris, *Varieties of Human Values*, Chicago: University of Chicago Press, 1956; Allen Barton, *Measuring the Values of Individuals*, New York: Bureau of Applied Social Research, cited in the reference in note 48 above.

97. 'The Interaction of Social Values and Political Responsibility: A Pilot Cross Cultural Study of the Integration of Political Communities', p. 10.

98. *Ibid.*, p. 16.

99. *Ibid.*, p. 11.

100. J. Ruesch, Annemarie Jacobsen, and M. B. Loeb, 'Acculturation and Illness', *Psychological Monographs* (1948) **62**:1–40.

101. Leonard W. Doob, *Patriotism and Nationalism: Their Psychological*

Foundations, New Haven, Conn.: Yale University Press, 1964. See especially the chapter entitled, 'The Organization of Values'.

102. Charles E. Osgood, G. J. Suci, and P. H. Tannenbaum, *The Measuring of Meaning*, Urbana, Ill.: University of Ill. Press, 1957. For an excellent and recent use of Osgood's approach, see Sheldon G. Levy and Robert Hefner, 'Multidimensional Scaling of International Attitudes', *Papers, Peace Research Society* (1964) 1:129–165.

103. Solomon Kobrin, 'The Conflict of Values in Delinquency Areas', *American Sociological Review* (1951) 16:653–661.

104. Milton L. Barron, 'Juvenile Delinquency and American Values', *American Sociological Review* (1951) 16:208–214.

105. Kobrin, *op. cit.*, p. 657, note 11.

106. Barron, *op. cit.*, p. 209.

107. *Ibid.*, p. 211. Our own references to Sellin's *Culture Conflict and Crime* suggest our agreement with Barron on this point.

108. Denis Szabo, Francyne Goyer, Denis Gogne, 'Jugements moraux et milieu socio-culturel: étude-pilote' (mimeographed), Department of Criminology, University of Montreal, December 1964. Mr Richard Gould, former research assistant from the Center of Criminological Research University of Pennsylvania, Philadelphia, was helpful in providing a critique of this study in seminar.

109. Thorsten Sellin and Marvin E. Wolfgang, *The Measurement of Delinquency*, New York: Wiley, 1964; especially Chapters 15–20.

110. G. T. Fechner, *Elemente der Psychophysik*, Leipzig: Breitkopf und Hartel, 1860.

111. L. L. Thurstone, 'A Law of Comparative Judgment', *Psychological Review* (1927) 34:273–286.

112. S. S. Stevens, 'Mathematics, Measurement and Psychophysics', in S. S. Stevens (ed.), *Handbook of Experimental Psychology*, New York: Wiley, 1951, p. 23.

113. *Ibid.*

114. For a fuller description, see Harold Gulliksen and Samuel Messick (eds.), *Psychological Scaling: Theory and Applications*, New York: Wiley, 1960, pp. 49–66.

115. Sellin and Wolfgang, *The Measurement of Delinquency*, pp. 224–225.

116. The IQ score, for example, is not a ratio scale; among other things, there is no zero point. Therefore, an IQ of 100 is not to be considered twice as high as 50. In the Sellin–Wolfgang scale, the zero point is an act that is not a crime. This problem would have to be examined if assumptions of a ratio scale are to be made for a scale of cultural and subcultural values.

117. Leslie T. Wilkins has made this suggestion. See his *Social Deviance*, London: Tavistock Publications; Englewood Cliffs, N.J.: Prentice-Hall, 1964.

118. Sellin and Wolfgang, *op. cit.*, pp. 286–287.

119. Saul Rosenzweig, 'Levels of Behavior in Psychodiagnosis with Special Reference to the Picture-Frustration Study', *American Journal of Orthopsychiatry* (1950) 20:63–72.

120. *Ibid.*, p. 63.
121. Eugene Galanter, 'The Direct Measurement of Utility and Subjective Probability', *American Journal of Psychology* (June, 1962) 75:212–213.
122. Possibly other diagnostic techniques of the projective type, and analysis of differential perceptual habits, can be used in conjunction with the scaling of values, thus enhancing the validity and reliability of the data. Moreover, the effort by Mylonas to scale attitudes of prisoners toward the legal system that convicted and incarcerated them represents a study of persons not originally grouped together. See Anastassios D. Mylonas, 'Prisoners' Attitudes Toward Law and Legal Institutions', Unpublished Ph.D. Dissertation, Ohio State University, 1962; 'Prisoners' Attitudes Toward Law and Legal Institutions', *Journal of Criminal Law, Criminology and Police Science* (December, 1963) 54:479–484.
123. It may be profitable to study 'middle-class' murder – the episodic, planned, rational murder – from the same perspective that Cressey uses in examining embezzlement (Donald Cressey, *Other People's Money*, Glencoe, Ill.: The Free Press, 1953). Paraphrasing Cressey's final revised postulate and applying it to 'middle-class' murder, we might say: These persons conceive of themselves as having a problem which is non-shareable, are aware that this problem can be secretly resolved by violation of the middle-class norms, and are able to apply to their own conduct in that situation rationalizations which enable them to adjust their conceptions of themselves as law-abiding persons with their conceptions of themselves as slayers.
124. Karl Menninger, *Love Against Hate*, New York: Harcourt, Brace and World, 1942.
125. R. Waelder, 'Critical Discussion of the Concept of an Instinct of Destruction', *Bulletin of the Philadelphia Psychoanalytic Association*, (1956) 6:97–109.
126. Franz Alexander, 'The Psychiatric Aspects of War and Peace', *American Journal of Sociology* (1941) 46:504–520.
127. H. Hartmann, E. Kris, and R. Loewenstein, 'Notes on the Theory of Aggression', *Psychoanalytic Study of the Child* (1949) 3:9–36.
128. L. S. Saul, *The Hostile Mind*, New York: Random House, 1956.
129. S. Glueck and E. Glueck, *Physique and Delinquency*, New York: Harper and Brothers, 1956, pp. 98–99. If, however, we hypothesize that the acquisition of violence values is determined by a learning process identifiable with early conditioning, we must keep in mind the typological differences which influence the differential readiness and resistance to conditioning. (An up-to-date discussion of this problem, according to Eysenckian theory, can be found in Gordon Trasler, *The Explanation of Criminality*, London: Routledge and Kegan Paul, 1962, Chapter III.) In a given subcultural exposition to conditioning violent stimuli, introverts will acquire more effective and permanent values than extroverts. The individual's position upon

the introversion–extroversion continuum is considered as partly determined by genetic factors (Trasler, *ibid.*, p. 63).

130. E. B. McNeil, 'Psychology and Aggression', *The Journal of Conflict Resolution* (1959) **3**:195–293.

131. Saul Rosenzweig, 'An Outline of Frustration Theory', in J. McV. Hunt (ed.), *Personality and the Behavior Disorders*, New York: Ronald Press, 1944.

132. Leonard Berkowitz, *Aggression*, New York: McGraw-Hill, 1962.

133. *Ibid.*

134. *Ibid.*

135. John Dollard, L. W. Doob, N. E. Miller, O. H. Mowrer, R. R. Sears, C. S. Ford, C. I. Hovland, R. T. Sollenberger, *Frustration and Aggression*, New Haven, Conn.: Yale University Press, 1939.

136. See:

N. Pastore, 'The Role of Arbitrariness in the Frustration–Aggression Hypothesis', *Journal of Abnormal and Social Psychology* (1952) **47**:728–731.

A. R. Cohen, 'Social Norms, Arbitrariness of Frustration and Status of the Agent of Frustration in the Frustration–Aggression Hypothesis', *Journal of Abnormal and Social Psychology* (1955) **51**:222–226.

Also:

Paul Rothaus and Philip Worchel, 'The Inhibition of Aggression under Nonarbitrary Frustration', *Journal of Personality* (1960) **28**:108–117.

John J. Kregarman and Philip Worchel, 'Arbitrariness of Frustration and Aggression', *Journal of Abnormal and Social Psychology* (1961) **63**:183–187.

Eugene Burnstein and Philip Worchel, 'Arbitrariness of Frustration and Its Consequences for Aggression in a Social Situation', *Journal of Personality* (December, 1962) **30**:528–540.

Worchel has also studied personality factors relevant to the problem: Philip Worchel, 'Personality Factors in the Readiness to Express Aggression', *Journal of Clinical Psychology* (1958) **14**:355–359.

137. G. Patterson, 'A Nonverbal Technique for the Assessment of Aggression in Children', *Child Development* (1960) **31**:4:643–653.

138. Julius H. Masserman, 'The Biodynamic Approaches', Chapter 83 in Silvano Arieti (ed.), *American Handbook of Psychiatry*, Vol. 2, New York: Basic Books, 1959, p. 1684.

139. See, for example:

Aubrey J. Yates, *Frustration and Conflict*, London: Methuen; New York: Wiley, 1962.

Neal E. Miller, 'Comment on Theoretical Models Illustrated by the Development of a Theory of Conflict Behavior', *Journal of Personality* (September, 1951) **20**:82–100.

Philip Worchel, 'Hostility: Theory and Experimental Investigation', in D. Willner (ed.), *Decisions, Values and Groups*, Vol. I, pp. 254–266.

Philip Worchel, 'Status Restoration and the Reduction of Hostility', *Journal of Abnormal and Social Psychology* (September, 1961) **63**:443–445.

Seymour Feshbach, 'The Influence of Drive Arousal and Conflict Upon Fantasy Behavior', in Jerome Kagan, *Contemporary Issues in Thematic Apperceptive Methods*, Springfield, Ill.: C. C. Thomas, 1961.

Donald J. Veldman and Philip Worchel, 'Defensiveness and Self-Acceptance in the Management of Hostility', *Journal of Abnormal and Social Psychology* (September, 1961) **63**:319–325.

Albert Pepitone, *Attraction and Hostility*, New York: Atherton, 1963; London: Tavistock Publications, 1966.

140. Leonard Berkowitz, *Aggression*, 1962; see also Leonard Berkowitz, 'The Expression and Reduction of Hostility', *Psychological Bulletin* (September, 1958) 55:257–271. For a careful and detailed critical analysis of Berkowitz's work, see the review of *Aggression* by Albert Pepitone, 'Old Bottles, New Wine', *Contemporary Psychology* (August, 1963) 8:306–308.

141. Henry and Short, Jr., *Suicide and Homicide*, 1954.

142. Palmer, *A Study of Murder*, 1960.

143. For Reckless's analysis of Henry and Short's book, see Walter C. Reckless, *The Crime Problem*, Third Edition, New York: Appleton-Century-Crofts, 1961, pp. 138–140.

144. J. L. McCary, 'Ethnic and Cultural Reactions to Frustration', *Journal of Personality* (1949–1950) **18**:3:321–326; J. L. McCary, 'Reactions to Frustration by Some Cultural and Racial Groups', *Personality: Symposia in Topical Issues* (1951) **1**:84–102.

145. For a critical review of the concept of frustration which covers the major theoretical and experimental writings, see Reed Lawson, *Frustration, the Development of a Scientific Concept*, New York: Macmillan, 1965, which contains an anthology of relevant papers. Other writings which should be consulted include:

Saul Rosenzweig, 'Frustration as an Experimental Problem, Part I: The Significance of Frustration as a Problem of Research', *Character and Personality* (1938) 7:2:126–128.

Saul Rosenzweig, 'Frustration as an Experimental Problem. Part VI: A General Outline of Frustration', *Character and Personality* (1938) 7:2:151–160.

Saul Rosenzweig, *An Outline of Frustration Theory* in J. McV. Hunt (ed.), *Personality and the Behavior Disorders*, New York: Ronald Press, 1944.

R. J. McCaldon, 'Aggression', *Journal of the Canadian Psychiatric Association* (1964) **9**:6:502–511, cited in *Excerpta Criminologica* (1965) p. 664.

146. Walter C. Reckless, *The Crime Problem*, New York: Appleton-
     Century-Crofts, Third Edition, Chapter 18; also, Walter C. Reck-
     less, 'A Non-Causal Explanation: Containment Theory', *Excerpta
     Criminologica* (1962) 2:131–134; Guy Houchon, 'Définition et
     éléments constitutifs de l'état dangereux prédélictuel', General Re-
     port to the Third French Congress of Criminology, Aix-en-Provence,
     October, 1962.
147. Fritz Redl and David Wineman, *Children Who Hate*, Glencoe, Ill.:
     The Free Press, 1951.
148. See, for example, Simon Dinitz, Frank R. Scarpitti, and Walter C.
     Reckless, 'Delinquency Vulnerability: A Cross-Group and Longitu-
     dinal Analysis', *American Sociological Review* (August, 1962) 27:515–
     517.
149. See Chapter III, note 136. Also:

     Berkowitz, *Aggression*, 1962, Chapter 9, for an extensive review of
         available experimental literature.
     Seymour Feshbach, 'The Stimulating Versus Cathartic Effects of a
         Vicarious Aggressive Activity', *Journal of Abnormal and Social
         Psychology* (1961) 63:381–385.
     Paul Mussen and E. Rutherford, 'Effects of Aggressive Cartoons on
         Children's Aggressive Play', *Journal of Abnormal and Social
         Psychology* (1961) 62:461–464.
     A. Bandura, D. Ross, and S. A. Ross, 'Transmission of Aggression
         Through Imitation of Aggressive Models', *Journal of Abnormal
         and Social Psychology* (1961) 63:575–582.
     O. I. Lovaas, 'Effect of Exposure to Symbolic Aggression on Aggres-
         sive Behavior', *Child Development* (1961) 32:37–44.
     Leonard Berkowitz, James A. Green, and Jacqueline R. Macaulay,
         'Hostility Catharsis as the Reduction of Emotional Tension',
         Psychiatry (1962) 25:23–31.
     R. H. Walters, E. L. Thomas, and C. W. Acker, 'Enchancement of
         Punitive Behavior by Audio-Visual Display', *Science* (1962)
         136:872–873.
     D. L. Larder, 'Effect of Aggressive Story Content on Nonverbal
         Play Behavior', *Psychological Reprints* (1962) 11:1:14.
     E. A. Bergler, 'A Basic Oversight in the Discussion of Violence on
         TV', *Diseases of Nervous System* (1962) 23:5:267–269.
     Albert Bandura, Dorothea Ross, and Sheila A. Ross, 'Imitation of
         Film-Mediated Aggressive Models', *Journal of Abnormal and
         Social Psychology* (1963) 66:1:3–11.
     L. D. Eron, 'Relationship of TV Viewing Habits and Aggressive
         Behavior in Children', *Journal of Abnormal and Social Psycho-
         logy* (1963) 67:2:193–196.
     Leonard Berkowitz and E. Rawlings, 'Effects of Film Violence on
         Inhibitions against Subsequent Aggression', *Journal of Abnor-
         mal and Social Psychology* (1963) 66:5:405–412. Leonardo
         Ancona and M. Bertini, 'Effet de fixation de l'aggressivité

provoqué par des films à contenu émotif élevé', *IKON* (1963) **15**:33–44.

Leonard Berkowitz, 'The Effect of Observing Violence', *Scientific American* (1964) 210–35–41.

Leonardo Ancona and Mario Fontanesi, 'La dinamica dell'aggressività in un gruppo di criminali', *Quaderni di· Criminologia Clinica* (1965) **7**:1:3–30.

A recent book on research designs on television effects includes two very interesting research projects on the effects of portrayal of aggression, one by Seymour Feshbach and another by Arthur J. Brodbeck and Dorothy B. Jones.

150. S. Rosenzweig and L. Rosenzweig, 'Aggression in Problem Children and Normals as Evaluated by the Rosenzweig P-F Study', *Journal of Abnormal and Social Psychology* (1952) **47**:683–687.

151. Albert Bandura, 'Social Learning Through Imitation', *Nebraska Symposium on Motivation*, 1962, Lincoln, Nebraska: University of Nebraska, 1962.

Albert Bandura and R. H. Walters, *Adolescent Aggression*, New York: Ronald Press, 1959.

Albert Bandura and A. C. Huston, 'Identification as a Process of Incidental Learning', *Journal of Abnormal and Social Psychology* (1961) **63**:311–318.

Albert Bandura, D. Ross, and S. A. Ross, 'Imitation of Film-Mediated Aggressive Models', *Journal of Abnormal and Social Psychology* (1963) **66**:3–11.

152. R. R. Sears, 'Survey of Objective Studies of Psychoanalytical Concepts', *Bulletin* **51**, New York: Social Science Research Council, 1943.

153. O. I. Lovaas, 'Effect of Exposure to Symbolic Aggression on Aggressive Behavior', *Child Development* (1961) **32**:37–44.

154. Following is a brief listing of recent papers on child-rearing and adolescent aggression:

E. K. Beller and J. L. B. Turner, 'Dependency and Aggression. Six Differences in "Normal" and "Emotionally Disturbed" Pre-School Children', *American Psychologist* (1962) **17**:6:300.

S. B. Chorost, 'Parental Child-Rearing Attitudes and Their Correlates in Adolescent Hostility', *Genetic Psychology Monographs* (1962) **66**:1:49–90.

Jacob Chwast, 'The Malevolent Transformation', *The Journal of Criminal Law, Criminology and Police Science* (1963) **54**:1:42–47.

A. T. Dittman and D. W. Goodrich, 'A Comparison of Social Behavior in Normal and Hyperaggressive Preadolescent Boys', *Child Development* (1961) **32**:2:315–327.

L. D. Eron, L. O. Walder, R. Taigo, and M. M. Lefkowitz, 'Social Class', Parental Punishment for Aggression and Child Aggression', *Child Development* (1963) **34**:4:849–867.

J. C. Finney, 'Some Material Influences on Children's Personality and Character', *Genetic Psychology Monographs* (1961) 63:2:199-278.

L. E. Hewitt and R. L. Jenkins, *Fundamental Patterns of Maladjustment: The Dynamics of Their Origin*, Springfield, Ill.: State of Illinois, 1946.

S. Jegard and R. H. Walters, 'A Study of Some Determinants of Aggression in Young Children', *Child Development* (1960) 31:4:739-747.

D. Lebo, 'Aggressiveness and Expansiveness in Children', *Journal of Genetic Psychology* (1962) 100:2:227-240.

R. Lynn, 'Personality Characteristics of the Mothers of Aggressive and Unaggressive Children', *Journal of Genetic Psychology* (1961) 99:1:159-164.

J. McCord, W. McCord, and A. Howard, 'Family Interaction as Antecedent to the Directions of Male Aggressiveness', *Journal of Abnormal and Social Psychology* (1963) 66:3:239-242.

J. McCord, W. McCord, and E. Thurber, 'Some Effects of Paternal Absence on Male Children', *Journal of Abnormal and Social Psychology* (1962) 64:5:361-369.

E. B. McNeil, 'Patterns of Aggression', *Journal of Child Psychology* (1962) 3:2:65-77.

J. D. Noshpitz and P. Spielman, 'Diagnosis: A Study of the Differential Characteristics of Hyperaggressive Children', *American Journal of Orthopsychiatry* (1961) 3:111-112.

A. Roland, 'Persuasibility in Young Children as a Function of Aggressive Motivation and Aggression Conflict', *Journal of Abnormal and Social Psychology* (1963) 66:5:454-461.

Charlotte Schenk-Danziger, 'Social Difficulties of Children Who Were Deprived of Maternal Care in Early Childhood', *Vita Humana* (1961) 4:229-241.

R. E. Schulman, D. J. Shoemaker, and I. Moelis, 'Laboratory Measurement of Parental Behavior', *Journal of Consulting Psychology* (1962) 26:2:109-114.

R. R. Sears, 'Relation of Early Socialization Experience to Aggression in Middle Childhood', *Journal of Abnormal and Social Psychology* (1961) 63:3:466-492.

Ph. E. Slater, 'Parental Behavior and the Personality of the Child', *Journal of Genetic Psychology* (1962) 101:1:53-58.

D. Weatherley, 'Maternal Permissiveness toward Aggression and Subsequent T.A.T. Aggression', *Journal of Abnormal and Social Psychology* (1962) 65:1:1-5.

D. Weatherley, 'Maternal Response to Childhood Aggression and Subsequent Anti-semitism', *Journal of Abnormal and Social Psychology* (1963) 66:2:183-185.

C. L. Winder and L. Rau, 'Parental Attitudes Associated with Social Deviance in Preadolescent Boys', *Journal of Abnormal and Social Psychology* (1962) 64:6:418-424.

155. Anna Freud, *The Ego and the Mechanisms of Defence*, London, Hogarth; New York: International Universities Press, 1936.
156. Bandura and Huston, *op. cit.*
157. L. S. Saul, *The Hostile Mind*, New York: Random House, 1956.
158. Bandura and Walters, *Adolescent Aggression*, New York: Ronald Press, 1959.
159. William N. Schoenfeld, 'Learning Theory and Social Psychology', in Otto Klineberg and Richard Christie (eds.), *Perspectives in Social Psychology*, New York: Holt, Rinehart & Winston, 1965, pp. 117–135.
160. C. R. Jeffery, 'Criminal Behavior and Learning Theory', *Journal of Criminal Law, Criminology and Police Science* (1965) **56**:294–300.
161. H. J. Eysenck, *Crime and Personality*, Boston: Houghton Mifflin Co., 1964; H. J. Eysenck, 'Conditioning and Personality', *British Journal of Psychology* (1962) **53**:3:299–305.
162. C. N. Franks, 'Recidivism, Psychopathy and Personality', *British Journal of Delinquency* (1955–1956) **6**:192–201.

Allen A. Bartholomew, 'Extraversion–Introversion and Neuroticism in First Offenders and Recidivists', *British Journal of Delinquency* (1959) **10**:2:120–129.

N. McConaghy, 'The Inhibitory Index in Relation to Extraversion–Introversion', *American Journal of Psychiatry* (1962) **119**:6:527–533.

E. M. Hetherington and E. Klinger, 'Psychopathy and Punishment', *Journal of Abnormal and Social Psychology* (1964) **69**:1:112–115.

163. Gordon Trasler, *The Explanation of Criminality*, London: Routledge & Kegan Paul, 1962.
164. O. H. Mowrer, *Learning Theory and Behavior*, New York: Wiley, 1960, p. 404.
165. Albert Bandura and Richard H. Walters, *Adolescent Aggression*, New York: Ronald Press, 1959.

Albert Bandura and Richard H. Walters, *Social Learning and Personality Development*, New York: Holt, Rinehart & Winston, 1963.

Albert Bandura, 'Behavior Theory and Identificatory Learning', *American Journal of Orthopsychiatry* (1963) **33**:4:591–601.

166. For a recent concise restatement of Eysenck's theory in relation to criminality, see Renato Canestrari and M. W. Battacchi, *Strutture e dinamiche della personalità nella antisocialità minorile*, Bologna: Edizioni Malipiero, 1963, pp. 98–101.

For an example of experimentation in social learning and aggression, see 'Application of Role and Learning Theories to the Study of the Development of Aggression in Children', *Psychological Reports* (1961) **9**:2:292–334. This is a reference to seven studies from the Rip van Winkle Foundation, Hudson, New York. Authors of the studies are L.D. Eron, J. H. Lanlicht, L. O. Wallace, I. E. Farber, J. P. Spiegel.

One interesting recent research design following the social-learning approach may be found in Robert D. Hare, 'A Conflict and Learning Theory Analysis of Psychopathic Behavior', *Journal of Research in Crime and Delinquency* (1965) **2**:1:12–19.

A clinical exposition is made by George C. Curtis, in 'Violence Breeds Violence: Perhaps?', *American Journal of Psychiatry* (1963) **120**:4:386–389, which could, with slight modifications, be reformulated within the frame of learning theory.

One of the best and most succinct statements we have encountered on learning theory and aggression is that contained in J. R. Thurston, N. F. Feldhusen, J. J. Benning, 'An Approach to Theory Explaining Classroom Aggression', Chapter 10 from *Eau Claire County Youth Study*, Wisconsin State Department of Public Welfare, United States Department of Health, Education, and Welfare, National Institute of Health, NIMH Grant No. 5–R11 MH 00672–03.

167. Bandura and Walters, *op. cit.*, 1959, 1963; also Albert Bandura 'Psychotherapy as a Learning Process', *Psychological Bulletin* (1961) **58**:143–195; and J. M. Grassberg, 'Behavior Therapy: A Review', *Psychological Bulletin* (1964) **62**:2:73–88; Joseph Wolpe, Andrew Salter, and Leo J. Reyna, *The Conditioning Therapies: The Challenge in Psychotherapy*, New York: Holt, Rinehart & Winston, 1964. For an excellent critique of conditioning therapies, see the review of the Wolpe, Salter, Reyna book by L. Breger in the *Journal of Projective Techniques and Personality Assessment* (1965) **29**:2:252–255. More detailed discussion of the combined notions of learning theory, subcultures, and therapy appear in Chapter V, note 129.

168. Leon Festinger, *A Theory of Cognitive Dissonance*, 1957; reissued, Stanford: Stanford University Press; London: Tavistock 1962.

Dana Bramel, 'A Dissonance Theory Approach to Defensive Projection', *Journal of Abnormal and Social Psychology* (1962) **64**:121–129.

Arnold H. Buss and Timothy C. Brock, 'Repression and Guilt in Relation to Aggression', *Journal of Abnormal and Social Psychology* (1963) **66**:4:345–350.

Philip Worchel and Betty L. McCormick, 'Self-Concept and Dissonance Reduction', *Journal of Personality* (1963) **31**:4:588–599.

169. Ross Stagner, The 'Psychology of Human Conflict', Chapter 3 in Elton B. McNeil (ed.), *The Nature of Human Conflict*, Englewood Cliffs, N. J.: Prentice-Hall, 1965, pp. 60–61.

170. Charles E. Osgood, *An Alternative to War or Surrender*, Urbana, Ill.: University of Illinois Press, 1962.

171. Ross Stagner, *Psychology and Personality*, Third Edition, New York: McGraw-Hill, 1961, p. 71. For other references relating perceptual theory to crime and aggression, see: Stagner, 'The Psychology of Human Conflict', *op. cit.*, *passim*; Stagner, *Psychology of Industrial Conflict*, New York: Wiley, 1956, *passim*.

Ross Stagner, 'Le teorie della personalità', *Rassegna di Psicologia Generale e Clinica* (1957) **2**:34–48.

H. H. Toch and R. Schulte, 'Readiness to Perceive Violence as a Result of Police Training', *British Journal of Psychology* (1961) **52**:4:389.

Hans H. Toch, 'The Stereoscope: A New Frontier in Psychological Research', *The Research Newsletter* (December, 1961) **3**:3–4:18–22.

Ernest L. V. Shelley and Hans H. Toch, 'The Perception of Violence as an Indicator of Adjustment in Institutionalized Offenders', *Journal of Criminal Law, Criminology and Police Science* (1962) **53**:4:463–469.

Paul S. D. Berg and Hans H. Toch, 'Impulsive and Neurotic Inmates: A Study in Personality and Perception', *Journal of Criminal Law, Criminology and Police Science* (June, 1946) **55**:230–234.

172. Hanan C. Selvin, 'Durkheim's *Suicide* and Problems of Empirical Research', *American Journal of Sociology* (1958) **63**:607–619.

173. Robert K. Merton, *Social Theory and Social Structure*, Glencoe, Ill.: The Free Press, 1949, pp. 131–194.

174. E. H. Powell, 'Occupational Status and Suicide: Toward a Redefinition of Anomie', *American Sociological Review* (1958) **23**:131–139. See also the latest book publication which discusses the major notions, research, and inferences of anomie: Marshall Clinard (ed.) *Anomie and Deviant Behavior: A Discussion and Critique*, New York: The Free Press of Glencoe, 1964.

175. What is meant by psychological anomie can be a number of different constructs. For example, MacIver gives a psychological definition of anomie which describes psychopathological syndromes resulting from loss of sense of social cohesion [R. M. MacIver, *The Ramparts We Guard*, New York: Macmillan, 1950]. Ansbacher (H. L. Ansbacher, 'Anomie, the Sociologist's Conception of Lack of Social Interest', *Ind. Psychol. Newsletter* (1956) **5**:11–12, 3–5) has equated this to Adler's lack of social interest [A. Adler, *Social Interest*, New York: Putnam, 1939]. Merton defines psychological anomie as a counterpart of, and not a substitute for, sociological anomie [Merton, *op. cit.*], and, indeed, it would be difficult to exclude a psychological correlate to such a pervading concept as sociological anomie. The difficulty rests with its integration into other meaningful personality constructs and with its reliable measurement. Srole's scale [L. Srole, 'Anomie, Authoritarianism and Prejudice', *American Journal of Sociology* (1956) **62**:63–67; L. Srole, 'Social Integration and Certain Corollaries: An Exploratory Study', *American Sociological Review* (1956) **21**:709–716] has had so far a very limited application and its use is difficult in groups characterized by low educational level.

For an expository analysis of anomie as a psychological concept, see Stephen H. Davol and Gunars Reimanis, 'The Role of Anomie as a Psychological Concept', *Journal of Individual Psychology* (1959) **15**:215–225.

176. Marvin E. Wolfgang, *Patterns in Criminal Homicide*, Philadelphia, Pennsylvania: University of Pennsylvania Press, 1958.
177. A Pigliaru, *La vendetta barbaricina come ordinamento giuridico*, Milano: Giuffrè, 1959.
  For an amazing report on the whole small town, Albanova, near Rome, that is devoted to the use of violence, see Giulio Frisoli, 'La pistola regalo di battesimo', *Epoca* (February 27, 1965), and Giulio Frisoli and Pietro Zullino, 'Il segreto di Albanova', *Epoca* (March 7, 1965).
178. G. Guzman Campos, O. Fals Borda, and E. Umaña Luna, '*La Violencia en Colombia: Estudio de un proceso social*', Bogotá: Tercer Mundo, 1962.
179. Wolfgang, *Patterns in Criminal Homicide*, pp. 188–189.
180. We have elsewhere, in Chapter II, referred to the many studies of delinquency that discuss these matters. For recent items, see especially Lewis Yablonsky, *The Violent Gang*, New York: Macmillan, 1962; also, Dorothy Hayes and Russell Hogrefe, 'Group Sanction and Restraints Related to Use of Violence in Teenagers', paper read at the 41st annual meeting of the American Orthopsychiatric Association, Chicago, Illinois, March 20, 1964.
181. For an especially insightful comment that aided our thinking on this topic, see Otto Pollak, 'Our Social Values and Juvenile Delinquency', *The Quarterly of the Pennsylvania Association on Probation, Parole and Correction* (September, 1964) **21**:12–22.
182. There is an abundant literature on the combined topics of child-rearing practices, physical aggression, and social class. Among the earlier works, particularly useful are R. R. Sears, *Survey of Objective Studies of Psychoanalytical Concepts*, Bulletin 51, New York: Social Science Research Council, 1943; A. Davis and R. J. Havighurst, 'Racial Class and Color Difference in Child Rearing', *American Sociological Review* (1946) **11**:698–710; J. H. S. Bossard, *The Sociology of Child Development*, New York: Harper and Brothers, 1948.
  Several specific references of special use in our concern with the transmission of values related to violence or physical aggression include:

Charles McArthur, 'Personality Differences Between Middle and Upper Classes', *Journal of Abnormal and Social Psychology* (1955) **50**:247–254.
Clyde R. White, 'Social Class Differences in the Use of Leisure', *American Journal of Sociology* (1955) **61**:145–151.
O. G. Brim, 'Parent–Child Relations as a Social System: I. Parent and Child Roles', *Child Development* (1957) **28**:342–364.
Joel B. Montague and Edgar G. Epps, 'Attitudes Toward Social Mobility as Revealed by Samples of Negro and White Boys', *Pacific Sociological Review* (1958) **1**:81–84.
Lawrence Kohlberg, 'Status as Perspective on Society: An Interpre-

tation of Class Differences in Children's Moral Judgments', paper delivered at the Society for Research in Child Development Symposium on Moral Process, Bethesda, Maryland, March 21, 1959.

Melvin L. Kohn, 'Social Class and Parent–Child Relationships: An Interpretation', *American Journal of Sociology* (1963) **68**:471–480.

Louis Kriesberg, 'The Relationship Between Socio-Economic Rank and Behavior', *Social Problems* (1963) **10**:334–353.

Hyman Rodman, 'The Lower-Class Value Stretch', *Social Forces* (1963) **42**:205–215.

John C. Leggett, 'Uprootedness and Working-Class Consciousness', *American Journal of Sociology* (1963) **68**:682–692.

C. R. Roger, 'Toward a Modern Approach to Values: The Valuing Process in the Mature Person', *Journal of Abnormal and Social Psychology* (1964), **68**:160–167.

Leigh Minturn and William W. Lambert, *Mothers of Six Cultures*, New York: Wiley, 1964, especially Chapter 7, 'Aggression Training: Mother-Directed Aggression', pp. 136–162.

Kathryn P. Johnson and Gerald R. Leslie, 'Methodological Notes on Research in Childrearing and Social Class', paper presented to the annual meeting of the American Sociological Association, Montreal, August, 1964.

Excellent summaries of the literature in current works are found in Paul Henry Mussen (ed.) *Handbook of Research Methods in Child Development*, New York: Wiley, 1960; in Martin L. Hoffman and Lois W. Hoffman, *Review of Child Development Research*, Vol. I, New York: Russell Sage Foundation, 1964; and in the rich bibliography noted in John J. Honigmann and Richard J. Preston, 'Recent Developments in Culture and Personality', Supplement to *The Annals of the American Academy of Political and Social Science* (July, 1964) **354**:153–162.

All of the recent literature we have been able to examine from anthropology, psychology, and sociology buttressed the general position of our thesis regarding class, punishment, and aggression.

183. Martin Gold, 'Suicide, Homicide and the Socialization of Aggression', *American Journal of Sociology* (May, 1958) **63**:651–661.

184. *Ibid.*

185. This is different from the 'strength of the relational system' discussed by Henry and Short in their provocative analysis (Andrew F. Henry and James F. Short, Jr., *Suicide and Homicide*, Glencoe, Ill.: The Free Press, 1954, pp. 16–18, 91–92, 124–125). Relative to the Henry and Short suggestion, see Wolfgang, *Patterns in Criminal Homicide*, pp. 278–279. The attempt of Gibbs and Martin to measure Durkheim's reference to 'degree of integration' is a competent analysis of the problem, but a subculture of violence integrated around a given value item or value system may require quite different indices of

integration than those to which these authors refer (Jack P. Gibbs and Walter T. Martin, 'A Theory of Status Integration and Its Relationship to Suicide', *American Sociological Review* (April, 1958) 23:140–147.

186. Robert J. Smith, 'The Japanese World Community: Norms, Sanctions, and Ostracism', *American Anthropologist* (1961) 63:522–533. Withdrawal from the group may be by the deviant's own design and desire, or by response to the reaction of the group. Cf. Robert A. Dentler and Kai T. Erikson, 'The Functions of Deviance in Groups', *Social Problems* (Fall 1959) 7:98–107.

187. Ross Stagner, *Psychology of Industrial Conflict*, New York: Wiley, 1956.

188. See, for example, John Paul Scott, *Aggression*, Chicago: University of Chicago Press, 1958, pp. 44–64.

189. For the concept of subculture to have psychological validity, psychologically meaningful differences should, of course, be evident in subjects belonging to the subculture of violence. From a diagnostic point of view, a number of signs and indicators, of both psychometric and projective type, can be used. The differential perception of violent stimuli can be used as an indicator. Partial studies in this direction are those of Shelley and Toch (E. L. V. Shelley and H. Toch, 'The Perception of Violence As an Indicator of Adjustment in Institutionalized Offenders', *Journal of Criminal Law, Criminology and Police Science*, (1962) 53:463–469).

190. The Philadelphia study (Wolfgang, *Patterns in Criminal Homicide*) showed that 65 per cent of the offenders and 47 per cent of the victims had a previous police record of arrests and that 75 per cent of these arrests were for aggravated assaults. Here, then, is a situation in homicide often not unlike that of combat in which two persons committed to the value of violence come together and in which chance often dictates the identity of the slayer and of the slain.

191. A recent study (L. G. Schultz, 'Why the Negro Carries Weapons', *Journal of Criminal Law, Criminology and Police Science* (1962) 53:476–483) on weapon-carrying suggests that this habit is related, within the colored population, to lower-class status, rural origin from the South, and prior criminal record.

192. As previously mentioned, differential reactions to conditioning may be the cause of differential adherence to the subculture by equally exposed subjects.

193. Alternative hypotheses make use of the concept of differential association (Edwin H. Sutherland and Donald R. Cressey, *Principles of Criminology*, Philadelphia: Lippincott, 1955).

194. Differential identification has been presented as a more psychologically meaningful alternative to simple association (Daniel Glaser, 'Criminality Theories and Behavioral Images', *American Journal of Sociology* (1956) 5:433–444).

195. A. H. Buss, *The Psychology of Aggression*, New York: Wiley, 1961, pp. 1–2.

196. *Ibid.*, pp. 2–4.
197. *Ibid.*, Chapter 1, *passim*.
198. For an analysis of relevant literature on diagnostic psychological instruments, see Buss, *op. cit.*, Chapters VIII and IX. For discussion of a preventive psychiatric system, see Leon D. Hankoff, 'Prevention of Violence', paper read at the annual meeting of the Association for the Psychiatric Treatment of Offenders, New York, May 7, 1964.
199. *The Sociology of Georg Simmel* (translated, edited, and with an introduction by Kurt H. Wolff), Glencoe, Ill.: The Free Press, 1950; *Georg Simmel, 1858–1918* (edited by Kurt H. Wolff), Columbus, Ohio: Ohio State University Press, 1959; Georg Simmel, *Conflict and the Web of Group Affiliations* (translated by Kurt H. Wolff and Reinhard Bendix), New York: The Free Press of Glencoe, 1964 paperback edition; Lewis Coser, *The Functions of Social Conflict*, Glencoe, Ill.: The Free Press, 1956; *The Nature of Human Conflict*, (edited by Elton B. McNeil) Englewood Cliffs, N.J.: Prentice-Hall, 1965.
200. The issues of *The Journal of Conflict Resolution* are, of course, pertinent. Relative to our main concern with violence, see especially Rolf Dahrendorf, 'Toward a Theory of Social Conflict', *Journal of Conflict Resolution* (1958) **2**:170–183; the entire issue entitled 'The Anthropology of Conflict', *Journal of Conflict Resolution* (1961), Volume V, Number 1.
201. For an early provocative discussion of violence from a sociological viewpoint and as a tool of social protest against the Establishment, as a proletarian technique to threaten the existing institutions of society, see Georges Sorel, *Reflections on Violence* (the original French text appeared in 1906).

For recent general references to the sociology of violence, see:

Joseph S. Rouček, 'The Sociology of Violence', *Journal of Human Relations* (1957) **5**:9–21.
David Marlowe, 'Commitment, Contract, Group Boundaries and Conflict', reprinted from *Science and Psychoanalysis* (Masserman), New York: Grune & Stratton, 1963, pp. 43–55.
E. V. Walter, 'Violence and the Process of Terror', *American Sociological Review* (1964) **29**:248–257.
Jessie Bernard, 'Some Current Conceptualizations in the Field of Conflict', *American Journal of Sociology* (1965) **70**:442–454.
Austin L. Porterfield, *Cultures of Violence*, Fort Worth, Texas: Leo Potishman, 1965.

There is a growing concern in peace research with what has been called 'the sociology of nonviolence'. For a review of these ideas, see Martin Oppenheimer, 'Towards a Sociology of Nonviolence', paper read at the Eastern Sociological Society meeting, Boston, April 11, 1964.

IV · Biological, Psychiatric, and Psychometric Perspectives on a Subculture of Violence from Studies on Homicide

In the preceding chapters we have discussed the need for integration in criminology and the concept of subculture as an integrating construct. We have focused our analysis on the subculture of violence and have presented some of its theoretical implications. We shall now direct our attention to the existing literature on violence, especially homicide, in an attempt to note convergences and divergences between existing criminological facts and our theoretical formulation.

The literature on violence is very extensive; we can only attempt to trace its main trends. Criminological studies of violent and assaultive behavior have been conducted in many disciplines, ranging from biology to sociology, and have employed many different approaches. A systematic examination of this literature suggests a classification of existing studies into biological researches, 'animal' studies, psychiatric and clinical investigations, psychological, psychometric, and sociological studies. Following such a disciplinary classification does some injustice to the multidisciplinary character of several studies and may misclassify a portion of the existing data. However, keeping this and other inherent difficulties in mind, we shall follow a broad 'disciplinary' classification for the sake of clarity and parsimony of presentation, keeping a focus on our aim of integration by trying to pull together material related to our integrated thesis. The scope and aim of our analysis are limited by our theoretical approach, which will determine the degree of emphasis we shall place on each of the groups of studies. Our primary focus is on criminology, and more specifically on criminal violence in its most reportable form, homicide.

Much of the general literature, particularly of a psychological character, deals with violence and aggression from a descriptive, atomistic viewpoint and has only a marginal bearing on an integrated socio-psychological theory of a subculture of violence. Many studies, on account of design, content, or interpretation of the data, have little relevance to our approach. These we shall exclude from any detailed consideration, occasionally grouping them into categories that may not be discrete but are convenient for expository purposes. It should be remembered that it is not our purpose to examine all psychological theories of aggression except to the extent to which they bear on our problem. Aggression and violence are here viewed as synonymous, and the reader interested in more basic discussions of these phenomena may elsewhere find useful reviews, such as those by McNeil,[1] Buss,[2] and Berkowitz.[3]

THE CLASSIFICATION OF HOMICIDE AND HOMICIDE STUDIES

Among crimes against the person, violence and homicide are by a long way those which cause the most severe public reaction. Much attention has traditionally been given to the causes and phenomenological aspects of these crimes as well as to the disposition of violent offenders. Homicide remains a topic of paramount interest in criminology, although relative to other offenses the actual number of homicides is not great. As von Hentig has remarked, social reactions to the taking of human life have always been characterized by emotionality and much irrationality,[4] probably because homicide is considered almost everywhere to be the most serious of all crimes.

In a recent German book, Middendorff[5] recalls the opinion of Reiwald[6] who maintains that homicide is generally viewed as the 'first crime', the original or 'natural crime'. Repression of aggressive impulses and inhibition of individual aggression have led to an advanced and progressive 'collective conscience' against violence and homicide. Obviously, to maintain a state of equilibrium, any social system must have proscriptions against intragroup violence and slaying; and every new case of violent crime is proof that the cultural transmission of those prohibitions, or the proper socialization of an individual, has failed and the outbreak will evoke negative emotional reactions in the public.

Although all legal systems punish homicide, there are wide differences in classification, terminology, juridical concepts, and forms of sanctions. These differences make difficult the task of trying to compare statistical data internationally. Even within the same country, different juris-prudential approaches may cause many problems for trend analyses. Examining legal differences in the definition of violent crimes falls within the field of comparative criminal law and generally is outside the range of our present interest. By excluding the more strictly legal discussions, we have somewhat reduced our task of analysis and classification, although we realize the need for a comparative study of the law of homicide. Even with this exclusion, the general literature on violence and homicide is dispersed in an abundant number of professional journals and is vast in quantity.[7]

Murder and homicide present a great variety of situations, motives, and manner of execution (*modus operandi*), ranging from brutal killing in the course of a trivial quarrel to the skillfully planned, almost 'perfect' and undetectable premeditated crime for purely financial reasons. This variety may explain the legal confusion of terms and the objective difficulty facing anyone who attempts a statistical analysis of homicides. The need for unification of terminology and for more detailed statistics has often been pointed out,[8] but the present picture is still confusing.

From our point of view, interest is focused on criminal homicide and includes all degrees of murder and some types of manslaughter in the Anglo-Saxon criminal system. Homicide due to negligence, as in the case of traffic offenses, is excluded from our area of study.[9] The discriminating factors between criminal and noncriminal homicide seem to be the intention to kill or to inflict harm upon the victim, and the anticipation of the noxious results. From a psychological viewpoint, the legal distinction between 'attempted' and completed criminal homicide is difficult to defend because the victim's survival is often the result of chance, accident, or the availability of medical care, and these factors may in themselves have a considerable effect on criminal statistics.[10] Still, the bulk of psychological literature is concerned with murder, not with attempts at it, and serious doubts may be raised about the validity of the categories used. The psychological differences between attempted and completed homicides are probably minimal, although society's attitude toward the successful homicide offender is certainly different from its approach to the man who failed in his homicidal attempt. This fact in itself would probably constitute an interesting area of research, but so far it has not been the subject of detailed study by criminologically oriented psychologists.

The psychiatric and psychological literature on murderers is extensive and will be examined later in more detail. Although mentally ill criminals are generally the province of psychiatrists, rarely have their individualistic explanations been able to generate useful generalizations. Much more empirical research is needed before generalizations based on one case or a handful of cases can be accepted as valid. Moreover, we must restrict our discussion at this stage to criminal homicides committed by people who are not legally insane. Psychopathological homicide will be briefly discussed in another section of this chapter.

We must emphasize again that the group of 'normal' homicides may show two basic kinds of behavior: (a) premeditated, felonious, intentional, planned, and rational murder; and (b) slaying in the heat of passion, or killing as a result of intent to do harm, but without a specific intent to kill. Probably less than 5 per cent of all known killings are premeditated, planned, and intentional. The individuals who commit them are most likely to be episodic offenders who never had serious prior contacts with the police or criminal courts. As a result, these offenders may have a greater chance of remaining undetected. These cases are of limited numerical interest and should be differentiated from the group of passionate, unpremeditated killers. Many authors fail to distinguish between these two basic types of murderers. In the present analysis we shall keep the two groups separated and concentrate attention on the 'passionate' killer.

For a long time criminologists have been concerned to construct a consistent typology of the criminal population, and many ingenious classifications have emerged.[11] Of particular interest for us is the fact that, in almost all the proposed classifications, the passionate homicide, the emotional, unplanned, rage killer has been included. When analysis is made of the distribution of homicides, this type of offender is found to be numerically important, usually constituting the largest group. Seelig,[12] for example, described the category of 'aggressive criminals' as a group characterized by high emotionality and a tendency toward motor discharge, coupled with a weakness of inhibitory mechanisms. In the homicidal types described by Ferri,[13] the 'instinctive', the 'occasional', and the 'passion' types appear to belong to this hyperthymic, emotional group. In Ferri's early opinion, persons 'born' to commit homicide were characterized by moral insensibility, ferocity, apathy, a weak power of resistance to criminal desires, exaggerated sensibility, sanguine or nervous temperament, and observable anthropomorphic differences from the general criminal population.[14]

In his analysis of 96 Wisconsin murderers, Gillin[15] found that most of these killings were 'crimes of passion, explosive reactions to difficult situations'. Clinard[16] differentiated between murders which resulted from a long period of hostility, those which occurred during sudden anger, and those in which subcultural factors played an important role. In his general classification of homicides, Gemelli[17] included passionate killing, homicidal impulsivity, and alcoholic impulsivity. As we shall later see, some of these distinctions are frequently more apparent than real.

In considering the distribution of passionate murders, it should also be remembered that alcohol functions to release emotions and lower cortical control over manifestations of anger. Intoxication was found to be associated with homicide in one-third of the cases examined by Gillin.[18] In the cases studied by Wolfgang in Philadelphia,[19] alcohol was present in 64 per cent of the homicide situations, either in the victim or in the offender, or in both. In a Puerto Rican study, Toro Calder also found a high rate of alcoholic intoxication among violent offenders.[20]

Following the initial taxonomic efforts of a primarily intuitive character, the development of typologies in criminology resulted in a tendency to replace general theories that tried to explain all criminal behavior with separate theories for specific patterns of crime. Gibbons and Garrity[21] have discussed this problem in detail and indicate the criteria for the 'goodness of fit' of proposed typologies. Some of the necessary procedural guides to be followed are briefly outlined by these authors, who claim that an adequate criminal typology should:

1. include a major part of the offender population;
2. describe and discriminate between offender types at any given point in the lives of the subjects;
3. describe the developmental history and provide an etiological description of each type;
4. make it possible to classify actual offenders within the typology with clarity, reliability, and precision;
5. be as parsimonious as possible.

Some of these requisites are obviously difficult to meet. In a more structured classification, Gibbons[22] lists two types who could be identified with our 'passion murderer': the 'one time loser, personal offense',

and 'the psychopathic assaultist'. Although classifications are sometimes considered to be purely descriptive devices, without much value
for individual case examination and disposition, they serve to underline
the existence of a type of homicide characterized by sudden violent
explosions of aggressive behavior, by the easy evocation of anger, by
facilitation of aggressive responses.

Von Hentig[23] attempted to classify homicides according to motives,
which were identified as follows: 'profit', 'conflict', 'to cover up', 'sex',
and 'absurd'. This last category is very similar to the 'motiveless'
murder which we shall discuss in the section on psychiatric literature.
Most authors, however, prefer a classification based on behavioral,
phenomenological characteristics, such as those we have listed in the
preceding pages. Peterson and others,[24] in a study of police records in
St Louis, Missouri, have shown the consistency of violent or nonviolent offenses in criminals. Offenders, they point out, tend to commit
one or the other type of crime, but rarely both.

Homicides have been studied from almost every conceivable point of
view. Some studies are of very marginal relevance to our analysis; many
of these and others will be mentioned here only to provide a relatively
comprehensive list of the literature. Many different factors, even
weather, have been analyzed, in an attempt to find some explanation for
homicidal behavior.[25] Some authors deal with the condemned murderers' evaluations of their own acts[26] or with the murderers' attitudes
toward death.[27] These latter studies are of some interest in a psychological analysis of the murderer's rationalizations of his motives. Finally,
many authors have studied the relationship between the murderer and
his victim.[28] The relationship between offender and victim in crimes of
violence is especially important to the issue of public compensation for
victims of violent crime.[29]

From this general statement on the types of studies that have been
made, we now seek to provide a reasonably systematic analysis of the
literature that is relevant to our focus on violence, with special emphasis on criminal homicide and the subculture of violence.

THE BIOLOGY OF VIOLENCE

The biological analysis of violent behavior can be undertaken from
various viewpoints, including the comparative, neurological, endocrinological, and anthropometrical. The contributions assembled in the

following discussion represent a fairly large sample of the pertinent literature, although some selection has proved necessary from among the widely dispersed published papers and monographs. The different hypotheses and research results are often contradictory, and, in spite of some recent efforts[30] in interdisciplinary research, the gaps between specialists, as, for example, between ethologists and endocrinologists, are often difficult to bridge. We shall save for later discussion the psychoanalytic approaches to violence, as well as the other psychological and psychopathological hypotheses, in spite of the obvious links between the 'biological', instinct-oriented hypotheses and the 'innate', aggressive-motive conception of orthodox psychoanalysts.

AGGRESSION VIEWED AS INNATE INSTINCT OR LEARNED RESPONSE

Two main and clearly opposed hypotheses have been formulated about the biological basis of violence and aggression. One considers this behavioral manifestation to be an innate instinct, inborn in animals, including men, whereas the other views aggression as a learned response for which no biological pre-formed basis exists. The first hypothesis has received support from such well-known authors as Konrad Lorenz.[31] He states that intraspecific aggression (the most relevant type of violent behavior) has important functions, such as the spacing of individuals of the same species over their available territory, the selection of the fittest individual, and the establishment of social rank, which permits the younger generation to have the benefit of experience from the aged. Interspecific aggression must be distinguished from predatory activity and seems to be stronger in species that show small taxonomic differences. There is, of course, the possibility of an overspill of intraspecific aggression to interspecific violence. The 'lust for hatred and destruction' was advanced by Einstein (with Freud's support) as the explanation for war.[32] And a recent popular book by Ardrey[33] postulates that man's development and evolution are due to his inborn aggressive, killing attitudes and his love for weapons, which Ardrey traces back, mostly on Raymond Dart's anthropological evidence,[34] from the bone weapons of Australopithecus to the knife of the modern juvenile delinquent. This opinion is shared by Derek Freeman, who recently reviewed much of the relevant literature.[35]

This evolutionary viewpoint, however, appears to be sharply opposed by the majority of biologists and comparative psychologists. The thesis of an innate aggressive instinct has never been satisfactorily proved. In his review of the existing evidence,[36] Scott has stated that there is no need for fighting, either aggressive or defensive, apart from what happens in the external environment. The study of animals has not yet uncovered evidence that aggression is a product of an instinctive, innate urge in the organism. McNeil[37] recently stated that it is improbable that such a conclusion will ever be reached. This opinion is echoed by Buss[38] and by Berkowitz,[39] who contend that, although the capacity to be aggressive is characteristic of every form of life, aggressiveness is fashioned from experience. This view does not contradict the possibility of individual differences in conformity to experience or of individual susceptibility to the learning process of violence. Perhaps it should be mentioned that Eibl-Eibesfeldt[40] has denied Scott's conclusions on the basis of experiments conducted on Norwegian rats. However, Eibl-Eibesfeldt has also focused attention on the ritual, non-killing characteristics of intraspecific fighting.

A number of comparative studies were reported at a session of the American Association for the Advancement of Science in Philadelphia in 1962. They concur with the statement of McK. Rioch, who denied the existence of any occult force pushing people to violence, and instead consider violence as a pattern which may be reasonably used, or may be resorted to, in situations of uncertainty or under conditions of social disorganization.[41] Of specific interest are the studies conducted by L. D. Clark[42] on the *Onychomys leucogaster*. This is an unusually aggressive mouse, originally found in Utah; he is stocky, small, and well equipped for killing. Even this highly aggressive animal, although showing a genetic predisposition to aggression, may never exhibit aggressive behavior if he does not meet external, environmental threats to his security (pain, fear, anxiety-generating stimuli). Aggression is influenced by learning, reinforced by successful fights, and decreased by defeats. In Clark's conclusions, aggression is not an instinct or even a drive; it can remain forever latent, and, even if developed, can be eliminated or altered in favor of non-aggressive solutions.

The 'Osteodontokeratic' culture of the Australopithecines is still a matter of discussion among anthropologists. The bones which some authors have interpreted as weapons were, according to others including K. P. Oakley, broken to extract marrow as food. Uncontroversial evidence for the existence of tooled weapons relates to much more recent ages, and organized warfare dates back only to the Neolithic period.[43]

The thesis of aggression as a learned motive has, as Russell recently stated at the symposium of the London Institute of Biology, received important support from carefully controlled studies conducted on primates by H. F. Harlow and his associates. Rhesus monkeys reared in isolation from their mothers and from one another exhibited grossly disturbed behavior and rejected their offspring. Obviously and objectively seriously frustrated by 'bad' mothers in their attempts to obtain bodily contacts in early life, these offspring showed more aggression than any other experimental groups. [44]

In a more general vein, and from a strictly behavioristic standpoint, Hebb has emphasized rejection of the concept of instinct. He has proposed the substitution of the term 'instinctive behavior', keeping in mind that no special activity or part of the brain exists for the construct called 'instinct'. He also emphasized the importance of perceptual learning for the acquisition of instinctive behavioral patterns, which in higher animals are a function of the perception of environmental objects and events. Normal perceptual development depends on exposure to the normally present stimulus patterns of the early environment. [45] This kind of hypothesis is, of course, in full agreement with a subcultural approach.

THE NEUROPHYSIOLOGICAL BASIS

In a comprehensive analysis of the neurophysiological basis for drives and motives, Stellar [46] reviewed the different contributions to our present and still rather limited knowledge of the underlying structures and mechanisms. He also carefully analyzed the behavioristic evidence opposed to the concept of instinct and discussed the complex relationships between learning and motivation. Obvious 'rage-controlling' centers have been demonstrated. However, Stellar's conclusion emphasizes the importance of the various sensory avenues and states: 'An often neglected, but nevertheless important factor is learning, for previously neutral stimuli can, through experience, come to contribute to the arousal and satiation of motivated behavior, and various new instrumentalities and goals may be learned in the execution of motivated behavior.' [47] Another area of interaction with the basic neurophysiological structures is outlined by Stellar: 'A second neglected problem has to do with perceptual changes in motivated behavior. We have discussed only the relatively nonspecific role of different systems in the arousal of motivation, but the motivated organism is highly specific and selective in its perception of the environment, as many ethological and psychological studies show. Unfortunately, we have very little physiological evidence relevant to this problem.'[48]

The subjective experience of free will and self-determination appears to contradict the hypotheses of existing underlying motivational structures. MacKay[49] has tried to resolve this conflict, and in his view motivation is identical with positive and negative affects and desires. It constitutes the subjective correlate of neuronal activities determined by biological drives of original and acquired needs. The needs, originally primal and unconditioned, undergo elaboration owing to the addition of other derivative and conditioned needs through the impact of experience. In a universe of varying circumstances, conflicting needs lead to conflicting drives towards alternative actions and offer to the organism a choice, the resolution of which is accomplished when neuronal activity follows preponderant habitual paths. The differences between unconditioned and conditioned needs are, in MacKay's hypothesis, small and artificial. With few variations, the same conceptualization could be extended to cover social motivation.

Of interest are the studies on anthropometric differences between violent and nonviolent, or less violent, human subjects. Evidence on the heredity of violence and aggressiveness is contradictory, and has never overcome the 'nature-versus-nurture' methodological problem. Thorne[50] has studied their epidemiological transmission. Folklore and tradition claim there are differences in the predisposition of given national and ethnic groups towards violence, but no objective proof is available. In criminological studies, Eyrich[51] in 1930 found a prevalence of leptosomes and athletics in a small group (34 subjects) of murderers. In a larger and more recent study of 500 delinquents and 500 nondelinquents, Sheldon and Eleanor Glueck found that hostility, although closely associated with delinquency, did not differ significantly among the four Sheldonian somatotype categories.[52]

Studies on the physiology of anger have a direct relevance to the object of our analysis. They are, however, controversial, and in spite of the time and effort which physiologists and endocrinologists have devoted to them, no final conclusion has been reached. Since the pioneer work of Cannon,[53] several neurological and endocrinological structures and mechanisms have been discovered which are closely linked with the expression of anger and fear. The available knowledge has been summarized by Funkenstein,[54] Scott,[55] and Buss,[56] among others. Neurologically, aggression appears to be controlled by the hypothalamus and the neocortex. The amygdala also control rage and their unilateral destruction produces long-lasting rage reactions.[57] But, again, the evidence is quite contradictory, and, in effect, stereotaxis amygdalotomy has been used to control behavior disorders.[58] These different structures appear to balance each other in a continuous interplay of excitation and inhibition.

Even if the hypothalamus overcomes central inhibition, and rage expressions occur, control is quickly restored, following prevailing outside stimulation. However, Hess[59] has produced long-lasting rage effects in rats through electrical stimulation of the hypothalamus. Scott[60] tends to interpret these results as due to technical differences in the procedures used.

Cannon first showed the importance of adrenalin secretion in the physiology of anger. Since his original work, available evidence points to the existence of two[61] and possibly three[62] adrenal medullary hormones. Since Selye's[63] description of the stress reaction, an adrenal-cortical hormone, cortisone, has also been found to be of paramount importance in the endocrinology of aggressive emotional states. All these substances have clear neurovegetative effects. But in terms of autonomic reactions, it is very difficult to differentiate between fear and anger in humans. It is also difficult to attribute emotion-specific functions to the different hormonal substances which, after central neurological stimulation, originate in the adrenal cortex and medulla. The fear pattern seems to correspond to that elicited by adrenalin; the anger pattern is similar to that caused by both adrenalin and nonadrenalin together. Ax[64] tried to distinguish fear from anger reactions by means of objective polygraphic measurements of neurovegetative-controlled manifestations. Still, Hebb[65] has more recently asserted that fear and anger are so intimately related and similar in observable terms that it is impossible to discuss one without the other. In both emotions there is a disruption of coordinated cerebral activity and perhaps the two emotions cannot be distinguished. Flight and aggression, still according to Hebb, are two different modes of reaction tending to restore the dynamic equilibrium or stability of cerebral processes. In some situations it appears to be a matter of chance whether aggression or flight dominates behavior.

Although the underlying neurological mechanisms are of modest importance for the study of homicidal behavior, they help to throw some light on the neuropathology that can result in homicidal aggression. The importance of central neurological lesions due to traumas, infections, or congenital anomalies has been pointed out by several authors. Bachet has isolated a special syndrome which he defines as 'criminogenic encephalosis'.[66] And Papez, in a review of psychiatrically relevant neuroanatomical data, has stated that irritative lesions in the sub-callosal gyrus and in the medial frontal cortex produce aggressive and uncontrolled activities. In experimental animals, anger, rage, and fights are recorded. In men, patients who show a proclivity towards this behavior frequently present sclerosis (resulting in a decreased blood supply) of the branches of the anterior cerebral arteries which supply, among other areas, the medial frontal cortex. It may be that the medial forebrain bundle provides the hypothalamic reactions which support aggressive behavior.[67]

Denis Hill[68] recalls the frequent occurrence of marked destructiveness and impulsiveness, combined with primitive aggressive and sexual impulses of both an auto- and etero-directed character, which followed recovery in children who suffered from encephalitis lethargica in the 1920 pandemic. This disease affected the basal ganglia, the hypothalamus, and the pereiaqueductal grey matter. However, no focal pathology has yet been found for specific conduct disorders. Patients with lesions in the limbic system, or with temporal lobe epilepsy (where lesions are found in the temporal lobe – the amygdala, uncal, hyppocampal areas), due to atrophic, neoplastic, or postinfective damage, show, in about 50 per cent of the cases, a low threshold for aggressive behavior, intolerance of frustration, impulsiveness, and irritability. It is interesting to note that ordinary psychosurgical procedures which sever the connections between the thalamus and the frontal cortex reduce self-directed violence but have little or no effect on externally directed violence. The inhibitory action of the cortex is removed. Hill notes that aggressiveness is frequent in children and declines with age, with the exception of psychopaths, for whom electroencephalographic (EEG) analysis reveals patterns of immaturity resembling childhood EEGs. With age, both the E.E.G. patterns and violent behavior decrease, even in the psychopaths, who appear to be clear-cut cases of retarded maturation. According to Hill, about 10 per cent of murderers are in this category. However, Hill emphasizes the importance of the environment, particularly therapeutic surroundings, in the development and maintenance of violence. 'To the extent to which the mentally sick are treated with aggressiveness,' he says, 'to that extent they have difficulties in coping with their own aggressive tendencies.'[69] One could, it appears, postulate the existence of a violence-generating factor in pre-modern psychiatric treatment.

Central neurological lesions can, of course, be caused by a variety of etiological agents ranging from infections to neoplasms. It is quite possible that in children of lower social class and in developing countries where sanitary conditions, especially at childbirth, are inadequate, more organic causes are operative. One important group of lesions may be connected with perinatal anoxia. Kinberg,[70] some decades ago, spoke of the importance of 'microlesions' affecting behavior, but unfortunately they are often undetectable by ordinary neurological procedures. Head injuries are frequently found in the history of offenders exhibiting aggressive behavior, and a recent Czechoslovakian study noted that as many as 24 per cent of violent offenders had had such injuries.[71] Still, the main causes generally appear to be social in character.

The development of refined electroencephalographic techniques and the increased interest for electroneurophysiology have produced a concentration of studies on offenders, and these studies provide interesting background information on the biological correlates of aggressive behavior.[72] We shall discuss the aggressive aspect of epileptic disorders later, in the section that covers the psychiatric correlates of violence; at present we shall limit our presentation to those studies which deal with unspecific abnormalities of EEG recordings, i.e. other than those which are pathognomic of convulsive disorders.

A number of EEG researches have consistently demonstrated the existence of many different kinds of abnormality in juvenile and adult offenders who also had conduct disorders. But there has been no clear specificity in the diagnosis of aggressive and violent behavior. The frequency of cases exhibiting abnormalities varies from 55 per cent in an Italian study[73] to 70 per cent in an English study[74] that was conducted on 'motiveless' murders and murders with 'slight motives'. However, certain methodological difficulties inherent in electroencephalographic researches have never been satisfactorily solved. Even when cases of conduct disorder are shown to have a high incidence of EEG abnormalities, the relationship is never invariable or total. In carefully controlled studies conducted in England by Grunberg and Pond,[75] and by Hodge, Walter, and Walter,[76] the importance of environmental social factors both in epileptic children and in juvenile delinquents with EEG abnormalities has been strongly emphasized. As an analysis of the Grunberg and Pond study demonstrates, when environmental social factors were examined, epileptics and non-epileptics with conduct disorders had very similar backgrounds. Both groups suffered from disturbed parental emotional attitudes, marital disharmony of parents, sibling rivalry, restriction, and variations in environment. This finding suggests a causal relationship between conduct disorders and disturbed social background in epileptic children. In terms of abnormalities found in EEG recordings, they are unspecific (Delta and Theta slow waves, Alphoid rhythms, general indications of immaturity, etc.). The type of abnormality does not differentiate significantly between normal and aggressive offenders in any of the many studies devoted to this topic.[77]

One hypothesis of specificity regarding EEG signs and aggressive behavior has been formulated on scanty evidence (only two juvenile homicide offenders) by Woods.[78] It concerns the so-called '6-and-14 syndrome', which is a specific type of dysrhythmia. The syndrome was discovered by Frederic A. Gibbs and E. L. Gibbs and has been claimed by many others[79] to be associated with aggressive behavior. Woods postulated that the dysrhythmia was associated with homicide, although he admits that the dysrhythmia does not itself induce violence, but rather that it serves as a biologically determined stress on an already impoverished ego. This specificity has been firmly denied, however, by Frederic A. Gibbs and asserted recently with careful research data by others.[80]

Another area that has captured the attention of criminologists is the investigation of endocrinological disturbances connected with violent and aggressive behavior. In 1923 Di Tullio[81] pointed out the frequency of endocrinological disturbances of various types among criminals. More recently, Podolsky[82] has again listed a number of endocrinal pathological conditions among prisoners. However, no specificity of relationship between endocrinal malfunctioning and aggressive behavior can be claimed, with few exceptions. We have already mentioned the relationships between adrenal hormones and aggression. To this we should add a recent and interesting case of homicide which occurred during ACTH therapy. In the opinion of Train and Winkler,[83] the ACTH therapy caused impairment of the patient's ego controls and resulted in unconscious hostility.

The role of the male sex hormone in the development of aggressive behavior has been the object of lengthy discussions and even of therapeutic efforts.[84] There is little doubt about the different sex ratios in aggression, but male aggressiveness is, after all, also and perhaps primarily linked to role expectations and previously learned behavior patterns. It is interesting to note that the effect of gonadal hormones on aggression is more clear-cut in lower animal orders, where presumably the sex-role expectations are less differentiated. Scott relates an interesting experiment by Beeman[85] which throws some light on male sex hormones and aggressive behavior. If male mice trained to fight daily are given a rest after castration they may stop fighting altogether. If, instead, the fighting routine is maintained, they continue fighting regardless of castration. Scott[86] concludes that 'a strong habit of fighting will persist even without the presence of the male hormone', whose function, however, would be the lowering of the threshold of aggressive responses.

Other hormones, such as thyroid secretions, have been discussed as having a causal relationship to aggression.[87] Of special interest are the relationships between sugar metabolism, controlled by insulin, and violence. After a careful review of the literature, Wilder[88] lists many cases of aggressive acts presumably due to a hypoglycemic state; and Podolsky[89] refers to cases where a lowered blood-sugar level was postulated as releasing primitive impulsiveness and aggression. Little evidence, however, is ever presented in these studies and the possibility of social releasing factors is neither ruled out nor considered.

More recently, Barry Wyke has presented an interesting but still unconfirmed hypothesis which postulates, among other symptoms, that sudden aggressive behavior can be caused by 'relative cerebral hypoglycemia', determined by enzymatic deficiencies, or by the administration of hormones, such as thyroid extracts or cortisone. From a general analysis of 4,205 patients examined in the Neurosurgical Unit of the Brook General Hospital in Woolwich, 86 were identified as possibly affected by this syndrome. The blood-sugar level remained normal while the ability of the brain-tissue to utilize the available blood sugar decreased sharply. Raising the level of the blood sugar by about 50 per cent was the recommended treatment. This finding led to the suggestion that the existence of a number of cases of initially unrecognized and brain-localized hypoglycemia might have caused the aggressive acts. Further study of this specific hypothesis seems likely to be fruitful.[90]

We hope that this rapid excursus on biology and aggression serves to show the complexity of an etiological study of violence from a biological standpoint. Although some demonstrable correlations exist, we are compelled to conclude with Scott, McNeil, and Buss[91] that there is no basic need for fighting, either aggressively or defensively, unless adequate stimuli meet the organism from the external environment. In brief, there is no physiological evidence of any stimuli for fighting in a normal organism. 'The important fact,' says Scott,[92] 'is that the chain of causation in every [well-studied] case eventually traces back to the outside.' Although there may be individual differences in the reactivity to external stimuli evoking aggression, these inner characteristics do not by themselves explain aggressive behavior. This general conclusion, we find, is in agreement with a behavioral, subcultural approach.

PSYCHIATRIC ASPECTS
OF HOMICIDE AND VIOLENCE

THE PSYCHIATRIC LITERATURE

The psychiatric literature on homicide and violence is extensive. Social interest in violent behavior and the frequent use of medico-legal experts in homicide cases have drawn the attention of psychiatrists from every school and denomination. To organize this mass of literature into a meaningful pattern is not an easy task and it becomes even more complicated when analysis is conducted within a social science framework, oriented toward a subcultural approach.

Among the contributions from the field of psychiatry, there are many case reports which have been published for their training value. The publication of case studies follows an accepted tradition in the medical sciences; but in criminology these studies unfortunately have limited value unless they contain a broad, interdisciplinary perspective.[93]

Morris G. Caldwell[94] has discussed some criteria for an appropriate case-analysis method in the study of the personality of the offender. He emphasizes the following requisites, among others, if case analysis is to serve a useful scientific purpose: factor personality into its component elements, isolate the principal personality variables for study, establish scientific instruments for the measurement of these personality variables. None of these criteria appears to be commonly used by the authors of most case reports. Instead, the personality classifications and the nosographic systems used are inconsistent, and the instruments employed for personality assessment frequently belong to the intuitive, *Verstehen*-oriented approach. Moreover, preoccupation with the legal and medico-legal implications of a single case clouds the criminogenic and criminodynamic issues. The criteria for medico-legal assessment of responsibility are inconsistent from country to country and follow the prevailing legal interpretations in each. It is, for example, difficult to explain the fact that in England one-third to one-half of the homicide offenders are classified as legally insane, whereas in the United States, on the average,

H

only 2–4 per cent of homicide offenders are so classified.[95] The provisions for 'partial insanity' which exist in some countries further complicate the issue.[96]

In other countries, as Lamont[97] has pointed out for South Africa, racial and cultural differences affect criminal psychiatric phenomenology. When these 'case histories' are studied outside their specific medico-legal aspects, explanations given for assaultive behavior are so controversial that generalizations cannot easily be made. Of more value, perhaps, are the systematic and methodologically more consistent and comprehensive publications of case analyses which have been undertaken, for example, by Karpmann[98] and, more recently, by the diagnostic team at Rebibbia, Rome.[99]

Moving from single case reports to studies involving more cases, more elaborate description, and cross-sectional analysis, we shall now turn our attention to analyzing systematically the existing psychiatric literature on homicide.

The study of 'group homicide' or '*massen Mord*' has appeared in some German psychiatric literature, in a recent Japanese paper, and in some American studies.[100] 'Amok' has also been studied from this point of view.[101] This extreme manifestation of destructive behavior is rare and is almost consistently linked to psychotic disturbances. Equally pathological is the so-called 'sudden murderer'. Lamberti, Blackman, and Weiss have referred to this type of criminal as schizoid and passive-aggressive. His 'mask of adequacy', which explains the sudden, unexpected characteristics of his aggression, cannot be penetrated except through detailed psychiatric explorations.[102] Other specific areas of homicidal behavior, particularly those linked with different types of sexual abnormality, have been extensively investigated, but their relevance to our specific object of study is quite limited.[103] The same comment applies to other special studies, such as those of Meyers, Apfelberg, and Sugar[104] on homicides of women, and to the abundant literature produced by the wide medico-legal interest in psychiatric expert opinions of homicide cases.[105] These contributions have already been discussed and others will be considered when we examine the methodology of psychiatric examinations.

It should be noted that recent medico-legal writings have shown an increasing awareness of psychological and socio-psychological factors. A recent review by Lanzkron[106] divides 150 mentally ill homicide offenders into three main categories: (*a*) those for whom the homicide was the direct result of a delusion; (*b*) those declared insane who pos-

sessed 'some' motives (such as, for example, anger, revenge, etc.); and
(c) those in whom the insanity developed after the homicide, which was
committed for understandable motives. Groups (a) and (b) constitute the
prevailing area of interest of forensic psychiatry. Subcultural determinants of homicidal violence can, of course, enter with varying degrees
of intensity in the dynamics of all three groups. The importance of
intrafamily homicidal aggression, evident in some of the results of the
Wolfgang homicide study in Philadelphia, has also been discussed by
Kurland, Morgenstern, and Sheets, reporting on 12 cases, and by
Guttmacher, on 36 cases.[107]

Relatively large-scale case studies have been published and are continually appearing in professional journals. Often their usefulness does
not exceed that of providing statistical information about percentages of
the mentally ill (according to the legal definition, or according to a
psychiatric nosography) in a homicidal group. These 'criminological'
contributions from the field of psychiatry are, in general, of more limited
interest than the data on homicide and violence in different psychiatric
nosographies, which will be examined below.

Frequently, as Gibbens[108] remarked, the degree of aggressiveness
appears to be an indicator of the malignancy (in terms of psychotic
behavior) of the mental disease. However, the popular notion of the
serious aggressiveness of the mentally ill appears disproved by a recent
study by Brennan.[109] A contribution by Barron, Duncan, Frazier,
Litin, and Johnson,[110] unfortunately based on only six cases, stresses
the role of imitation and identification in the etiology of four non-
psychotic murders. This finding is of interest in connection with the
'social learning' process of the subculture of violence.

Some psychiatric contributions are in book form[111] and constitute
well-known items of criminological literature. They range widely in
scope, depth, and content; some are of a quasi-journalistic value while
others are medico-legal treatises. Consistently, however, they show little
or no awareness of etiological and dynamic factors in homicide other
than those which appeal to the particular psychiatric hypothesis upheld
by the author. The theoretical contributions are sometimes negligible
and often consist of a rewording of the basic tenets of Freudian ortho-
doxy. The generalizations are loose, and the practical treatment or
prevention techniques which are advocated are often shallow, un-
realistic, and contradictory. Moreover, the typologies presented are inconsistent and not mutually exclusive. The main contribution of these
items possibly is and has been that of generating some interest among

psychiatrists, physicians, and laymen in the importance and complexity of the problem of homicidal behavior. Their scientific value and their practical impact remain quite doubtful.

A relatively large group of publications refer to studies of the differential characteristics of young children and other juveniles who have committed homicides. Apart from the apparent increase in such crimes as part of the general increase in juvenile delinquency, many of these cases are directly traceable to highly specific psychiatric disturbances that cut across a variety of socio-psychological variables.[112]

The psychiatric literature we have so far analyzed offers only a limited contribution to our knowledge of homicide. One particular reason for this limitation is of specific interest to us in view of our earlier discussion[113] about the diverging schools of sociological and clinical criminology. Apart from the usual brief for integration in criminology, we must restate at this point our position concerning the need for theoretically integrated approaches. The lack of major contributions, either in theory or in practice, to our basic general knowledge about violent and homicidal behavior stems from the failure of many authors to recognize that meaningful integration is more than mere splicing of the diagnostic psychiatric and sociological labels, and more than a simple head-count of different psychiatric nosographic entities in a given and often poorly defined criminal population. No clinician today would maintain that psychopathology can explain (etiologically or phenomenologically) all criminal behavior. By the same token, no sociologist claims that socio-cultural forces can account for all antisocial acts. The real problem from the point of view of etiological theory construction, is how to deal with 'normal' (statistically, functionally, or normatively defined) criminals, and how to relate knowledge about the psychopathology of crime, in the varying percentages in which we find it, with data about the genesis of normal criminal behavior. Many of our difficulties originate from the vagueness of our concepts about 'normal' and 'pathological'. With these points in mind, it may be helpful, although partially distracting from our main theme, to review briefly the papers and books that discuss the incidence of criminal homicide in different psychiatric syndromes. We shall, of course, abstain from taking into consideration their medico-legal implications, which are important in the judicial treatment of the homicidal offender but have no role in an etiological study. Although we cannot engage here in any detailed discussion of the different nosographies used in psychiatry, which by themselves complicate the issue of any psychiatric epidemiological study of a criminal population, we shall follow major diagnostic classifications. Most of the reviewed literature deals with psychotic syndromes, a fact which is not surprising in view of the almost general exclusion of psychoneurotic disturbances from the group of mental illnesses whose presence exclude responsibility, and in view of the close link between psychiatric studies of homicides and medico-legal assessments of the offender's personality.

THE INCIDENCE OF CRIMINAL HOMICIDE IN DIFFERENT PSYCHIATRIC SYNDROMES

Homicide can be 'caused' by practically any type of major psychiatric illness, and it is more in the analysis of the homicidal motives than in the identification of the presence of a specific nosographic entity that clues to the establishment of causal relationships must be found. Neustatter[114] has published interesting case collections which demonstrate the variety of syndromes that can be linked with violent behavior. As Messinger and Apfelberg[115] have demonstrated in a recent large-scale study of a general criminal population, the number of psychotic subjects is small, the bulk of the cases being either normal or 'psychopaths' (in one of the many varieties of this encompassing and ill-defined category). One interesting schematic classification of pathological criminal homicide has been published by Guy Benoit,[116] again maintaining the ubiquity of homicide in the psychiatric nosography, but showing some differential phenomenological aspects from one syndrome to another. In a diagnostic typology of delinquents, Esman[117] has identified the aggressive delinquent with the 'antisocial', the schizophrenic, and the defective. And in a detailed analysis of 20 case histories, Stürup[118] found not less than seven different categories and restated the case against encompassing psychiatric generalizations.

Much of the psychiatric literature on homicide deals with this problem of the frequency of homicidal behavior in different schizophrenic nosologies. The nearly classic works of Willmans, Schipkowensky, *et al.* on this point are echoed by many recent papers. In view of the compelling diagnostic and medico-legal implications of a psychiatric label, particular importance has been given to homicide as the *Initialdelikt*, the initial symptom of an underlying schizophrenic process which can remain (before and after the act) undetected.[119] The disease, however, can usually be spotted through other symptoms (athymic behavior, delusions, etc.). Many of the 'specific' signs which are listed in the literature as pathognomic of the schizophrenic homicide have been rejected.

or can be explained in terms of alternative causes.[120] Calabrese and Semerari have recently criticized Willmans's *Initialdelikt* concept, emphasizing the need for a detailed, longitudinal 'diaphenomenic' study of the personality.[121]

Among the feeble-minded, homicide can occur quite unintentionally, but it may also be due to the specific vulnerability to irritation of defective subjects.[122] As we shall see in the section devoted to psychometric studies, homicidal subjects rate very low or lowest in a classification of mental endowment among prison populations.

In old age, the biological and psychological changes of senescence can cause many types of criminal, especially sexual, behavior. Violence and homicide are not frequent[123] except in cases with a clear-cut senile psychosis having manic[124] or paranoid characteristics.[125]

In epilepsy, aggression and homicide can occur, but their frequency appears to be no greater than that found in the normal population. In psychomotor epilepsy their occurrence is greater (and our previous section on biology has discussed some of the etiological hypotheses for this fact). A degree of automatism is often present in epilepsy and in epileptic equivalents.[126] Witton has recently maintained the value of narcoanalysis in bringing out unconscious conflicts and thus preventing automatic behavior.[127]

Alcoholism, whenever it reaches chronic pathological levels, can cause homicide through its violent motor outbursts or through its persecutory or jealousy delusional components.[128] We have already referred to the 'release' function of alcohol in non-pathological homicides.[129]

In manic psychosis, despite controversial opinions,[130] homicide is rare. It is more frequent in depressive states, either as a defense against the depression itself or as an actualization of death and other destructive delusions.[131]

The depressive psychosis must also be considered in relation to the links which appear to exist between homicide and suicide. Apart from the well-known sociological study of Henry and Short, the psychiatric literature on homicidal and suicidal behavior is abundant.[132] A favorite psychoanalytic explanation of homicide considers this behavior as an equivalent of suicide, caused by a drive for self-punishment.[133] The thesis seems to be useful in explaining some unique and very pathological cases, but is unsubstantiated by facts. The theory of indirect suicide has also been advocated because of the negative correlation that is commonly found in the statistics of homicides and suicides, but is contradicted in some countries like Denmark.[134] It is also supported by many speculative considerations, such as the decrease of murders in time of war. Von Hentig[135] has stated that 'murder and suicide are complementary phenomena: the total amount of available destructiveness is discharged in two psychologically similar, socially distinct *Gestalten*'.

Occasionally, we find data in support of the 'murder as indirect suicide' thesis.[136] A case in point is the epidemic of indirect suicides which took place in Norway and Denmark in the seventeenth and eighteenth centuries when depressed people committed murder presumably in order to be put to death, because they would not commit suicide for religious reasons. The cases were so frequent that a special law had to be passed excluding those individuals from the death penalty in order to stop this particular type of homicide.[137] However, these indirect suicides cannot prove the psychoanalytic hypothesis that the victim represents the murderer in the latter's unconscious.

Partially verified through sociological analysis is Wolfgang's hypothesis that an individual may commit an unorthodox form of suicide by provoking another person to slay him. The 'victim-precipitated homicides' represented 26 per cent of a total of 588 homicides studied in Philadelphia.[138] Data such as these, however, need to be verified by psychological analysis if they are to have a more direct general relation to the problem of the psychological aspects of the criminals who commit homicides.

Of great interest in this nosographic analysis is the obvious importance of the category of the so-called 'psychopathic personalities' (or character disorders) for violent, aggressive behavior. This large group is probably one of the most important in a psychopathological analysis of violence. However, the etiology is controversial, ranging from biological hypotheses to pure psychogenic ones, and the medico-legal treatment granted to this group is extremely inconsistent from country to country in accordance with the prevailing insanity tests (and psychiatric schools). These subjects can be classified into a number of different, often contrasting subcategories, many of which are characterized by violent, impulsive behavior as their main behavioral abnormality.[139] They may vary from a passive–aggressive typology to primitive, immature behavior, and to clearly established impulse disorders. Their basic aggression can be compensated and transformed into neurotic compulsive or psychosomatic symptoms or both; or can be 'acted out' into violence.[140] The influence of the environmental factors on the structural, endogenous aspects of the personality, and the importance of the resulting modifications in the so-called psychopathic developments have recently been emphasized by Di Tullio.[141]

Infanticide and child murder have attracted specific attention in criminological literature. In the case of infanticide, the special legal provisions and the particular 'honor' reasons for it make it such a specific type of criminal behavior that few generalizations can be added from its etiology and phenomenology to the general knowledge about homicidal behavior.[142] Child murder[143] is often linked to deep psychopathological causes, or may be the causal end-result of a much more widespread aggressive primitive behavior on the part of some parents. This latter has recently resulted in what is referred to as the 'battered child syndrome'. The proclivity to violence on the part of parents who engage in this type of offense can occasionally be subcultural. However, little objective research is available so far on the differential aspects of the parents of the 'battered child'.[144]

Some studies refer to homicidal behavior that appears to be almost automatic and followed by a claim of amnesia, which can be caused either by a somnambulistic type of aggressive behavior in specific mental illness or by a psychogenic defense mechanism.[145]

Buss[146] has reviewed the role of hostility and aggression in the development of psychopathology, analyzing the classification of aggressive reactions, their importance in psychotherapeutic treatment, the differences between normal and neurotic aggression, the different defense mechanisms which have an aggressive character, and the importance of aggression among the psychoses. Moreover, the role of aggressive punishment by parents in provoking rebellion and counter-aggression is maintained by Buss, and this aspect is, of course, important to the subcultural transmission of aggression. In Buss's analysis, one section is devoted to the relationship between the direction of aggression and prognosis.[147] The inhibition of aggression is seen as a result of motivation, and the growing child moves from extra-aggression to self-aggressive responses. In general, outward aggression in psychopathology is associated with poor prognosis, although the relationship is far from being linear and can be mediated by variables such as the reaction of the environment to the aggression exhibited by the patient, the attitude of the treatment staff, etc. In electroconvulsive therapy, intrapunitiveness is an indicator of a favorable prognosis, which is consistent with the better outcome of depressed patients undergoing this type of treatment.[148]

A few psychiatric papers analyze the prediction of violent aggressive behavior,[149] and MacDonald[150] has studied a series of 100 consecutive hospital admissions who had made homicidal threats. But the prediction of aggressive and homicidal behavior is not easy, and we are far from possessing adequate clinical or statistical data for doing so with success much above chance. However, efforts to predict should take into account subcultural elements of the violent act in order to allow for the prediction of 'normal' non-psychopathological violence.[151]

From the many psychiatric studies we have analyzed so far, very few valid general conclusions of interest to our subcultural approach can be drawn. The variety of the psychopathological criminogenesis and criminodynamics is enormous and seems to defy attempts at systematization. The percentages of 'mentally ill criminals' vary, not so much in accordance with demonstrated variations of the phenomenon, but in the nosographies and medico-legal norms employed and in the orientation of the examining psychiatrists. In the absence of a catch-all psychiatric explanation or of a unique nosographical identification, little is left to the psychiatrist but the categorization of the mentally ill subjects and efforts to provide a psychopathological explanation in terms of motivational analysis.

The analysis of the motives for murder has attracted considerable attention from psychiatrists, psychologists, lawyers, and criminologists. Economically determined, planned, rational murders are rare and are from a legal standpoint generally considered to be particularly vicious. Most homicides, as we have indicated, are unplanned, explosive, determined by sudden motivational bursts. However, the motives can generally be traced and assessed in terms of a normal–abnormal bipolarity. Even within the area of non-psychoanalytic psychiatry, motivational analysis remains a tool of paramount importance for the understanding of homicidal behavior and serves as a guideline for an evaluation of the etiology of the violent impulse. In general, the less clearly motivated a murder is (in the sense that it is impossible to comprehend the motives) the higher is the probability that the homicidal subject is very abnormal. The easier it is to 'understand' (in the sense of both emotional and rational understanding) the homicidal motives, the more normal the subject is likely to be.[152] In motivational analysis, a longitudinal and cultural perspective of the offender's personality is necessary, for frequently the normality or abnormality of a motive is linked to existing cultural or subcultural values.[153] Even in 'motiveless' murder, which is of particular psychopathological significance,[154] a violent family and a subcultural theme may be present, as in a group of homicides studied by Satten, Menninger, Rosen, and Mayman.[155] Another important value of motivational analysis lies in the help it affords in the identification of psychoneurotic criminal determinants.[156]

Analysis of motives can be conducted at a rational, cognitive, methodologically intuitive level, or can be extended to the unconscious strata of personality through psychoanalytic constructs and techniques. The interest of psychoanalysis in violent behavior is old, and part of basic psychoanalytic theory is closely connected with it. Extensive reviews of psychoanalytic contributions have recently been published by Buss,[157] MacNeil,[158] and Berkowitz.[159] We shall, therefore, limit ourselves only to those comments which are pertinent to our line of analysis.[160]

In examining the psychoanalytically oriented explanations of homicide, we find that they seem consistently to be based on unproven theories and often reach extremely obscure interpretative levels. Wertham's famous case, extensively reported in *Dark Legend: A Study in Murder*,[161] and the discordant interpretations of the Leopold and Loeb case,[162] are good examples of the dangers implicit in an uncritical acceptance of Freudian theories in criminology. The tautologies and unconfirmed statements which abound in psychoanalytic reports make it very difficult to accept many of their contentions unless one steps into the syllogistic circle of the doctrinal position. It is difficult for those outside this circle to accept the general hypotheses of the psychoanalytically oriented psychiatrists because of the unconfirmed and unconfirmable propositions that underlie them,[163] and the general disregard of cultural factors that appear to be so important in criminology.[164] As Vold has pointed out, the explanations given often have such a degree of peculiarity and specificity, to which are added the individuality of the therapist's approach and understanding, that no generalization is possible. As he has expressed it, 'This has little in common with the accepted idea of science as a body of generalizations going beyond the individual, particular case.'[165]

Methodologically, the psychoanalytic method of depth exploration through symbolic analysis lends itself to excessive subjectivism. A symbol is often identified with the object it symbolizes through an application of paleological thinking, as Hartung, quoting Arieti, has recently emphasized. Some physical relationship may be found between the symbol and its referent, and identity is too readily assumed. (Thus, both a tie and a Zeppelin may be male sexual symbols for opposite reasons.) This kind of 'proof' is indeed difficult to accept, and if a patient himself were to use it too often we should be likely to classify him as delusional. Repression, again according to Hartung, is an essential prerequisite of symbol analysis but still awaits quantitative experimental proof.[166] Very common in psychoanalytic thinking is an explanation of homicide conceived as the actualization of a so-called 'death instinct', a general aggressive instinctual drive. Freud maintained that a somatically based instinct toward aggression exists, 'an active instinct for hatred and destruction', which became labeled as the death instinct. This basic drive, for which Freud provided a fascinating, albeit unproven theoretical foundation, could, of course, be modified through its interaction with the opposite 'life-instinct' and through education, sublimation, and socialization of its objectives. However, its essentially teleological nature, and the tension-reducing characteristics of the behavior which it elicits, remain unvaried. Central to this formulation is the assumption of an innate aspect (for which, as we have seen, biology provides no foundation) and of the universality of the existence of the drive.[167]

After the initial formulation of Freud, psychoanalysts have taken varying positions. Some[168] have followed the original formulation of a death instinct. Others, like Alexander[169] and Hartmann, Kris, and Loewenstein[170] have accepted the instinctual aspects but rejected the general concept of a death instinct. Still others, like Saul,[171] do not accept the aggression instinct as innate. Outside orthodox Freudian circles, the death instinct has little currency in psychiatry and psychopathology, primarily because evidence of cultural differences in the handling of aggression and of its learned characteristics is overwhelming; and because diagnosis and treatment appear to function as well, or better, without use of the concept.

PSYCHOLOGICAL DIAGNOSIS OF
THE AGGRESSIVE HOMICIDAL PERSONALITY

We now turn our attention to an aspect of the problem of violence and homicide which has so far received little systematic consideration, despite the fact that its practical implications are of paramount relevance to any treatment and prevention program. In brief, the questions that we shall try to answer in this section are the following: How can a homicidal personality be diagnosed psychologically? Is the diagnosis valid and reliable? Given the array of instruments which are available to the psychologist in a clinical institutional setting, which would he choose or reject?

This diagnostic aspect of the problem of the homicidal subject derives its wealth of information mainly from two areas: studies on the assessment of aggression, and studies on the differential psychology of the violent offender. In principle at least, a wide range of instruments is provided by typological classifications, such as the one proposed by Don Gibbons[172] and the one in use in the California correctional system.[173] Anamnestic data profile examinations and behavioral ratings have often been proposed, but none has emerged to acceptable degrees of reliability and validity. Descriptions given of the violent offender are often refined and amenable to objectification, but, so far, a diagnostic extension of some of the theoretically oriented speculations has been lacking.[174] Many psychiatric evaluations are equally unpromising (outside the restricted area of psychopathology) because of the subjectivity of the results and their limited reliability.

Buss[175] carefully reviewed many different studies in the assessment of aggression through the use of projective techniques and questionnaires. The Rorschach and the TAT seem to be able to distinguish between extremely aggressive and extremely non-aggressive groups. What is measured, however, is behavioral and not projective aggression. The aggressive trends revealed in projective techniques seem to be those which the subject can, if asked, verbalize. This fact makes projective tools very useful for examining criminal, non-cooperative populations. What is being measured is the 'habit strength' of aggression. Questionnaires and inventories, although less studied, appear to be useful. The Buss–Durkee Inventory shows promising characteristics not only for assessing aggression, but also for a more refined classification of different types of aggressive behavior.[176]

Gemelli has stated that 'a psychological test has no value in itself; it can be a very useful diagnostic tool if it is integrated by the psychologist in the complex pattern of the total personality'.[177] This opinion, which is shared by most psychologists, should be kept in mind by criminologists engaged in psychometric investigations of violent offenders. In our opinion, both a meaningful personality theory and an adequate theoretical approach in criminology are necessary for an appropriate use of such diagnostic instruments.

The review by Buss does not consider the extensive literature on criminal aggression and restricts itself primarily to North American sources. We shall try, as much as possible, to examine additional contributions from criminological studies and from other countries and to integrate and supplement Buss's findings. In reviewing the psychological aspects of criminal homicide, the studies of offenders carried out with psychological tests should be examined in detail. Our attempt to trace and analyze such studies will be briefly discussed in the following pages. However, a few general considerations should first be outlined.

With few exceptions, the psychometric studies of homicides have failed to distinguish between different types of homicide. They have neglected to make use of control groups, they use inadequate statistical analyses, and often they do not emerge from testable hypotheses. Most of the studies on the differential psychology of homicide are of an exploratory, tentative nature.

In criticizing the studies on the personality characteristics of criminals, Schuessler and Cressey[178] note: 'In general, the studies examined are characterized by a tendency merely to apply a personality test without reference to a hypothesis about personality elements and criminal behavior.' With few exceptions, this criticism is valid for the existing studies of violent offenders and should be overcome before psychometric efforts can hope to make a real contribution to the psychology of criminal types.[179]

The oldest studies deal with the *intelligence* of murderers. Murchison in 1926 summarized his findings in the following way: 'In the case of each national group, the individuals committing crimes against property tend to rank higher in mental test scores than the individuals committing crimes against the person.'[180] These results have been confirmed by many writers, including Glueck,[181] Berg and Fox,[182] and more recently in studies conducted in the Rebibbia Observation Center in Rome[183] and on a large group of Puerto Rican convicts.[184] However, the differences are not discriminative, and the intragroup differences are larger than the differences between different criminal typologies. (This comment, as we shall see, applies to many of the psychometric researches on homicides.)

THE RORSCHACH TEST

As might be expected, the largest group of psychometric studies on homicidal cases uses the Rorschach Test. Studies on other types of offenders are, however, relevant to the problem of aggression. In 1952, Piotrowski and Abrahamsen[185] carried out a study of 100 sexual criminals. They found that, in 84 per cent of the cases, the individuals who produce more expansive and more spontaneous animal movement responses than human movement responses are likely to display a more active, and at times a more aggressive, attitude towards others when in a state of diminished consciousness (as, for example, under the influence of alcohol). This 'release function' of alcoholic intoxication, and particularly its potential assessment through the Rorschach Test, would seem to warrant further study.[186]

Schneider, in a Rorschach study of 18 homicide cases, found that 'murder could be a substitute for an epileptic fit, whereby the accumulated aggressive impulses are directed against another person instead of the subject himself'. He also discusses other psychopathological syndromes of homicides in relation to the Rorschach protocols.[187] Paolella,[188] in a Rorschach study of twenty homicides, has underlined the frequency of a coarctated or introversive personality type, contrasted with the empirical evidence of an extroversive, labile, impulsive effectivity. In these cases, evidence of inner conflicts was available.

In a study of twenty homicides utilizing Rorschach, TAT, Wechsler–Bellevue, and the Gleb, Goldstein, Weigl, and Scheerer tests for concrete and abstract thinking, Romano and Paolella found that hyperthymic homicide offenders displayed affect lability with egocentrism and impulsivity, exaggerated emotional reactivity, hyperactivity, nonconformism, and a psychopathic Wechsler–Bellevue pattern. However, offenders involved in 'cold' homicides were commonly found to have introverted affect, rigidity, egocentrism, irritability, low emotional reactivity, and a schizophrenic Wechsler–Bellevue pattern.[189]

Among thirty parricides, Tsuboi and Takemura[190] found evidence in Rorschach protocols of a 'refusal of human relations', of a difficulty in controlling inertia movements, and of the existence of both impulsive and explosive emotions.

Kohlmann,[191] in a Rorschach study of a group of 113 psychopaths (which included thirteen murderers), found disinhibition of the affective components of the personality structure and an increase of the mechanism of aggressive projection. Rabin,[192] in a longitudinal study of a homicide-attempted-suicide case, tested the subject before the homicide, in the course of a depressive episode, and found extreme tension and severe constriction. Six months after the crime, he found relaxation, personality dilatation, and affect release. These characteristics were also evident in a third Rorschach administered a year after satisfactory hospital adjustment. Perdue[193] studied 100 murderers at the Virginia State Penitentiary. He found a relatively high number of human content responses (a finding contradicted by other studies which will be examined later) and other differentiating signs which indicated 'an emotionally shallow and highly suggestible personality who appears narcissistic, immature, impulsive, socially retarded and whose general behavior, when faced with tension, stress or frustration is very unpredictable'. No general personality picture was found, however, and even different specific types of homicidal behavior, such as parricide, did not show differential traits. As did Banay,[194] Perdue states that the act of murder is so varied that we can diagnostically approach it only in individual terms. In a study of juvenile homicides, Schachter and Cotte[195] found similar difficulties in the establishment of a specific profile. Pakesch,[196] in a Rorschach and Szondi study of homicides, of robbers with violence, and of sexual criminals, had parallel conclusions for the first two groups.

Endara reported on several Rorschach investigations in criminology,[197] including those of Serebrinsky,[198] which used large groups and control data. He described the following findings:

1. In crimes against the person, after the coarctated group, the largest group is composed of extroversive egocentrics. The introversive are a minority.
2. Homicide offenders have a Rorschach pattern indicating low empathy and a deficit of conscious control. Their protocols show defective emotional control, with impulsive reactivity, a need for immediate gratification of impulses, affect lability, maladjustment, and egocentrism.
3. The most important finding, in Endara's opinion, is the fact that homicide offenders produce about half the number of human content (H + Hd) responses found in other criminals; this shows lack of empathy, hostility, and rebelliousness against authority among the former.
4. When the Orr scale,[199] which establishes the degree of degradation and devitalization of the maternal image, is applied to the Rorschach protocols of homicide offenders and homicide repeaters, it is noted that these offenders, more than other types, exhibit the most distinctive features of degradation and devitalization. This finding indicates that in the primary mother–son relationship they have been severely disturbed or depersonalized. The 'good mother' has been internalized by these subjects only as a source of frustration and anguish.

In a recent research, Rizzo and Ferracuti[200] attempted to test psychometrically some criminological hypotheses on a group of 160 authors of crimes against the person and 40 thieves. The control group was composed of 400 normal individuals. The first hypothesis postulated that the homicidal act is an expression of egocentrism and immaturity, which could be investigated by means of the Rorschach ratio between movement and color responses,[201] and through an analysis of the distribution of color responses.[202] In 33 per cent of the subjects who had committed murder or attempted murder, pure color and color-form responses were more frequent than form-color responses, while the percentage for the thieves was 25 per cent.

The second hypothesis postulated that both the inability to adjust and the rigidity of the subject are important determinants of his aggressive behavior. The ability to adjust can be expressed in the Rorschach test by the percentage of form-color responses.[203] Only 37 per cent of the perpetrators of crimes against the person had any FC responses versus 58 per cent in the group of thieves. The percentage of FC responses out of total responses for each subject was 0·5 for the perpetrators of crimes against the person, 0·8 for the thieves and 1·1 for the normals.

The third hypothesis stated that aggressive behavior is related to lack of empathy and a reduced capacity for social contact. In Rorschach terms, this hypothesis can be expressed, among other indicators, through the percentage of human content responses. These responses were 10 per cent for the authors of crimes against the person, 12 per cent for individuals involved in crimes against property, and 20 per cent for normals.[204]

Obviously, many other areas could be explored with the Rorschach Test, and the above studies can be considered as only tentative and initial. For example, content analysis in criminological research has been limited to the human content responses. Other types of content could be examined, following some of the interpretative norms outlined by Phillips and Smith[205] and often utilized in the different content scales which have been proposed by several authors.[206] The success of the content scales in identifying overt aggressive behavior, demonstrated, for example, by Towbin[207] in aggressive schizophrenic patients, could be extended to the study of the offender's personality. Towbin, following the opinion of several writers, has given an acceptable rationale for the diagnostic validity of the Rorschach Test relative to homicidal situations. This hypothesis postulates that the Rorschach protocol can be considered as a sample of behavior in a specific interpersonal situation, characterized by the mutual awareness and influence between the testee and the tester. This would imply that the responses are influenced by the perceived situation in the same way as the perceived situation determines behavior in other interpersonal settings. In comparable conditions, Rorschach responses and interpersonal behavior should be positively correlated. The importance of subcultural determinants in the perception of a social situation should, therefore, be equally reflected in the Rorschach protocol and in the actual behavior. An extension of the many cross-cultural Rorschach and other projective studies to subcultural dimensions would appear to be possible and desirable.[208]

It must be kept in mind that, because of its enlarged, inclusive, multifaceted approach to personality diagnosis, the Rorschach Test may present unusual difficulties in relation to the identification of valid diagnostic indicators. Some of these difficulties are well presented in Beck's discussion of the way different defensive mechanisms, including those which are referred to as 'symptomatic aggressiveness' and 'adaptive aggressiveness', reflect themselves in the protocols.[209]

From the Rorschach studies of the murderer, especially when compared with normal subjects, emerges a personality characterized by egocentrism and a lack of emotional control. He can also be described as an explosive, immature, hyperthymic person who is unable to establish social contact. He displays a deficit of conscious control and a strong need for the immediate gratification of impulses.

In some respects, these psychometric conclusions, based on studies of known homicide offenders, concur so completely with the criminal behavior that objective critics rather naturally become suspicious of the diagnoses and wonder what the Rorschach findings would be if the offenders had been diagnosed prior to the homicides or in a 'blind' procedure where the offenders were mixed with normal subjects. No objective studies using either of these methods have been available to us in the sources we have been able to consult.

OTHER PROJECTIVE TECHNIQUES

A wide range of other projective instruments has been used in the study of the homicidal personality. In a research with the Thematic Apperception Test, Paolella[210] found frequent 'heroes' of an antisocial type and a prevalence of themes of rebellion and impulsivity. In his careful study of an aggressive content scale applied to the TAT, Stone[211] found the scale to be objectively scorable and valid in identifying murder cases. Similar results have been obtained by Rizzo on homicides studied with the MAPS (Make-A-Picture Story) test, using the methodology proposed by Fine and Walker.[212] The validity of the MAPS test has been also studied by Goldenberg.[213] The use of the TAT and MAPS is often unreliable because the thematic wide-ranging protocols are difficult to score objectively. The 'rules' outlined by Piotrowsky for TAT interpretation are a good example of the problems facing objective research with these instruments.[214]

A few studies have been conducted with the Rosenzweig Picture-Frustration method, an obvious choice in view of its theoretical derivation from the frustration–aggression hypothesis. These studies, largely negative of the possibilities of identifying homicides, are also pertinent to our discussion of this hypothesis.[215] It can be stated here, however, that as in the case of other projective tests, one obvious difficulty is that of assessing whether the subject is responding to the test situation at a level of opinion, projection, or behavior.[216]

The Luesher Test was used by Coppola[217] who examined 14 homicides (7 normals and 7 insane). The normal cases had a tendency to extroversion and activity, whereas the mentally ill had a tendency to passivity. The Szondi Test has been used by several investigators. In separate studies and with isolated cases, Walder[218] and Brachfeld[219] indicated the presence of a negative E profile in murderers with this test.

In a study with the Draw-A-Person Test, Spadaro[220] found no relevant difference between persons who had committed crimes against the person and those who had committed crimes against property. Both groups showed inhibition and a tendency to escape reality. Schachter[221] found a peculiar drawing of the head separated from the body ('bonhomme décapité') in two adolescents charged with criminal aggression.

In a recent study with the 'Tree Test' given to 16 'hyperthymic' homicides, Vaccaro[222] found a prevalence of 'instinctual life', deficit of will control, lack of valid criticism of behavior, with exaggerated affect, abnormal reactivity to stimulation, and prevalence of uncontrolled impulses. Another projective instrument, the 'Hand Test', has recently been presented by Bricklin, Piotrowski, and Wagner[223] for the study of overt aggressive behavior. As yet, systematically collected data are scarce, but this test shows promising characteristics of validity and an ease of administration that should encourage further criminological researches.

A group of studies have been conducted with questionnaires; those concerned with aggression have been reviewed by Buss,[224] whose scale was used by Collins and Wrightman[225] in a study of maladjustment of adolescent and preadolescent boys, with a good level of agreement between inventory and bipolar ratings. Rosen found interesting correlations between MMPI aggression and Rorschach white space responses, another traditional indication of hostility.[226]

In a comprehensive study of social, psychiatric, and psychometric variables of a group of 15 homicides and 24 burglars, Kahn[227] found, with the Wechsler–Bellevue and the Rorschach test, that murderers have personalities which 'could permit characteristic impulsive breakthrough of sadistic hostility' and 'less personality resources for expression of their feelings'. In another paper on 43 murderers,[228] Kahn presented a factor-analytic study which included Rorschach and WAIS data. Both personality factors (as elicited from the Rorschach), on a psychotic/nonpsychotic factor, and intelligence factors emerged in the first five strongest factors. Kahn's papers are an exception to the general provincialism of psychometric studies and provide an attempt to integrate different sets of data.

Shelley and Toch[229] employed an interesting experimental technique involving nine sets of pictograms prepared according to Engel's experimental approach to the importance of content in binocular perceptions. Each pictogram, to be viewed through a stereoscope, included two structurally matched but mutually exclusive pictures, one with a crime-related or violent scene, and the other void of violent content. In the perceptual fusion process, one content prevails and this is assumed to be the one more consistent with stimuli which are familiar or congruent to the subjects. Violent and control nonviolent groups (according to number of 'violent' perceptions) were compared in respect to violence from other indicators. Other projective measures were used (TAT, Rorschach, and House-Tree-Person drawings) and a behavioral rating was included. The stereoscope technique appears to differentiate validly the violence-prone individuals. This result is particularly important for a subcultural hypothesis because the subcultural allegiance of the subject should involve a differential perception of violent stimuli and a perception of neutral stimuli as violent.

CONCLUSIONS

The collected evidence for a consistent personality pattern of the homicidal offender is scarce and unreliable. The several studies examined here confirm the fact that diagnosis remains a matter for the individual ability of the clinician. This negative answer to the questions outlined at the beginning of this section does not exclude the importance of a careful and comprehensive assessment of the psychological factors of the homicidal personality. The choice of instruments remains a problem to be solved in relation to the purpose of the examination. The psychometric results, in general, however, could be improved by refining the techniques, by better research designs, and by an awareness of both the biological and the sociological determinants of aggressive behavior.

NOTES AND REFERENCES

1. Elton B. McNeil, 'Psychology and Aggression', *Journal of Conflict Resolution* (1959) **3**:195–293.
2. Arnold H. Buss, *The Psychology of Aggression*, New York: Wiley, 1961.
3. Leonard Berkowitz, *Aggression*, New York: McGraw-Hill, 1962.
4. Hans von Hentig, *The Criminal and His Victim*, New Haven, Conn.: Yale University Press, 1948; and Hans von Hentig, *Zur Psychologie der Einzeldelikte*, Vol. II, *Der Mord*, Tübingen, 1956.
5. Wolff Middendorf, *Sociologia del delito*, Madrid: Revista de Occidente, 1961.
6. S. Reiwald, *Die Gesellschaft und ihre Verbrecher*, Zurich, 1948.
7. The following is a chronological list of major books and articles on homicide and violent offenses. Interest in this topic has been increasing in recent years:

Enrico Ferri, *L'omicidio nell'Antropologia Criminale*, Torino: Bocca, 1895.
P. Gast, 'Der Mörder', *Krim. Abh.* (1930) **2**:64.
H. C. Brearley, *Homicide in the United States*, Chapel Hill: University of North Carolina Press, 1932.
W. Winckelmann, *Beobachtungen an 50 Mörderinnen in der Strafanstalt zu Jauer*, Berlin: Schotz, 1934.
M. El-Rawi, 'Alkatlo'l Syasy', *Egyptian Journal of Psychology* (1947) **3**:207–214.
Agostino Gemelli, *Gli omicidi: saggio di interpretazione*, appendix to *La personalità del delinquente*, Milano: Giuffrè, 1948, pp. 248–300.
Colorado University, *Crimes of Violence* (Report of a Conference on Crime Sponsored by the University, August 15–18, 1949), Boulder: 1950.
L. H. Cohen, *Murder, Madness and the Law*, New York: World Publishing Co., 1952.
M. Finzi, *La intenzione di uccidere*, Milano: Giuffrè, 1954.
Albert Morris, *Homicide: An Approach to the Problem of Crime*, Boston: Boston University Press, 1955.
Hans von Hentig, *Zur Psychologie der Einzeldelikte*, Vol. II, *Der Mord*, Tubingen, 1956.
Hans von Hentig, *Probleme des Freispruchs beim Morde*, Tubingen: J. C. B. Mohr, 1957.
Hans von Hentig, 'Pre-murderous Kindness and Post Murder Grief', *Journal of Criminal Law, Criminology and Police Science* (1957) **48**:369–377.

Marvin E. Wolfgang, *Patterns in Criminal Homicide*, Philadelphia: University of Pensylvania Press, 1958.

H. F. Weatherly, 'Juvenile Violence', *Journal of the Association for the Psychiatric Treatment of Offenders* (1958) 2:1–2:6.

M. Shoda and M. Takahashi, 'Study on Sentences for Crime of Inflicting Death by Wounding', *Horitsujio* (January, 1959), pp. 87–100.

Paul J. Gernert, 'The Dangerous Offender', *Pennsylvania Chiefs of Police Association Bulletin* (1959) 20:28–29.

Hans von Hentig, 'Lustmord und Buschverstech der Beute', *Machr. Kriminol. u. Strafrechtsref.* (1960) 43:2:31–41.

Hans von Hentig, 'Der Mord auf homophiler Basis', *Kriminalistik* (1960) 8:342–344.

G. Bruchner, *Zur Kriminologie des Mordes*, Zurich: Kriminalistik Verlag, 1960.

Manfred Guttmacher, *The Mind of the Murderer*, New York: Farrar, Straus and Cudahy, 1960.

R. S. Banay, 'Violent Youth', *Journal of Social Therapy* (1960) 6:207–215.

Stuart Palmer, *A Study of Murder*, New York: Crowell, 1960.

Walter Bromberg, *The Mold of Murder*, New York: Grune and Stratton, 1961.

J. M. MacDonald, *The Murderer and His Victim*, Springfield, Ill.: C. C. Thomas, 1961.

T. Morris and L. Blom-Cooper, 'Murder in Microcosm', London: *The Observer*, 1961, pp. 3–26.

F. Labardini y Mendez, 'Las lesiones y el homicidio en los deportes', *Rev. Jr. Veracruz* (1961) 12:4:269–354.

T. Morris and L. Blom-Cooper, *A Calendar of Murder*, London: Michael Joseph, 1962.

C. Banks, 'Violence', *Howard Journal* (1962) 2:1:13–25.

C. Wilson and P. Pitman, *Encyclopedia of Murder*, New York: Putnam, 1962.

Samuel Wallace and José Canals, 'Socio-Legal Aspects of a Study of Acts of Violence', *The American University Law Review* (1962) 2:2:173–188.

Franco Ferracuti, 'The Psychology of Criminal Homicide', *Revista Juridica de la Universidad de Puerto Rico* (1963) 32:4:569–605.

F. H. McClintock, *Crimes of Violence*, London: Macmillan, 1963.

D. W. Elliott, 'Causation in Homicide', *Newcastle Medical Journal* (1964) 28:4:130–137.

Some of the increase in homicide literature is probably due to popular concern about the increase in violent crimes. (See, for example, the reports of the U.S. Senate Committee on the Judiciary, Subcommittee to Investigate Juvenile Delinquency; and the testimony of Herman Stark that criminals are becoming more violent in committing assault and battery, sex offenses, and robbery, in California Department of the Youth Authority, Activity Report to Governor, 1961, February 1.)

Several articles are devoted to special types of homicide, such as poisoning [H. T. Sanders, 'Zur Psychologie des Giftmordes durch Arzte', *Arch. f. Krimin.* (1930) **86**:33–35; R. Heindl, 'Das Weib als Morderin', *Arch. Crim. Anthrop.* (1934) **95**:61–63] and infanticide [H. Gummersbach, 'Zur Kriminologischen und rechtlichen Beurteilung der Kinderstotung', *Mschr. KrimBiol.* (1937) **28**:364; W. Tuteur and J. Glotzer, 'Murdering Mothers', *American Journal of Psychiatry* (1959) **116**:447–452; 'Murder of Infants by Parents in Situations of Stress', *Journal of Social Therapy* (1960) **6**:1:9 :17; H. Winnk and H. Horovitz, 'The Problem of Infanticide', *British Journal of Criminology* (1961) **2**:1:40–52.]

8. See, for example:

Trevor C. N. Gibbens, 'Psychiatry and the Abnormal Offender', *Medico-Legal Journal* (1956) **24**:4:142–162.

Albert Morris, *Homicide: An Approach to the Problem of Crime*, Boston: Boston University Press, 1955.

E. Roesner, 'Der Mord, seine Tater, Motive un Opfer nebst einer Bibliographie zum Problem des Mordes', *Z. Strafechtswiss*, (1936) **56**:327.

E. Roesner, 'Mörder in ihre Opfer', *Mschr. KrimBiol.* (1938) **29**:161–185 and 209–228.

E. Roesner, 'Internationale Mordstatistik', *Mschr. KrimBiol.* (1939) **30**:65–88.

9. Although, as a recent British study has demonstrated, the relationship between traffic offenses and criminal behavior, often of a violent type, is probably close and meaningful. See T. C. Willett, *Criminal on the Road*, London: Tavistock Publications, 1964.

10. Jayewardene has conducted an interesting study on the relationship between medical progress and homicide statistics. See, C. H. S. Jayewardene, 'L'influenza del progresso medico nell'andamento statistico degli omicidi', *Quaderni di Criminologia Clinica* (1961) **2**:162–180. For a theoretical discussion, see Marvin E. Wolfgang, *Patterns in Criminal Homicide*, pp. 116–119.

11. Many different classification systems in criminal typologies are available in the literature. See, for example:

H. E. Barnes and N. K. Teeters, *New Horizons in Criminology*, Englewood Cliffs, N.J.: Prentice-Hall, 1959, Third Edition; P. Gast, 'Der Mörder', *Krim. Abh.* (1930) **11**:64.

H. Gummersbach, 'Mordmotive und Motivmorde', *Arch. Krim.* (1935) **96**:58–76 and 143–155.

M. D. Pothast, 'A Personality Study of Two Types of Murderers' *Dissertation Abstracts* (1957) **17**:898–899.

12. E. Seelig, *Traité de Criminologie*, Paris: P.U.F., 1956.
13. Enrico Ferri, *L'omicidio nell'Antropologia Criminale*, Torino: Bocca, 1895.
14. Enrico Ferri, *Criminal Sociology*, Boston: Little, Brown, 1917, pp. 152–153.
15. J. L. Gillin, *The Wisconsin Prisoner*, Madison, Wisconsin: University of Wisconsin Press, 1946.
16. Marshall B. Clinard, *Sociology of Deviant Behavior*, New York: Rinehart, 1957.
17. Agostino Gemelli, *La personalità del delinquente nei suoi fondamenti biologici e psicologici*, Milano: Giuffrè, Second Edition. For an interesting discussion of the typology of homicides, see Herbert A. Bloch and Gilbert Geis, *Man, Crime and Society*, New York: Random House, 1962.
18. Gillin, *op. cit.*
19. Marvin E. Wolfgang and R. B. Strohm, 'The Relationship between Alcohol and Criminal Homicide', *Quarterly Journal of Studies of Alcohol* (1956) **17**: 411–425.
20. Jaime Toro Calder, 'Personal Crime in Puerto Rico', Master's Thesis, University of Wisconsin, 1950.
21. Don C. Gibbons and D. L. Garrity, 'Some Suggestions for the Development of an Etiological and Treatment Theory in Criminology', *Social Forces* (1959) **38**:1:51–58.
22. Don C. Gibbons, *Changing the Law-Breaker*, Englewood Cliffs, N.J.: Prentice-Hall, 1965, pp. 274–276.
23. Quoted by Middendorf, *op. cit.*
24. Richard A. Peterson, D. J. Pittman, and P. O'Neal, 'Stabilities in Deviance: A Study of Assaultive and Non-Assaultive Offenders', *Journal of Criminal Law, Criminology and Police Science* (1962) **53**:44–48.
25. Alex D. Pokorny and B. A. Fred Davis, 'Homicide and Weather', *American Journal of Psychiatry* (February, 1964) **120**: 806–808. No single significant relationship was found between 106 Houston homicides and 11 variables related to weather conditions. The same absence of significant relationship was found with time of the day, month, and season. However, 30 years earlier Mills found a definite time relationship between weather changes and suicides and homicides for the years 1924–1928. See C. A. Mills, 'Suicides and Homicides in Their Relation to Weather Changes', *American Journal of Psychiatry* (1934) **91**:669–677.
26. For example, see Tersiev, 'Die Bewertung ihrer Taten seitens der verurteilten Mörder', *Monatssch. f. Krimpsychol. u. Strafrechtsref.* (1930) **4**:198–207. The examination of 130 condemned murderers in a Moscow prison revealed that the great majority (87 per cent) condemned their own action.
27. P. Schilder, 'The Attitude of Murderers Towards Death', *Journal of Abnormal Social Psychology* (1936) **31**:348–363. The author has identified three main different attitudes toward death. In one group

the motives can be understood, although there are deep emotional disturbances. In another group, murder is linked with an abnormal preoccupation with death. In the third group, more important for our analysis of violence, the murderer is generally young, kills for futile motives, has no respect for life and no preoccupation with death. He kills in the course of quarrels or hold-ups.

28. This is linked to the emergence of 'victimology' in the study of crime, but is, in homicide, of particular relevance because of the importance of the victim's behavior in causing or sometimes initiating aggression. For a discussion of this topic, see Marvin E. Wolfgang, *Patterns in Criminal Homicide;* Hans von Hentig, *The Criminal and His Victim*, 1948; J. M. McDonald, *The Murderer and His Victim.* Rausch has recently conducted an interesting analysis of the dual relationship between victim and murderer (S. W. Rausch, *Tötung des Intimpartners*, privately distributed) focused mainly on middle-class murderers; K. Higuchi, 'The Victim of Homicide by Immediate Relations. A Contribution to Victimology', *Acta Criminol. Med. Leg. Jap.* (1960) **25:6**:2–7; B. Holist, 'Role ofiary w genezie zabójstwa', *Pánstwo i Prawo* (1964) **19:11**:746–755; O. Nakata, *Violent Crime in the Light of Victimology*, paper presented at the First Annual Meeting of the Japanese Association of Criminology, October 6, 1962.

29. For a discussion of this very important topic, see Stephen Schafer, *Restitution to Victims of Crime*, London: Stevens, 1960; Margery Fry and others, 'Compensation for Victims of Criminal Violence', *Journal of Public Law* (1959) **8:1**:191–253; and, more recently, Marvin E. Wolfgang, *Victim Compensation in Crimes of Personal Violence*, paper presented at the Annual Meeting of the A.A.A.S., Montreal, December 30, 1964 and published in the *Minnesota Law Review* (December, 1965) **50**: 223–241.

30. In recent years several efforts have been made to provide a balanced interdisciplinary approach to the study of violence and aggression. See, for example, John Paul Scott, *Aggression*, Chicago: University of Chicago Press, 1958; and the long article by Elton B. McNeil, 'Psychology and Aggression', *Journal of Conflict Resolution* (1959) **3:3**:195–293. On December 28 and 29, 1962, the Academy of Psychoanalysis and the Committee on Science in the Promotion of Human Welfare at the A.A.A.S. Philadelphia Meeting held a conference on the role of violence in human behavior. A brief account of the conference has been published by Alfred H. Rifkin, 'Violence in Human Behavior', *Science* (May, 1963) **140**:904–906. In London, an important symposium was held at the British Museum (Natural History) on October 21 and 22, 1963. The proceedings have been edited and published by J. D. Carthy and F. J. Ebling, *The Natural History of Aggression*, London: Academic Press, 1964.

31. See Konrad Lorenz, 'Ritualized Fighting', pp. 39–50, in J. D. Carthy and F. J. Ebling, *op. cit.*; also Konrad Lorenz, *On Aggression*, London: Methuen; New York: Harcourt Brace, 1966.

32. Leonard Berkowitz, *Aggression*, p. 4.
33. Robert Ardrey, *African Genesis*, New York: Atheneum, 1963.
34. Raymond A. Dart, 'The Predatory Transition from Ape to Man', *International Anthropological and Linguistic Review* (1953) 1:4. See also Raymond A. Dart, *Adventures with the Missing Link*, New York: Harper and Brothers, 1959.
35. Derek Freeman, 'Human Aggression in Anthropological Perspective', in J. D. Carthy and F. J. Ebling, *op. cit.*, 109–119.
36. John P. Scott, *Aggression*, Chicago: University of Chicago Press, 1958.
37. Elton B. McNeil, *op. cit.*
38. Arnold H. Buss, *op. cit.*
39. Leonard Berkowitz, *op. cit.*
40. Irenäus Eibl-Eibesfeldt, 'The Fighting Behavior of Animals', *Scientific American* (December, 1961).
41. See *supra*, note 30.
42. Lincoln D. Clark, 'A Comparative View of Aggressive Behavior', mimeographed.
43. See J. D. Carthy and F. J. Ebling, *op. cit.*, pp. 125–126.
44. W. M. S. Russell, in J. D. Carthy and F. J. Ebling, *op. cit.*, pp. 156–157.
45. Donald O. Hebb, *A Textbook of Psychology*, Philadelphia: W. B. Saunders, 1958.
46. Eliot Stellar, 'Drive and Motivation', Chapter LXII, in J. Field, H. W. Magoun and V. E. Hall, *Neurophysiology*, Washington: American Physiological Society, 1960, Vol. III, Section 1, pp. 1501–1527.
47. *Ibid.*, p. 1524.
48. *Ibid.*, p. 1525.
49. Roland P. MacKay, 'The Neurology of Motivation', *Archiv. Neurol.* (1959) 1:535–543.
50. Frederick C. Thorne, 'Epidemiological Studies of Chronic Frustration–Hostility–Aggression States', *The American Journal of Psychiatry* (1957) 113:8:717–721. In this clinical-genetic study of two families, Thorne emphasizes the fact that the outward phenomenology of anger involves other persons in establishing an epidemic of negative reactions. The end result can be a vicious situational psychopathy.
51. M. Eyrich, 'Kriminal-biologische und sociologische Untersuchungen an Mördern und Totschägern', *Bl. f. Gefängnisk.* (1930) 61:247–262.
52. Sheldon and Eleanor Glueck, *Physique and Delinquency*, New York: Harper, 1956.
53. Walter B. Cannon, *Bodily Changes in Pain, Hunger, Fear and Rage*, Boston: Branford, 1953, Second Edition. The First Edition of this classic volume appeared in 1929.
54. For a concise résumé of Funkenstein's work, see Daniel H. Funkenstein, 'The Physiology of Fear and Anger', *Scientific American* (May, 1955).
55. Chapter III in John P. Scott, *op. cit.*

56. Chapter 6 in Arnold H. Buss, *op. cit.*, is an up-to-date analysis of relevant physiological and psychophysiological literature.

57. See, for example, P. Bard, 'A Diencephalic Mechanism for Expression of Rage with Special Reference to Sympathetic Nervous System', *American Journal of Psychology* (1938) **84**:490.

58. One interesting account of this neurosurgical technique used on 60 patients who were epileptic or who had severe behavior disturbances appears in H. Narabayashi, T. Nagao, Y. Saito, M. Yoshida, and M. Nagahata, 'Stereotaxic Amygdalotomy for Behavior Disorders', *Arch. Neurol.* (July, 1963) **9**:1-16. Marked improvement was reported in 51 of the 60 cases (85 per cent) after neurosurgery.

59. Cited by J. P. Scott, *op. cit.*, p. 51.

60. J. P. Scott, *op. cit.*, p. 51.

61. Daniel H. Funkenstein, *op. cit.*

62. A recent and comprehensive discussion of this problem, with an analysis of the contrasting evidence, has been written by Arnold Klopper: 'Physiological Background to Aggression', in J. D. Carthy and F. J. Ebling (eds.), *op. cit.*, pp. 65-72.

63. On the adaptation and stress reaction, see, for example, the classical work of Hans Selye, 'The General Adaptation Syndrome and Diseases of Adaptation', *Journal of Clinical Endocrinology* (1946) **6**:**2**:217-230, and P. C. Constantidines and Niall Carey, 'The Alarm Reaction', *Scientific American* (March, 1949).

64. Albert F. Ax, 'The Physiological Differentiation between Fear and Anger in Humans', *Psychosomatic Medicine* (1953) **15**:**5**:433-442.

65. Donald O. Hebb, 'On the Nature of Fear', Chapter 10, in D. K. Candland (ed.), *Emotion: Bodily Change*, Princeton: D. van Nostrand, 1962, p. 164.

66. M. Bachet, *Les encephaloses criminogènes*, Paris: Éditions Foucher, 1930.

67. J. Papez, 'Neuroanatomy', Chapter 79 in S. Arieti, *American Handbook of Psychiatry*, Vol. II, New York: Basic Books, 1960, p. 1605.

68. Denis Hill, 'Aggression and Mental Illness', Chapter in J. D. Carthy and F. J. Ebling (eds.), *op. cit.*, pp. 91-99.

69. Denis Hill, *op. cit.*, p. 98.

70. Olof Kinberg, *Basic Problems of Criminology*, London: Heinemann 1935. A revised edition of this classic book has recently been reprinted in France: *Les problèmes fondamenteaux de la criminologie*, Paris: Cujas, 1960. A recent Italian study supports much of Kinberg's hypotheses: M. Zucchi and L. Stella, 'Lo sviluppo delle tendenze antisociali nel quadro delle anomalie del comportamento di tipo caratteriale del bambino e del ragazzo', *Rivista di Psicologia Sociale* (1960) **4**:235-269. See also D. H. Stott, *Studies of Troublesome Children*, London: Tavistock Publications, 1966.

71. I. Horvai, 'Head Injury in Forensic Psychiatry', *Acta Univ. Carol. Med.* (1962) **16**:131-132 (From *Excerpta Criminologica*, 1962, N. 1570).

72. See, for example:

A. U. Mundy Cutile, 'The E.E.G. in Twenty-Two Cases of Murder or Attempted Murder: Appendix on Possible Significance of Alphoid Rhythms', *Journal Nat. Inst. Personn. Res.* (1956) **6**:103–120. A. Sciorta and M. Zito, 'Correlazioni clinico-elettroencefalografiche nell'aggressività e criminalità epilettica', *Acta Neurol.* (1960) **1**:92–123. E. G. Winkler and G. J. Train, 'Acts of Violence with Electroencephalographic Changes', *Journal of Clinical and Experimental Psychopathology* (1959) **20**:223–230.

73. Giovanni Ricci, 'Rilievi elettroencefalografici su 484 detenuti', *Rassegna di Studi Penitenziari*, Atti del I Congresso Internazionale di Criminologia Clinica (1958) 470–472.

74. Cited by J. M. MacDonald, *Psychiatry and the Criminal*, Springfield, Ill.: C. C. Thomas, 1958. See also the original study, D. Hill and D. A. Pond, 'Reflections on One Hundred Capital Cases Submitted to Electroencephalography', *Journal of Mental Science* (1952) **98**:23–43.

75. F. Grunberg and D. A. Pond, 'Conduct Disorders in Epileptic Children', *Journal Neurol. Neurosurg. Psychiat.* (1957) **20**:65–68.

76. R. Sessions Hodge, V. J. Walter, and W. Grey Walter, 'Juvenile Delinquency: An Electrophysiological, Psychological and Social Study', *The British Journal of Delinquency* (1953) **3**:3:155–184.

77. The literature on the relationship of abnormal EEGs and aggressive behavior is extensive and can be found in specialized publications. Some of the more relevant papers are:

D. Hill, W. Sargant, and M. S. Heppenstall, 'A Case of Matricide', *Lancet* (1943) Part I, **244**:526–527.

D. Hill, 'Cerebral Dysrhythmia: Its Significance in Aggressive Behavior', *Proceedings R. Soc. Med.* (1944) **37**:317.

D. Silverman, 'The Electroencephalogram of Criminals', *Archives of Neurology and Psychiatry* (1944) **52**:1:38–42.

J. J. Michaels, 'The Relationship of Antisocial Traits to the E.E.G. in Children with Behavior Disorders', *Psychosomatic Medicine* (1945) **7**:41.

Maurice W. Laufer, Eric Denhoff, and Gerald Solomons, 'Hyperkinetic Impulse Disorders in Children's Behavior Problems', *Psychosomatic Medicine* (1957) **19**:38–49.

Jean Delay, J. Verdeaux, and R. Barande, 'Électroencephalographie et expertise médico-légale: étude clinique et électroencephalographique de 94 délinquents épileptiques adultes', *L'Encéphale* (1958) **47**:1–30.

Edward D. Schwade and Sara G. Geiger, 'Severe Behavior Disorders with Abnormal Electroencephalograms', *Dis. Nerv. System* (1960) **21**:616–620.

Masadoshi Ohtani, Keiichi Isozumi, Atzuo Yamamoto, Moriaki Ando, and Kiyoshi Fujioka, 'Electroencephalographic Study on Criminals, II', *Journal of Correctional Medicine* (1960) 9: Special Issue: 81–88.

Sara G. Geiger, 'The Organic Factors in Delinquency', *Journal of Correctional Medicine* (1960) 9: Special Issue: 221–233.

E. Podolsky, 'The Electrophysiology of Homicide', *Journal of Forensic Medicine* (1961) 8: 4: 161–164.

N. Yoshii, M. Shimokochi, K. Tani, 'The Electroencephalograms on Juvenile Delinquents', *Folia Psychiat. Neurol. Jap.* (1961) 15: 2: 85–91.

E. Podolsky, 'The Epileptic Murderer', *The Medico-Legal Journal* (1962) 30: 4: 176–179.

V. Ragina, E. A. Serafetidines, 'Epilepsy and Behavior Disorder in Patients with Generalized Spike and Wave Complexes', *Electroenceph. Clin. Neurophysiol.* (1962) 14: 376–382.

H. D. Kurland, C. T. Yeager and J. A. Ransom, 'Psychophysiologic Aspects of Severe Behavior Disorders, A Pilot Study', *Arch. Gen. Psychiat.* (1963) 8: 599–604.

M. Schachter, 'Cérébropathologie et dissocialité chez les jeunes, dans la perspective psycho-somatique', *Aggiornamento Pediatrico* (1964) 15: 6: 235–262.

For a general analysis of the relationship of electroencephalography to behavioral variables, see A. C. Mundy-Castle, 'An Appraisal of Electroencephalography in Relation to Psychology', *Journal of the National Institute for Personnel Research*, Monograph Supplement No. 2 (1958) p. 43. A recent survey of the relationship between schizophrenia and psychomotor epilepsy, two nosographic entities which frequently pose puzzling problems of differential diagnosis, has been published by Harold A. Treffert, 'The Psychiatric Patient with an E.E.G. Temporal Lobe Focus', *The American Journal of Psychiatry* (February, 1964) 765–771. A case study of 9 subjects showing prison psychosis and of their EEG records has been published by Muneaki Nagahama and Kei Matsumato. 'Prison Psychosis in Relation to Electroencephalogram', *Journal of Correctional Medicine* (1960) 9: Special Issue: 89–99.

78. Sherwyn M. Woods, 'Adolescent Violence and Homicide. Ego Disruption and the 6 and 14 Dysrhythmia', *Arch. Gen. Psychiat.* (1961) 5: 6: 528–534.

79. See, among others, the following source articles:

Frederic A. Gibbs, 'Clinical Correlates of 14 and 6 Per Second Positive Spikes', *Electroencephalography and Clinical Neurophysiology* (1956) 8: 149.

Peter Kellaway, F. J. Moore, and Nina Kagowa, 'The 14 and 6 Per Second Positive Spikes', *Electroencephalography and Clinical Neurophysiology* (1957) 9: 165.

R. D. Walter, E. G. Colbert, E. G. Koegler, J. O. Palmer, and F. M. Bond, 'A Controlled Study of 14 and 6 Per Second E.E.G. Pattern', *American Medical Association Archives of General Psychiatry* (May, 1960) **2**:559.
Frederic A. Gibbs and E. L. Gibbs, '14–6 Per Second Positive Spikes', *Electroencephalography and Clinical Neurophysiology* (1963) **15**:553–558.

80. See letter to *Time* by Frederic A. Gibbs, *Time*, January 19, 1962, p. 6. For a recent adequate study of the 6 and 14 syndrome, see: John T. Hughes, Eugene D. Means, Bernard S. Stell, 'A Controlled Study on the Behavior Disorders Associated with the Positive Spike Phenomenon', *Electroencephalography and Clinical Neurophysiology* (1965) **18**:4: 349–353. This study is based on 50 cases with 'positive spikes' compared with 2 control groups. The specificity of the syndrome appears demonstrated. See also the following older papers: E. D. Schwade and O. Otto, 'Homicide as a Manifestation of Thalamic or Hypothalamic Disorder with Abnormal Electroencephalographic Findings', *Wisconsin Medical Journal* (1953) **52**:171–174; E. D. Schwade and O. Otto, 'Matricide with Electroencephalographic Evidence of Thalamic or Hypothalamic Disorder', *Diseases of the Nervous System* (1953) **14**:18–20.

81. Benigno Di Tullio, 'L'endocrinologia e la morfologia costituzionale in Antropologia Criminale', *Zacchia* (July–October, 1923).

82. Edward Podolsky, 'The Chemical Brew of Criminal Behavior', *Journal of Criminal Law, Criminology and Police Science* (March–April, 1955) **45**:675–678.

83. G. J. Train and E. G. Winkler, 'Homicidal Psychosis while under ACTH Cortico-steroid Therapy for Pemphigus Vulgaris during Involution', *Psychosomatics* (1962) **3**:317–332.

84. Of specific interest are, for example, the efforts to utilize castration as treatment of aggressive drives in male psychopaths. This practice has been most consistently followed in the Scandinavian countries. Dr. Georg K. Stürup, Director of the Danish Institution for Criminal Psychopaths at Herstedvester, has collected a large number of cases. In this institution, however, castration is utilized in conjunction with psychotherapy and milieu therapy.

85. E. A. Beeman, 'The Effect of Male Hormone on Aggressive Behavior in Mice', *Physiol. Zool.* (1947) **20**:373–405, cited by John P. Scott, *op. cit.*, 71–76.

86. John P. Scott, *op. cit.*, p. 71.

87. Arnold Klopper, *op. cit.*, p. 71.

88. J. Wilder, 'Sugar Metabolism in Its Relation to Criminology', in R. M. Lindner and R. V. Seliger (eds.), *Handbook of Correctional Psychology*, New York: Philosophical Library, 1947, pp. 98–129.

89. Edward Podolsky, 'The Chemistry of Murder', *Pak. Med. Journal* (1964) **15**:6:9–14.

90. This study has been reported as a 'news' item in many medical journals. We have been unable to locate the original paper.
91. John P. Scott, *op. cit.*; Elton B. McNeil, *op. cit.*; Arnold H. Buss, *op. cit.*
92. John P. Scott, *op. cit.*, p. 62.
93. We have collected a large number of homicide case histories from the existing criminological literature. The bibliographical items listed below are included for their documentary and reference value:

T. Abe, 'A Case of Homicide. The Personality Pictures of Both Perpetrator and Victim and the Psychological Explanation of the Criminal Act', *Hanzaigaku Zasshi* (1960) **26**:1:26–30.

P. Abely, 'Démence précoce à évolution rapide. Impulsion homicide: première symptome', *Ann. Méd. psychol.* (1929) **87**:2:345–357.

Anon., 'Matricide and Schizoid Personality', *Rev. del Inst. de Investigaciones y Docencia Criminologica* (1959) **3**:119.

G. Antonini and E. Bravetta, 'Perizia medico-legale sullo stato di mente di Renzo Pettine', *Arch. di antrop. crim.* (1928), 48.

C. A. Bambarén and J. F. Valega, *Esquizofrenia y cuádruple homicidio*, Lima, Peru, 1945.

R. S. Banay, 'Study of a Murder for Revenge', *J. Crim. Psychopath.* (1941) **3**:1–10.

E. Berne, 'Cultural Aspects of a Multiple Murder', *Psychiat. Quart. Suppl.* (1950) **24**:250–269.

M. Bonaparte, 'The Case of Madame Lefebvre', *Arch. Crim. Psychodynamics* (1955) **1**:148–197.

P. A. Bovard, 'A propos de l'affaire Jaccoud', *Rev. Sci. Crim. Pén. Comparé* (1960) **15**:3:431–446.

P. E. Bowers, 'William Edward Hickman', *Med. J. and Rec.* (1929) **130**:79–82; 139–142.

R. J. Brabdt, 'Aus der Analyse eines Mörders,' *Psyche. Heidel.* (1958) **12**:18–32.

H. Brennecke, 'Ein casuistischer Beitrag zur Psychologie des Mörders', *Monatssch. f. Krimpsychol. u. Strafrechtsref.* (1932) **23**:402–415.

K. Bretzfeld, 'Jugendliche Massenmörder', *Arch. Kriminol.* (1935) **97**:205–210; (1936) **98**:57–70.

O. Bridgman, 'Four Young Murderers', *J. Juv. Res.* (1929) **13**:90–96.

W. Bromberg, 'A Psychological Study of Murder', *Int. J. Psycho-Anal.* (1951) **32**:117–127.

E. Brongersma, 'The Baarn Murder Case', *Ned. T. Criminol.* (1964) **6**:1:18–20; **6**:2:33–47.

J. H. Brown, 'Homosexuality as an Adaptation in Handling Aggression', *J. La. med. Soc.* (1963) **115**:9:304–311.

D. J. Carek and A. W. Watson, *Case Presentation of Undetermined Fratricide. I: Treatment of a Family Involved in Fratricide*, 40th Annual Meeting of the American Orthopsychiatric Association, Washington D.C., March 6–9, 1963.

G. M. Carstairs, 'The Case of Thakur Khuman Singh: a Culture Conditioned Crime', *Brit. J. Delinquency* (1953) 4:14–25.

C. Citterio, 'Delirio erotomaniaco e criminalità: il tentato omicidio dell'oggetto amato da parte dell'erotomane', *Folia psychiat.* (1964) 7:4:545–555.

A. Cuevas Tamariz, 'Análisis psicológico retrospectivo en un caso de homicidio por emoción violenta', *Archivos de Criminología, Neuro-psiquiatría y Disciplinas Conexas* (1956), 70–77.

A. Cuevas Tamariz, 'Paranoia y Homicidio', *Rev. Arch. de Neuro-psiquiatría y Disciplinas Conexas* (1964) 12:48:607–621.

A. K. Deb, 'Suicide and Homicide in Relation to Sexual Difficulties', *Ind. Med. Rec.* (1946) 66:134.

G. Dede and F. Pasolini, 'Congenito-lues ed imputabilità', *Ann. Neurol. Psichiat.* (1962) 56:1–26.

B. Di Tullio, 'Studio sulla criminalità di un minorenne', *Riv. di dir. peniten.* (1934) 1:270.

P. Dogliani, E. F. Inga and V. Micheletti, 'Considerazioni sul concetto di reazione a corto circuito', *Quad. Criminol. clin.* (1960) 2:47–79.

M. Doi, 'Die Tat einer mandschurischen Haufrau infolge von Besessenheirswahn', *Arb. Psychiat. Inst. Sendai* (1940) 7:18–39.

F. Dostoevsky, 'A Simple Affair?' *Psychoanal. Rev.* (1950) 37:164–171.

J. Drechsler, 'Erziehungsschuld und Elternmord', *Psychol. Rdsch.* (1957) 8:136–144.

K. Dreyfuss, 'Der Fall Wieland', *Int. Z. Psychoanal.* (1934) 20:210–240.

G. A. Ehrenreich, 'Headache, Necrophilia and Murder', *Bull. Menninger Clinic* (1960) 24:6:273–287.

W. Eliasberg, 'The Murdered to get Hanged: A Pre-analytical Case History of 1783', *Psychoanal. Rev.* (1952) 39:164–167.

A. Ellis, 'A Young Woman Convicted of Manslaughter', *Case Rep. Clin. Psychol.* (1951) 2:1:9–34.

O. Elo, 'Casistic Contribution to the Question of Grounds for Mercy in Infanticide', *Acta. Soc. Med. Doudecim* (1940) 28:1:243.

J. Endara, 'Homicidio, personalidad psicopática', *Arch. de Criminología, Neuro-psiquiatría y Disciplinas Conexas* (1957) 76–95.

L. Engelhardt, 'Der Gardien de la Paix Prévost', *Arch. f. Krim.* (1931) 89:177–190.

T. Erisman, 'Die psychologischen probleme im Fall Halsmann', *Ber. Kongr. Dtsch. Ges. Psychol.* (1932) 12:322–331.

N. Fenton, 'The Diagnosis "Hickman"', *Survey* (1929) 57:349–350.

E. Ferri, 'La personalidad de Violet Gilson', *Rev. de Crim.* (1927) 14:259–268.

V. Fontes, 'Un caso de homicidio voluntario realizado por un menor de 14 años', *Criança portug.* (1942) 1:131–140.

V. Fontes and O. de Assis Pacheco, 'Un caso de clínica psico-social.

Morte de dois menores por una criança de onze años', *Criança portug.* (1953–54) **13**: 129–142.

A. N. Foxe, 'Post-homicidal Contrition and Religious Conversion', *Psychiat. Quart.* (1943) **17**: 565–578.

J. A. Galvin and J. M. McDonald, 'Psychiatric Study of a Mass Murderer', *Amer. J. Psychiat.* (1959) **115**: 1057–1061.

F. Gonçalves, 'Experiencia penosa durante la infancia, esquizoidía y crimen', *Rev. Neurobiol.* (1939) **1**: 332–337.

F. González García, 'Estudio psiquiátrico de un parricida', *Rev. med. Legal Colombia* (1947) **9**: 111: 124.

L. A. Graeter, 'Mord wegen einer Mark', *Kriminalistik* (1960) **8**: 349–352.

A. R. Grant and S. M. Allan, 'Post-epileptic Automatism as a Defence in a Case of Murder', *J. Ment. Sci.* (1929) **75**: 311.

J. E. Greene, 'Motivation of a Murderer', *J. Abnor. soc. Psychol.* (1948) **43**: 526–531.

J. E. Greene, J. E. Moore, and T. F. Staton, 'Inferences Concerning the Motivation of a Murderer: A Psychological Study of "Displaced Aggression" ', *Amer. Psychologist* (1948) **3**: 335.

C. Greenland, 'L'Affaire Shortis and the Valleyfield Murder', *Cand. Psychiat. Ass. J.* (1962) **7**: **5**: 261–271.

A. Grossmann, 'Zur Psychologie und dynamischen Situation eines Mordes', *Schweiz. Med. Woch.* (1929) **59**: 1405–1411.

M. Guttmacher, 'Pseudopsychopathic Schizophrenia', *Arch. Crim. Psychodyn.* (1961), 502–508.

W. H. Haines and R. A. Esser, 'Case History of Ruth Steinhagen', *Amer. J. Psychiat.* (1950) **106**: 737–743.

H. Helweg, 'Du meurtre comme crime émotionnel "normal" ', *Acta Psychiat. et neurol.* (1932) **7**: 201–216.

A. Hellwig, 'Kritiken des Gattenmordes', *Krim. Monatsh.* (1930) **4**: 62–63.

R. Herbertz, 'Mord aus Wahrheitsfanatismus', *Psychol. Rundschau* (1930) **2**: 279–284.

R. Herbertz, 'Der morder will g'astimiert werden!', *Psychol. Berater gesunde prakt. Lebensgestalt* (1952) **4**: 434–439.

K. E. Hinsie, 'A Contribution to the Psychopathology of Murder. Study of a Case', *J. Crim. Psychopath.* (1940) **2**: 1–20.

E. Holler, 'Ein Jugendlicher Mordertypus', *Bl. f. Gefangniskunde* (1930) **61**: 60–75.

K. Hoppe, 'Persecution, Depression and Aggression', *Bull. Menninger Clinic* (1962) **26**: **4**: 195–203.

C. H. S. Jayewardene, 'Murder and Sexual Assault of an Old Woman', *Zacchia* (1963), 4.

A. Jüngling, 'Kasuistische Beiträge über mehrfachen Kindsmord mit Betrachtungen über die Psychologie and strafrechtliche Würdigung des Kindsmordes im allgemeinen', *Erlangen-Bruck: Krahl* (1935), 53.

D. M. Kahn, *Case Presentations of Undetermined Fratricide: II.*

I

Undetermined Fratricide, 40th Annual Meeting of the American Orthopsychiatric Association, Washington, D.C. March 6–9, 1963

M. W. Kahn, 'Psychological Test Study of a Mass Murderer', *J. Proj. Tech.* (1960) **24**:148–160.

B. Karpman, 'A Psychoanalytic Study of a Case of Murder', *Psychoanal. Rev.* (1951) **38**:139–157; 245–270.

B. Karpman, 'Dream Life in a Case of Uxoricide', *Arch. Crim. Psychodynamics* (1957) **2**:597–675; 866–925.

B. Karpman, 'Uxoricide and Infanticide in a Setting of Oedipal Jealousy', *Arch. Crim. Psychodynamics* (1957) **2**:339–401.

F. Kennedy, H. R. Hoffman, and W. H. Haines, 'Psychiatric Study of William Heirens', *J. Crim. Law Crim.* (1947) **38**:311–341.

K. Kiehne, 'Ein schizophrener Serienverbrecher', *Arch. fur Kriminol.* (1959) **124**:25.

O. Kinberg, 'Familienmord av schizoid under emotionellt omotö kningstillstand', *Svenska. Läkartidn.* (1934) **31**:489–512.

O. Kinberg, 'Mord a eget barn beganget av kvinna i tilstand av hoggrading psychologisk missanpassning', *Svenska Läkartidn.* (1934) **31**:969–987.

O. Kinberg, 'Drasforsok beganget av ung man mot hans fastmo under omtockning av medvetandet', *Svenska Läkartidn.* (1934) **31**: 1321–1338.

O. Kinberg, 'Mord a eget barn utom aktenskapet av achizoid kvinna i tilstad av psychologisk missanpassning', *Svenska Läkartidn.* (1935) **32**:582–596.

A. Kogler, 'Uber jugendliche Mörder', *Mschr. Krimbiol.* (1941) **32**:73–103.

K. Kolle, 'Der Fall Voller', *Monatssch. f. Krimpsychol. u. Strafrechtsref.* (1930) **4**:226–236.

K. Krekeler, 'Über den Fall R., einen paranoiden schizophrenen Totchläger', *Allg. Z. Psychiat.* (1936) **105**:79.

R. Kuhn, 'Mördversuch eines depressiven Fetischisten und Sodomisten und einer Dirne', *Mschr. Psychiat. Neurol.* (1948) **116**:66–124.

G. R. Lafora, 'Análisis psicopatológico del estrangulador Gregorio Cárdenas', *Criminalia* (1942) **9**:106–117.

H. Landmann, 'Der Frauenwürger B.', *Kriminalistik* (1960) **14**:7:326–329.

J. Lange, 'Einige kriminologische Lehren des Falles Seefeld', *Mschr. Krimbiol.* (1937) **28**:37.

G. Leggeri and A. Castellani, 'Contributo antropoanalítico allo studio del comportamento criminale', *Neopsichiatria* (1962) **28**:2.

M. Levin, *Compulsion*, New York: Simon and Schuster, 1956.

J. Lévy-Valensi and D. Rigot, 'Louvel le magnicide', *Hygiène mentale* (1929) **24**:125–150.

A. Lima and F. Guerner, 'Paranoico homicida', *Rev. Neurol. Psychiat.* (1935) **1**:232–237.

O. Lippuner, 'Die Schrift des Mörders Irniger', *Beih. Schweiz. Z. Psychol. Anwend.* (1945) **6**:66–72.

P. A. Llinas, 'Un homicida minor de edad; influencia del cinematógrafo y del ambiente hogareño y social', *Rev. Med. Leg. Colombia* (1943) **6**:40–47.

L. S. London, 'Psychopathologic Aspects of Murder', *J. Crim. Psychopath.* (1944) **5**:795–812.

W. Lüdtke, 'Zur Psychologie eines Mörders', *Kriminalistik* (1939) **13**:106–108.

A. M. Marx, 'Mord im hysterischen Dämmerzustand', *Arch. f. Krim.* (1929) **85**:4.

H. Mezger, 'Der Fall Julius Zell in Zweifelsberg', *Arch. f. Krim.* (1931) **89**:207–215.

M. F. Molina, 'Study of a Psychopathic Personality in Guatemala', *Psychiatry* (1947) **10**:31–36.

Mönkemöller, 'Der Fall Hopp', *Arch. f. Krim.* (1932) **90**:196–231.

G. G. Montesino, 'Asasinato y personalidad epileptoidea', *Archivos de Criminología, Neuro-psiquiatría y Disciplinas Conexas* (1953) **4**:497–512.

N. A. Neiberg, 'Murder and Suicide', *Arch. Crim. Psychodyn.* (1961) **4**:2:253–268.

Oertel, 'Der Raubmord an dem Rentenempfänger Todt', *Arch. f. Krimin.* (1928) **83**:3:4.

J. Ortíz Velázquez, 'Estudio psicológico de una homicida por celos', *An. Acad. Med. Medelin.* (1945) **1**:639–643.

A. E. Petrowa, 'Eine Mordtat in der Pubertätsperiode vollbracht', *Monatssch. f. Krimpsychol. u. Strafrechtsref.* (1930) **21**:592–607.

M. Pfister-Amende, 'Deux cas d'infanticide à l'examen psychiatrique', *Schweiz. Arch. Neurol. Psychiat.* (1937) **39**:2.

P. Plaut, 'Eine dreizehnjahrige Kindesmörderin', *Krim. Monatsh.* (1931) **5**:221–224.

Polke, 'Der Massenmörder Denke', *Arch. Krim. Anthrop.* (1934) **95**:8–30.

G. Ponti, 'La causa d'onore nel delitto di infanticidio', *Quaderni di Criminologia Clinica* (1962) **4**:4:397–444.

I. Popescu-Sibiu, 'Un cas rare d'inversion sexuelle criminelle', *Ann. méd. psychol.* (1958) **2**:2:279–285.

D. E. Price, 'Necrophilia Complicating a Case of Homicide', *Med. Sci. Law* (1963) **3**:3:121–131.

Reg. v. Podola, 'Symposium on April 4, 1960', *Med. Leg. J.* (1960) **28**:3:117–131.

K. H. Raizen, 'A Case of Matricide–Patricide', *Brit. J. of Delinquency* (1960) **10**:4:277–296.

R. Raskovsky, 'El parricidio', *Arch. med. leg.* (1945) **15**:115–141.

K. N. Remy, 'Der Fall "Tripp". Ein Beitrag zur Kriminalpsychologie des Lustmordes', *Heide in Holstein. Heider Anzeiger* (1934).

G. Rosapepe, 'Sullo stato di mente di Dina Natali, imputata di omicidio aggravato', *Annali di Neuropsichiatria e Psicoanalisi* (1958) 3:283–299.

G. J. Rose, 'Screen Memories in Homicidal Acting Out', *Psychoanal. Quart.* (1960) 29:328–343.

S. Rosenzweig, 'Unconscious Self-Defense in an Uxoricide', *J. Crim. Law Crim.* (1956) 46:791–795.

S. Rosenzweig, B. Simon, and M. Ballou, 'The Psychodynamics of an Uxoricide', *Amer. J. Orthopsychiat.* (1942) 12:283–294.

E. C. Rowe, 'A Case of Educational Futility', *J. Abnorm. Soc. Psychol.* (1935) 30:237–255.

L. Salzman, 'Psychodynamics of a Case of Murder', *Comprehensive Psychiatry* (1962) 3:3:152–169.

M. Schachter and S. Cotte, 'Étude clinico-psychologique d'un mineur oligophrène criminel', *Criança Portug.* (1946–1947) 6:61–70.

E. Schilf, 'Beitrage zur Kinderpsychologie. II. Zwei Kinder als Mörder', *Psychiat. Neurol. Med. Psychol.* (1953) 5:316–328.

E. Schmidt, 'Vorgeschichte eines Attentats', *Int. Zsch. f. Indiv.-Psychol.* (1931) 5:358–367.

J. Schottky, 'Uber dern Mordversuch eines Jugendlichen bei geplantem Selbstmord. Beitrag zur kriminalbiologischen Beurteilung asozialer Psychopathen', *Mschr. KrimBiol.* (1941) 32:1–32.

E. Seelig, 'Jugendliche Mörder', *Zsch. f. Jugendkd.* (1932) 2:112–119.

H. Sheeman-Dare, 'Homicide during a Schizophrenic Episode', *Int. J. Psycho-Anal.* (1955) 36:43–52.

A. Sizaret and J. Bastie, 'Impulsion homicide. Symptôme initial d'une démence précoce à évolution rapide', *Bull. Soc. Clin. Méd. Ment.* (1929) 22:166–169.

A. Smykal and F. C. Thorne, 'Etiological Studies of Psychopathic Personality. II. Asocial Type', *J. Clin. Psychol.* (1951) 7:299–316.

S. R. Spencer, *A Companion to Murder*, London: Cassel, 1960.

Spielmeyer, 'Das Gehirn des Massenmörders Peter Kürten', *Arch. f. Krim.* (1932) 90:252–253.

G. Störring, 'Gutachten in dem Halsmann Prozess', *Arch. f. d. ges. Psychol.* (1932) 84:372–385.

H. Stotz, 'Tueur et pilleur international de banques: Donald Brown Hume', *Rev. Int. Pol. Criminelle* (1961) 16:144:15–21.

R. Topping, 'Case Studies of Aggressive Delinquents', *Amer. J. of Orthopsychiat.* (1941) 2:485–492.

O. Tumlirz, 'Der Fall Manasse Friedlander', *Manns Pad. Mag.* (1930) 1314:45–49.

G. Uribe Cualla, 'Personalidad psicopática de un homicida', *Rev. med. Legal Colombia* (1946) 8:45–46; 146–159.

K. Von Kothe, 'Aus der Verhaltenpsychologie: Fall eines jugendlichen Mörders', *Psychiatrie, Neurologie and Medizinische Psychologie* (1964) 16:1:24–27.

PERSPECTIVES · 237

A. H. Williams, 'A Psycho-Analytic Approach to the Treatment of
the Murderer', *Int. J. Psycho-anal.* (1960) 41:4–5:532–539.
J. M. Williams, *Hume: Portrait of a Double Murderer*, London:
Heinemann, 1960.
M. Winkler, 'Der Zahn des Brüderchens, Kurzbeitrag zur Frage der
Beziehungen zwischen Aggression und Angst', *Prox. Kinder-
psychol.* (1960) 9:5:171–175.
F. Wiseman, 'Psychiatry and Law: Use and Abuse of Psychiatry in a
Murder Case', *Amer. J. Psychiat.* (1961) 118:4:289–299.
P. Wittman and M. Astrachan, 'Psychological Investigation of a
Homicidal Youth', *J. Clin. Psychol.* (1949) 5:88–93.
F. Wolff, 'Der Fall Neckermann', *Monatssch. f. Krimpsychol. u.
Strafrechtref.* (1930) 4:212–226.
L. Wurmser, 'Ein schizophrener Muttermörder', *Kriminalistik*
(1959) 13:5:206–210.
J. R. Zubizarreta Peris, 'Esquizofrenia y delito', *Arch. de Criminol.,
Neuro-psiquiatría y Disciplinas Conexas* (1963), 42.

94. Morris G. Caldwell, 'Case Analysis Method for the Personality
Study of Offenders', *Journal of Criminal Law, Criminology and
Police Science* (1954–55) 45:291–298.
95. For a statement on this point, see Marvin E. Wolfgang, *Patterns in
Criminal Homicide*, pp. 314–315, note 7.
96. Some recent surveys of legal 'insanity' provisions may be found in:
Cesare Gerin, Franco Ferracuti, and Aldo Semerari, 'Evaluation
médico-légale de l'imputabilité dans les anomalies et dans les
maladies psychiques: ses répercussions criminologiques', *Zacchia*
(1963) 38:1–2; 3–40; and Gösta Rylander, *Forensic Psychiatry in
Relation to Legislation in Different Countries. An International Review*, in Hans W. Gruhle, R. Jung, Wilhelm Mayer-Gross, and Max
Muller, *Psychiatrie der Gegenwart, Band III, Soziale und Ange-
wandte Psychiatrie*, Berlin: Springer Verlag, 1961, pp. 397–451.
97. A. M. Lamont, 'Forensic Psychiatric Practice in a South African
Mental Hospital', *South African Medical Journal* (1961) 35:40:833–
837.
98. See, for example, Benjamin Karpman, *Case Studies in the Psychopathology of Crime*. Vol. III, Cases 10–13, Washington: Medical
Science Press, 1948, p. 834, and Benjamin Karpman, *Case Studies
in the Psychopathology of Crime*, Vol. IV, Cases 14–17, Washington:
Medical Science Press, 1948, p. 875.
99. Since 1959, the diagnostic team of the Observation Institute of the
Italian Ministry of Justice, in Rebibbia, Rome, has published in the
quarterly *Quaderni di Criminologia Clinica* a full case in each issue,
with all the relevant data. The cases are of young adult offenders and
often include homicide or other violent offenses. Occasionally,
cases from other diagnostic centers, in Italy and abroad, have been
published.
100. Alfred Hoche, *Handbuch der gerichtlichen Psychiatrie*, Berlin:

Springer, 1934, 3rd Edition. Also, some of von Hentig's monographs discuss this phenomenology. A recent paper on mass-mur-
derers, based on an unusually large series of cases, has been published by K. Nakamura, 'Kriminal-biologische Untersuchungen an
86 Massenmörden', *Japanese Association of Criminology* (1964), pp.
172–189 (from *Excerpta Criminologica*, 1965, p. 397). A full discussion of mass-murder, with a listing of major historical cases and an
analysis of a recent airplane bombing case, is included in Chapters 7
and 8 from John M. MacDonald, *The Murderer and His Victim*,
Springfield, Ill.: C. C. Thomas, 1961.

101. M. Pamir, 'Psicopatici nelle Indie Nederlandesi. Loro importanza
forense (l'assassinio Atjese e l'Amok)', *Archivio di Antropologia
Criminale* (1936) **56**: 571–579.

102. J. W. Lamberti, N. Blackman, and J. M. A. Weiss, 'The Sudden
Murderer: A Preliminary Report', *Journal of Social Therapy* (1958)
4: 2–15. See also, Nathan Blackman, M. A. James, J. M. A. Weiss,
and J. W. Lamberti, 'The Sudden Murderer', *Arch. Gen. Psychiat.*
(March, 1963) **8**: 289–294.

103. See, among others, the following studies:

G. Morf, 'Zur Psychologie des Lustmörders', *Psychol. Rundschau*
(1930) **2**: 143–144.

Hans von Hentig, 'Die Kriminalität des Homophilen', *Beitrage zur
Sexual-Forschung* (1960), 20.

R. Camba and S. Barra, 'Alterazione della personalità morale e
sociale con manifestazioni delinquenziali sessuali ed ulteriore
decadimento intellettivo globale da traumi infortunistici cranio-
cerebrali', *Sicurezza Sociale* (1960), 9.

Hans von Hentig, 'Lustmord und Buschversteck der "Beute" ',
Mschr. Kriminol. u. Strafrechts. ref. (1960) **43**: 2: 31–41.

Hans von Hentig, 'Der Mord auf homophiler Basis', *Kriminalistik*
(1960) **8**: 342–344.

K. Kaiser and E. Schramm, 'Der homosexuelle Mann als Opfer von
Kapitalverbrechen', *Kriminalistik* (1962) **16**: 6: 255–260.

Eugene Revitch, 'Extreme Manifestations of Sexual Aggression',
The Welfare Reporter (1965) **16**: 1: 10–16.

104. A. F. Meyers, B. Apfelberg, and C. Sugar, 'Men Who Kill Women,
Part I', *Journal of Clinical Psychopathology* (1946) **7**: 441–472; and
A. F. Meyers, B. Apfelberg, and C. Sugar, 'Men Who Kill Women,
Part II', *ibid.* (1947) **8**: 481–517.

105. A complete listing of this literature would be forbidding, and medico-
legal considerations are contained in many papers and books already quoted, such as the numerous case studies reported in note 93.
The following are papers which have a definite criminological
interest:

Gregory Zilboorg, 'Some Sidelights on Psychology of Murder',
Journal of Nervous and Mental Diseases (1935) **81**: 442–443.

A. T. Baker, 'A Clinical Study of Inmates Sentenced to Sing Sing Prison for Murder—First Degree', *American Journal of Psychiatry* (1935) **91**:783–790.

J. H. Cassidy, 'Personality Study of 200 Murderers', *Journal of Clinical Psychopathology* (1941) **2**:296–304.

A. J. Rosanoff, 'Thirty Condemned Men', *American Journal of Psychiatry* (1943) **99**:484–495.

Ralph S. Banay, 'A Study of Twenty-two Men Convicted of Murder in the First Degree', *Journal of Criminal Law and Criminology* (1943) **34**:106–111.

David Abrahamsen, 'The Dynamic Connection Between Personality and Crime and the Detection of the Potential Criminal Illustrated by Different Types of Murder', *Journal of Clinical Psychopathology* (1944) **5**:481–488.

G. M. Davidson, 'Psychiatric Aspects of the Law of Homicide', *Psychiatric Quarterly Supplement* (1946) **20**:30–49.

G. McDermaid and E. G. Winkler, 'Psychiatric Study of Homicide Cases', *Journal of Clinical Psychopathology* (1950) **11**:93–146.

H. Binder, 'Über den Mord', *Schweizer Archiv. für Neurologie und Psychiatrie* (1951) **67**:245.

B. A. Cruvant and F. N. Waldrop, 'The Murderer in the Mental Institution', *Annals of the American Academy of Political and Social Science* (1952) **284**:35–44.

Groves B. Smith, 'Situational Murder Due to Emotional Stress', *Journal of Social Therapy* (1958) **4**:173–181.

E. Podolsky, 'The Psychodynamics of Criminal Behavior', *Journal of Forensic Medicine* (1959) **6**:79.

W. Lindesay, Neustatter, 'Psychiatric Aspects of Diminished Responsibility in Murder', *Med. Leg. J.* (1960) **28**:2:90–101.

Two recent studies are based on a large series of cases, 50 in D. Borzych and Z. Falicki, 'Zabójstwa ze Stanowiska psychiatryczego', *Neurol. Neurochir. Psychiat. Pol.* (1964) **14**:4:589–592, and 298 in A. Merland, H. Fiorentini, and E. Y. Bourdoncle, 'Considérations sur l'homicide d'après l'étude de 298 expertises psychiatriques pour assassinants, meurtres, homicides volontaires et tentatives d'homicides', *Ann. Méd. Lég.* (1964) **44**:3:289–297.

106. See the following two papers: J. Lanzkron, 'Murder and Insanity. A Survey', *American Journal of Psychiatry* (1963) **119**:8:754–758; and J. Lanzkron, 'Psychopathology of the Homicidal Patient', *Correctional Psychiatry* and *Journal of Social Therapy* (1946) **10**:3:142–154.

107. See Wolfgang, *Patterns in Criminal Homicide, passim.*; A. A. Kurland, J. Morgenstern, and C. Sheets, 'A Comparative Study of Wife Murderers Admitted to a State Psychiatric Hospital', *Journal of Social Therapy* (1955) **1**:2:5–15; Manfred S. Guttmacher, 'Criminal Responsibility in Certain Homicide Cases Involving Family Members', in Paul H. Hoch and J. Zubin, *Psychiatry and the Law*, New York: Grune & Stratton, 1955, Chapter 6, pp. 73–96.

108. Trevor C. N. Gibbens, 'Sane and Insane Homicide', *Journal of Criminal Law, Criminology and Police Science* (1958) **49**:2:110–115.

109. John J. Brennan, 'Mentally Ill Aggressiveness, Popular Delusion or Reality', *American Journal of Psychiatry* (1964) **120**:**12**:1181–1184.

110. A. J. Barron, G. M. Duncan, S. H. Frazier, E. M. Litin, and A. M. Johnson, 'Etiological Factors in First-Degree Murder', *Journal of the American Medical Association* (1958) **168**:1755–1758.

111. We have limited the following examples to those works which have appeared in book form. Their value, as stated above, is uneven and generally limited. They are, however, a definite expression of interest from the field of psychiatry, and some of the authors are highly reputed clinicians, with a wide experience in the medico-legal and psychiatric field:

A. Bjerre, *The Psychology of Murder*, New York: Longmans, Green, 1927.

H. Dearden, *The Mind of the Murderer*, New York: Sears, 1930.

David Abrahamsen, *Crime and Human Mind*, New York: Columbia University Press, 1944.

Walter Bromberg, *Crime and the Mind*, Philadelphia: J. B. Lippincott Co., 1948.

Robert Block, *The Will to Kill*, New York: Ace Books, 1954.

David Abrahamsen, *The Psychology of Crime*, New York: Columbia University Press, 1960. (Homicide is discussed in several chapters.)

Manfred Guttmacher, *The Mind of the Murderer*, New York: Farrar, Straus, and Cudahy, 1960.

Walter Bromberg, *The Mold of Murder: A Psychiatric Study of Homicide*, New York: Grune & Stratton, 1961.

John M. MacDonald, *The Murderer and His Victim*, Springfield, Ill.: C. C. Thomas, 1961.

An interesting study, by a non-psychiatrist, but based largely on medico-legal sources provided by Alfonso Quiroz Cuaron and Jose Gomez Robleda, is the analysis of a well-known political assassin, responsible for Trotsky's death: Isaac Don Levine, *The Mind of an Assassin*, New York: Signet Books, 1960. A book by James Reinhardt, *The Psychology of Strange Killers*, Springfield, Ill.: C. C. Thomas, 1962, is based on the analysis of 9 individual cases.

112. An early paper refers to psychiatric observations on 8 cases: M. W. MacDonald, 'Criminally Aggressive Behavior in Passive-Effeminate Boys', *American Journal of Orthopsychiatry* (1938) **8**:70–78. Other psychiatric papers are the following:

Lauretta Bender and F. J. Curran, 'Children and Adolescents Who Kill', *Journal of Clinical Psychopathology* (1940) **1**:297–322.

M. L. Karr, 'A Study of Adolescents Who Kill', *Smith Coll. Stud. Soc. Work.* (1941) **12**:199–200.

R. M. Patterson, 'Psychiatric Study of Juveniles Involved in Homicide', *American Journal of Orthopsychiatry* (1943) **13**:125–130.

M. Schachter and S. Cotte, 'Homicides et tentatives d'homicide chez des mineurs', *Rivistadi Pediatria Pratica* (1949) **20**: 1.

C. H. Growdon, *A Group Study of Juvenile Homicide*, Columbus, Ohio: State Bureau of Juvenile Research, Dept. of Public Welfare, 1950.

A well-known monograph by Bender presents the psychodynamic approach: Lauretta Bender, *Aggression, Hostility and Anxiety in Children*, Springfield, Ill.: C. C. Thomas, 1953. The same author presents a detailed analysis of 33 cases of boy and girl murderers: Lauretta Bender, 'Children and Adolescents Who Have Killed', *American Journal of Psychiatry* (1959) **116**: 510–513. A study of 3 cases is presented by Melitta Schmideberg, 'The Child Murderer', Chapter 15 in H. A. Bloch (ed.), *Crime in America*, New York: Philosophical Library, 1961, pp. 202–210. A paper by W. M. Easson and R. M. Steinhilber ('Murderous Aggression by Children and Adolescents', *Archives of General Psychiatry* (1961) **4**: 1: 1–7) based on 8 cases from the Mayo Clinic, submits the hypothesis that children and adolescent murders are fostered by parents, sometimes unconsciously. This conclusion is denied on grounds of unsufficient analysis of 'psychosomatic dispositions' by Joseph J. Michaels, 'Enuresis in Murderous Aggressive Children and Adolescents', *Archives of General Psychiatry* (1961) **5**: 490–493. More general books and articles have been written by:

Lucy Freeman and Wilfred C. Hulse, *Children Who Kill*, New York: Berkley Publishing Corporation, 1962.

Charlotte Banks, 'Violence', *Howard Journal* (1962) **11**: 1: 13–25.

N. Schipkowensky, 'L'omicidio dei familiari commesso da minorenni', *Quaderni di Criminologia Clinica* (1963) **5**: 4: 425–460.

E. Podolsky, 'Children Who Kill', *Acta Criminol. Med. Leg. Jap.* (1964) **30**: 2: 31–42.

113. See Chapter 2, *passim*.

114. See W. Lindesay Neustatter, *The Mind of the Murderer*, New York: Philosophical Library, 1957; and W. Lindesay Neustatter, *Psychological Disorders and Crime*, London: C. Johnson, 1953.

115. Emanuel Messinger and Benjamin Apfelberg, 'Rapporti esistenti tra comportamento criminale e psicosi, debolezza mentale e tipi di personalità', *Quaderni di criminologia clinica* (1960) **3**: 269–315.

116. Guy Benoit, *Conférences de Psychiatrie, Fascicule III, Psychiatrie Médico-Légale*, Paris: Doin, 1964. More specifically limited to an aggression study of different psychiatric nosographies is Ben Karpman, 'Aggression', *American Journal of Orthopsychiatry* (1950) **20**: 694–718. The emphasis of this latter paper is on an orthodox psychoanalytic approach.

117. Aaron H. Esman, 'Diagnostic Categories of "Delinquency" ', *National Probation and Parole Association Journal* (1955) **1**: 2: 113–117.

118. Georg K. Stürup, *Homicides*, Mimeographed Report, presented at

the XIV International Congress of Applied Psychology, Copenhagen, 1961. See also Georg K. Stürup, 'The Psychology of Murderers', *Journal of the Irish Medical Association* (1964) **54**:**319**:27–32.
119. Following are some of the classic writings on this topic:

Nikola Schipkowensky, *Schizophrenie und Mord*, Berlin: Springer,
1938.

K. Willmanns, 'Über Mord im Prodromalstadium der Schizophrenie', *Z. Ges. Neurol. u. Psychiat.* (1940) **170**:583–662.

H. Helweg, *Den retslige psykiatri*, Copenhagen: 1949.

E. Szansky, 'Das Initialdelikt', *Arch. Psychiat.* (1950) **185**:395.

S. Reichard and C. Tillman, 'Murder and Suicide as Defenses
Against Schizophrenic Psychosis', *Journal of Clinical Psychopathology* (1950) **2**:149–163.

E. Podolsky, 'The Paranoid Murderer', *Samiksa* (1956) **10**:65–69.

Nikola Schipkowensky, 'Psychose und Mord', *Wien. Med. Wschr.*
(1957) **2**:54–57.

Nikola Schipkowensky, *Schizophrenie und Mord*, Congress Reports
IV, 433–443, II International Kongress f. Psychiatrie, Zurich,
1957.

John M. MacDonald, *The Murderer and His Victim*, Springfield,
Ill.: C. C. Thomas, 1961, Chapter 10, pp. 224–233.

Irving Kaufmann, 'Crimes of Violence and Delinquency in Schizophrenic Children', *Journal of the American Academy of Child
Psychiatry* (1962) **1**:269–283.

Irving Kaufmann, Harry Durkin, Thomas Krank, Lora W. Heims,
Dorothea B. Jones, Zelda Ryter, Edward Stone, and John
Zilbach, 'Delineation in Two Diagnostic Groups Among
Juvenile Delinquents: The Schizophrenic and the Impulse-
Ridden Character Disorder', *Journal of the American Academy
of Child Psychiatry* (1963) **2**:292–318.

S. Kuroda and H. Nagamori, 'On Several Cases of Murder Committed by Psychotics', *Acta Criminol. Med. Leg. Jap.* (1964)
30:**1**:22–23.

120. Several authors are critical of the *Initialdelikt* hypothesis. Bürger
Prinz has stated the difficulty of differential diagnosis and the low
incidence of real schizophrenia in murder cases: H. Bürger Prinz,
'Schizophrenie und Mord, I Beitrage', *Mschr. Krim. Psychol.*
(1940) **31**:28, and 'II Beitrage', *Mschr. Krim. Psychol.* (1941)
149:32. Dukor, quoting Wyrsch, expresses a similar opinion: B.
Dukor, 'Aus dem Grenzgebiet zwischen Psychiatrie and Recht',
Schweiz. Juristen Z. (1946), 198.
    J. Wyrsch, *Psychopathologie und Verbrechen*, Innsbruck: Tyrolia,
1949. See also, Aldo Semerari, 'Sui rapporti tra le malattie mentali
e i comportamenti criminali', chapter in Benigno Di Tullio,
Principi di Criminologia Clinica, Roma: Istituto di Medicina Sociale
1963. In a survey of 57,000 criminal subjects examined over a
period of 25 years, Messinger and Apfelberg (*op. cit.*, pp. 272–273)

found an incidence of psychosis which rarely was higher than 1 per cent. Although their cases included all types of criminal behavior, the incidence of psychosis was strikingly low.

121. Aldo Semerari and Achille Calabrese, *Considerazioni critiche sul concetto di 'omicidio schizofrenico'*, Roma: La Tipografica, 1963.

122. For a complete listing of relevant psychometric and psychiatric papers and monographs, see Franco Ferracuti, *Intelligenza e criminalità, Bibliografia*, Milano: Giuffrè, 1966, which includes about one thousand items. Recent articles are: E. Culbertson, G. M. Guthrie, A. J. Butler and L. Gorlow, 'Patterns of Hostility Among the Retarded', *American Journal of Mental Deficiency* (1961) **66**:**3**:421–427; Nikola Schipkowensky, 'On Delinquency in Mental Defectives', *International Annals of Criminology* (1964) **2**:390–396. MacDonald, *op. cit.*, 1961, Chapter 14, pp. 271–277, discusses 'Mental Deficiency and Murder'. In the Messinger and Apfelberg paper, quoted in note 120, the authors found that only around 2 per cent of this general criminal population were mentally defective. On the general problem of feeblemindness and criminality, see Nikola Schipkowensky, *Schwachsinn und Verbrechen*, Jena: Fischer, 1962.

123. See H. Bürger Prinz and H. Lewrenz, *Die Alterskriminalität*, Ferdinand Enke Verlag, 1961, for a recent review of this topic, which contains a plea for special penal considerations for old-age criminality, along the same lines used for juvenile offenders. Also, M. E. Adams and C. B. Vedder, 'Age and Crime: Medical and Sociologic Characteristics of Prisoners over 50', *Geriatrics* (1961) **16**:**4**:177–181.

124. A. Ferraro, 'Senile Psychoses', Chapter 51 in Silvano Arieti, *American Handbook of Psychiatry*, Vol. II, New York: Basic Books, 1959.

125. John Lanzkron, 'Murder as a Reaction to Paranoid Delusions in Involutional Psychosis and Its Prevention', *American Journal of Psychiatry* (1961) **118**:**5**:426–427.

126. General discussions of epilepsy and murder are included in many major treatises. See, for example, W. Lindesay Neustatter, *op. cit.*, 1953, and John M. MacDonald, *op. cit.*, 1961, Chapter 11. Recent papers are: Ralph S. Banay, 'Criminal Genesis and the Degrees of Responsibility in Epilepsies', *American Journal of Psychiatry* (1961) **117**:**10**:873–876; L. E. Keating, 'Epilepsy and Behavior Disorder in School Children', *Journal of Mental Science* (1961) **107**:**446**:161–180. On the basis of a large case collection (15,000 cases) Livingston states that the incidence of crime in epileptics is no greater than among non-epileptics: S. Livingston, 'Epilepsy and Murder', *Journal of the American Medical Association* (1964) **188**:**2**:172.

The role of organic brain injury has already been discussed in the previous section of this chapter. Other relevant references include:

Sol Levy, 'Post-Encephalitic Behavior Disorder. A Forgotten Entity. A Report of 100 Cases', *American Journal of Psychiatry* (1959) **115**:1062–1067.

Asenath Petrie, Rook McCulloch, and Phoebe Kazdin, 'The Perceptual Characteristics of Juvenile Delinquents', *Journal of Nervous and Mental Diseases* (1962) **134**:415–421.

Th. B. Kraft, 'Afasie, verbale onbekwaamheid en lichamelijk agresief gedrag', *Ned. J. Geneesk* (1903) **107**:43:1964–1967.

Franz Petersohn, 'Les lésions cérébrales criminogènes', *International Annals of Criminology* (1964) **2**:373–389.

127. K. Witton, 'Automatism and Narcoanalysis', *Dis. Nerv. Syst.* (1962) **23**:12:695–697.

128. Guy Benoit, *op. cit.*, 1964, p. 146; J. McGeorge, 'Alcohol and Crime', *Med. Sci. Law* (1963) **3**:2:27–48.

129. Marvin E. Wolfgang and Rolf B. Strohm, 'The Relationship between Alcohol and Criminal Homicide', *Quarterly Journal of Studies on Alcohol* (1956) **17**:411–425.

130. E. Podolsky, 'The Manic Murder', *Correctional Psychiatry and Journal of Social Therapy* (1964) **10**:4:213–217.

131. See W. Lindesay Neustatter, *Depression as a Defence to Murder*, Report presented at the Quatrième Congrès de l'Académie Internationale de Médecine Légale et de Médecine Sociale, Genova: 1955; J. C. Batt, 'Homicidal Incidence in the Depressive Psychoses', *Journal of Mental Science* (1948) **94**:782–792; H. L. Burks and S. I. Harrison, 'Aggressive Behavior as a Means of Avoiding Depression', *American Journal of Orthopsychiatry* (1962) **32**:3:416–422.

132. See *infra* Chapter V, note 13. Additional references include:

A. Raven, 'Murder and Suicide as Marks of an Abnormal Mind', *Sociological Review* (1929) **21**:3.

R. G. Gordon, 'Certain Personality Problems in Relation to Mental Illness with Special Reference to Suicide and Homicide', *British Journal Med. Psychol.* (1929) **9**:60–66.

M. Levi-Bianchini, 'Il suicidio e l'omicidio degli alienati internati negli ospedali psichiatrici', *Arch. Gen. di Neurol. Psichiat. e Psicoanal.* (1933) **14**:205–278.

Karl Menninger, 'Psychoanalytic Aspects of Suicide', *International Journal of Psychoanalysis* (1933) **14**:376–390.

S. Ravicini, 'Omicidio e suicidio', *Difesa Sociale* (1934) **7**:367–374.

M. Grzywo-Dabrowska, 'Samobojstwo wspolne oraz z samoboitwen zlaczone', *Hig. psychiczn.* (1936) **2**:75–98.

G. Elsässer, 'Zur Frage des Familien- und Selbstmordes', *Allg. Z. Psychiat.* (1939) **110**:207–219.

Nikola Schipkowensky, 'Mitgehen und Mitnehmen in den Tod', *Psychiatrie Neurologie und Medizinische Psychologie* (1963) **15**:6–7; 226–234.

J. Cohen, 'Forme di suicidio e loro interpretazione', *Triangolo* (1965) **7**:1:2–8.

133. This is, for example, Abrahamsen's interpretation of the Leopold and Loeb case. See D. Abrahamsen, *op. cit.*, 1944, 1960, note 111.

For another psychoanalytic interpretation of the same case in novel form, see Meyer Levin, *Compulsion*, New York: Simon & Schuster, 1956.

134. Saverio Siciliano, 'Risultati preliminari di una indagine sull'omicidio in Danimarca', *La Scuola Positiva* (1961) 4: 718–729.

135. Hans von Hentig, *The Criminal and His Victim*, New Haven, Conn.: Yale University Press, 1948.

136. W. Eliasberg, 'The Murdered to Get Hanged: A Pre-analytical Case History of 1783', *Psychoanalytic Review* (1952) 39: 164–167.

137. See D. Abrahamsen, *op. cit.*, 1944, and S. Hurwitz, *Criminologia*, Firenze: Macrí, 1954.

138. Marvin E. Wolfgang, 'Suicide by Means of Victim-Precipitated Homicide', *Journal of Clinical and Experimental Psychopathology and Quarterly Review of Psychiatry and Neurology* (1959) 20:4:345–349.

139. For recent classifications of the psychopathic group, see Emanuel Messinger and Benjamin Apfelberg, *op. cit.*, 1960; also, John M. MacDonald, *op. cit.*, 1961, Chapter 12, pp. 247–260.

140. See, among others, the following:

A. Rorsch, *Mord und Mordversuch bei Psychopathie*, Giessen: Meyer, 1934.

F. Wertham, 'The Catathymic Crisis', *Arch. Neurol. and Psychiat.* (1937) 37: 974–978.

Joseph J. Michaels, 'Psychobiologic Interpretation of Delinquency', *American Journal of Orthopsychiatry* (1940) 10:3: 501–509.

F. Wertham, *The Show of Violence*, Garden City, N.Y.: Doubleday, 1949.

J. Frosh and S. B. Wortis, 'A Contribution to the Nosology of the Impulse Disorders', *American Journal of Psychiatry* (1954) 3:2: 133–138.

Richard G. Singer and C. C. Shaw, 'The Passive-Aggressive Personality', *U.S. Armed Forces Medical Journal* (1957) 8: 62–69.

Joseph J. Michaels, 'Character Structure and Character Disorders', Chapter 19 in S. Arieti (ed.), *American Handbook of Psychiatry*, Vol. I., New York: Basic Books, 1959.

N. Masor, 'Psychopathology of the Social Deviate', Chapter in J. S. Rouček, *Sociology of Crime*, New York: Philosophical Library, 1961, pp. 93–137.

Elizabeth S. Mackay and Edleff H. Schwaab, 'Some Problems in the Differential Diagnosis of Antisocial Character Disorders in Early Latency', *Journal of the American Academy of Child Psychiatry* (1962) 1: 414–430.

John N. Rosen, 'Acting-out and Acting-in', *American Journal of Psychotherapy* (1963) 17: 390–403.

141. Benigno Di Tullio, 'Sulle reazioni abnormi e sugli sviluppi psico-patici di maggiore interesse nel campo criminologico', *La Scuola Positiva* (1959) 1: 85–108.

142. J. C. M. Matheson, 'Infanticide', *Med. Leg. Rev.* (1941) 9:135–152.
Gladys McDermaid and Emil Winkler, 'Psychopathology of Infanticide', *Journal of Clinical and Experimental Psychopathology and Quarterly Review of Psychiatry and Neurology* (1955) 16:22–41.
    H. M. Klingler, 'Zum Problem der Kindesmörderin', *Kriminalistik* (1959) 13:5:192–194.
    A. H. Chapman, 'Obsession of Infanticide', *AMA, Arch. Gen. Psychiat.* (1959) 1:12–16.
    R. Holzer, 'Ein Beitrag zum mütterlichen Kindesmord', *Dtsch. Z. Ges. gerichtl. Med.* (1961), 51:1:1–6.

143. Lauretta Bender, 'Psychiatric Mechanisms in Child Murderers', *Journal of Nervous and Mental Diseases* (1934) 80:32–47.
    J. H. Morton, 'Female Homicides', *Journal of Mental Science* (1934) 80:64–74.
    Groves B. Smith, 'Murder of Infants by Parents in Situations of Stress', *Journal of Social Therapy* (1960) 6:1:9–17.
    L. Adelson, 'Slaughter of the Innocents, A Study of Forty-six Homicides in Which the Victims were Children', *New England Journal of Medicine* (1961) 264:26:1345–1349.
    R. Gatti, 'L'omicidio del fanciullo', *Minerva Medico-Legale* (1963) 5:134–141.

144. For a recent review of the abundant literature on this syndrome and an analysis of three cases, see Franco Ferracuti, Mario Fontanesi, Giorgio Legramante, and Ezio Zilli, 'La sindrome del bambino maltrattato. Rassegna della letteratura ed esemplificazione clinica', *Quaderni di Criminologia Clinica* (1966) 2.

145. For recent papers on this topic, see B. A. O'Connel, 'Amnesia and Homicide', *British Journal of Delinquency* (1960) 10:4:262–276, based on 50 cases; and E. Podolsky, 'Somnambulistic Homicide', *Medicine, Science and the Law* (1961) 1:3:260–265; E. Podolsky, 'Somnambulistic Homicide', *American Journal of Psychiatry* (1964) 121:2:191–192.

146. Arnold H. Buss, *op. cit.*, 1961, Chapter 11, pp. 207–220.

147. *Ibid.*, pp. 217–219.

148. L. G. Carpenter, 'Relation of Aggression in the Personality to Outcome with Electro-Convulsive Shock Therapy', *Journal of General Psychology* (1957) 57:3–22 (cited by Buss).

149. See, for example:

    Leon Michaux, 'L'aggressivité, facteur d'état dangéreux', in Jean Pinatel (ed.), *Deuxième Course Int. de Criminologie, Le Problème de l'état dangereux*, Paris: 1953, pp. 161–168.
    T. Tsuboi, 'Study on the Recidivism of Violence', *Psychiat. et Neurol. Jap.* (1959) 61:16.

K. Jarosch, 'Aggression', Paper presented at the 5th Congress of the International Academy of Legal Medicine and of Social Medicine, Wien: May, 1961.

W. Tuteur, 'Can Violent Behavior be Predicted?' *Correctional Psychiat. and Journal of Social Therapy* (1963) 9:1:39–43. John J. Brennan, *op. cit.*, 1964.

The supposed dangerousness of murderers should lead to use of violence, with assaults and killing, in prison. Data on six American prisons deny such dangerousness: C. H. S. Jayewardene, 'Are Murderers Dangerous?' *Prob. and Child. Care Journal* (1962) 2:1:33–35. See also a recent survey of assaults in prison reported by Thorsten Sellin, 'Homicides and Assaults in American Prisons, 1964', *Acta Criminologiae et Medicinae Legalis Japonica* (1965) 31:4:1–5.

150. John M. MacDonald, 'The Threat to Kill', *American Journal of Psychiatry* (1963) 120:2:125–130.

151. Franco Ferracuti and Marvin E. Wolfgang, 'The Prediction of Violent Behavior', *Corrective Psychiatry and Journal of Social Therapy* (1964) 10:6. For other 'prediction' approaches, linked to treatment, see the California Program (*infra*, Chapter V, note 125). Several memoranda on this program have been made available to us by John Conrad. The preliminary plan includes an analysis of violent behavior which is in accord with a subcultural hypothesis. Other 'predictive' statements, again in relation to a treatment program, are included in Carlton M. Orchinik, *The Aggressive Delinquent*, Philadelphia: County Court, Institute on Juvenile Delinquency, 1961.

152. The study of homicidal motives has always been an object of interest for psychiatric literature. Many of the 'cases' listed in note 93, *supra*, are based on such a type of analysis. The following papers should also be consulted:

F. Holtzendorff, 'Die Psychologie des Mörders', *Samml. gemeinverst. Wissenschaft* (1875) 10:232.

H. Frenkel, 'Der Mörder der nicht aus Gewinnsucht handelt', *Monatssch. f. Krimpsychol. u. Strafrechtsref.* (1929) 20:607–617.

H. Puyn, 'Beiträge zur Psychopathologie von Mord und Totschlag', *Allg. Zsch. f. Psychiat.* (1931) 93:1–2.

H. Többen, *Untersuchungsergebnisse an Totschlägern*, Berlin: Heymann, 1932.

H. Gummersbach, 'Affektbetonte Morde', *Krim. Monatsch.* (1934) 8:124–128 and 175–179.

H. Gummersbach, 'Mordmotive und Motivmorde', *Arch. Crim.* (1935) 96:58–76 and 145–155.

E. Roesner, 'Der Mord, seine Tater, Motive und Opfer nebst einer Bilbiographie zum Problem des Mordes', *Z. Strafrechtswiss.* (1936) 56:327.

P. Mohr, 'Psychologische Grundlagen zum Delikt des Mordes und des Totschlages', *Schweiz. Arch. Neurol. Psychiat.* (1938) 41:22.

L. H. Cohen and T. E. Coffin, 'The Pattern of Murder in Insanity: A Criterion of the Murderer's Abnormality', *Journal of Criminal Law and Criminology* (1947) **37**: 262–287.

Enrico Altavilla, *La dinamica del delitto*, Vol. II. Torino: U.T.E.T., 1953.

R. Pilmes, 'Frauen als Anstifterinnen', *Nervenarzt* (1953) **24**:248–251.

Motive analysis in juvenile homicide has been studied by Aldo Semerari and Maria Sciarra, 'L'omicidio nei minori. Parte I. I Motivi', *Infanzia Anormale* (1954) **9**:681–692; Aldo Semerari and Maria Sciarra, 'L'omicidio nei minori. Parte II. Casistica', *Infanzia Anormale* (1956) **19**:447–461.

Jealousy as a specific motive has been studied by S. Di Frisco, 'Lo stato di dubbio e lo stato di certezza in rapporto al delitto per gelosia', *Arch. Antrop. Crim.* (1934) **54**: 708–713; G. Langfeldt, 'The Erotic Jealousy Syndrome', *Acta Psychiat. Scand.* (1961) **36**:151; Bruno M. Cormier, 'Psychodynamics of Homicide Committed in a Marital Relationship', in Israel Drapkin (ed.), *Proceedings of the 12th International Course in Criminology, The Causation and Prevention of Crime in Developing Countries*, Vol. II, Part 2, Jerusalem: The Hebrew University of Jerusalem, 1963, pp. 371–383. This last paper examines the general problem of uxoricide.

153. For a detailed discussion of motivational analysis from the viewpoints of the psychometric and the phenomenological approaches in offenders, see Franco Ferracuti and Aldo Semerari, *Analisi dei motivi nella valutazione della personalità dell'imputato*, Roma: Istituto di Medicina Legale e delle Assicurazioni, 1963 (Reprinted from *Zacchia*, 1963, 1–2).

154. On 'motiveless' murder the following papers should be consulted:

P. Guiraud, 'Les meurtres immotivés', *L'Évolution Psychiatrique* (1931), 23–24.

E. Podolsky, 'Notes on Motiveless Murder', *International Journal of Social Psychiatry* (1956) **1**:4: 42–45.

A. W. Stearns, 'Murder by Adolescents with Obscure Motivation', *American Journal of Psychiatry* (1957) **114**:303–305.

R. Herren, 'Der Mord ohne Motiv', *Psychol. Rdsch.* (1958) **9**:273–290.

R. Herren, 'Gibt es Morde ohne Motiv', *Kriminalistik* (1960), 509.

155. Joseph Satten, Karl Menninger, Irwin Rosen, and Martin Mayman, 'Murder Without Apparent Motive: A Study in Personality Disorganization', *American Journal of Psychiatry* (1960) **116**: 48–53.

156. Tullio Bazzi and Mario Fontanesi, 'Il delitto nevrotico', *Quaderni di Criminologia Clinica* (1962) **1**: 47–61.

157. Arnold H. Buss, *op. cit.*, 1961.

158. Elton B. McNeil, *op. cit.*, 1959.

159. Leonard Berkowitz, *op. cit.*, 1962.

160. The psychoanalytic approach to violence has been briefly mentioned in Chapter III. A listing of additional relevant references is provided below:

Sigmund Freud, *The Ego and the Id*, London: Hogarth, 1927.

Anna Freud, *The Ego and the Mechanisms of Defence*, London: Hogarth, 1937.

P. R. Lehrman, 'Uber einige unbewusste Komponenten beim Mord', *Int. Z. Psychoanal.* (1937) 23:527–535.

P. R. Lehrman, 'Some Unconscious Determinants in Homicide', *Psychiat. Quart.* (1939) 13:605–621.

F. Wertham, 'The Matricidal Impulse: Critique of Freud's Interpretation of Hamlet', *Journal of Criminal Psychopathology* (1941) 2:455–464.

T. Reik, *The Unknown Murderer*, New York: Prentice-Hall, 1945.

Robert M. Lindner, 'The Equivalents of Matricide', *Psychoanalytic Quarterly* (1948) 17:4:453–470.

K. L. Eissler, *Searchlights on Delinquency*, New York: International Universities Press, 1949.

Anna Freud, 'Aggression, Normal and Pathological', in *The Psychoanalytic Study of the Child*, Vols. III–IV, London: Imago; New York: International Universities Press, 1949.

B. Rank, 'Aggression', in *The Psychoanalytic Study of the Child*, Vols. III–IV, London: Imago; New York: International Universities Press, 1949.

A. Aichhorn, *Wayward Youth*, London: Imago, 1951.

Robert M. Lindner, *Prescription for Rebellion*, New York: Grove Press, 1952.

Rudolf M. Loewenstein (ed.), *Drives, Affects, Behavior*, New York: International Universities Press, 1953 (see particularly the papers by Heinz Hartmann, Ernst Kris, and Rudolph M. Loewenstein, René A. Spitz, Jeanne Lampl de Groot, Anna Freud, Grete L. Bibring).

Gregory Zilboorg, *The Psychology of Criminal Act and Punishment*, New York: Harcourt, Brace, 1954.

Evoelin N. Rexford and Suzanne Taets von Amerongen, 'The Influence of Unsolved Maternal Oral Conflicts upon Impulsive Acting Out in Young Children', *American Journal of Orthpsychiatry* (1957) 27:75–87.

E. Glover, *The Roots of Crime*, Vol. II, London: Imago, 1960.

A. H. Williams, 'A Psycho-analytic Approach to the Treatment of the Murderer', *International Journal of Psycho-Analysis* (1960) 41:4–5.

A. C. Cain, 'The Pre-superego Turning-Inward of Aggression', *Psychoanalytic Quarterly* (1961) 30:2:171–208.

D. M. Lipshutz, 'Some Dynamic Factors in the Problem of Aggression', *Psychiatric Quarterly* (1961) 35:1:78–87.

H. H. Hart, 'A Review of the Psychoanalytic Literature on Passivity', *Psychiatric Quarterly* (1961) **35**:2:331–352.

P. C. Kuiper, 'Probleme der psychoanalytischen Technik in Bezug auf die passiv-feminine Gefühlseinstellung des Mannes das Verhältnis der beiden Odipuskomplexe und die Aggression', *Psyche* (1962) **16**:6:321–344.

G. Gero, 'Sadism, Masochism and Aggression: Their Role in Symptom-formation', *Psychoanalytic Quarterly* (1962) **31**:31–42.

For a recent, extensive, and balanced analysis of psychoanalytical literature on crime and aggression, see Renato Canestrari and M. Walter Battacchi, *Strutture e dinamiche della personalità nella antisocialità minorile*, Bologna: Malipiero, 1963.

161. F. Wertham, *Dark Legend: A Study in Murder*, New York: Duell, Sloan & Pearce, 1941; also, Jimenez de Asua, *infra*, note 163.

162. See *supra*, note 133.

163. R. R. Sears, *Survey of Objective Studies of Psychoanalytical Concepts*, New York: Social Science Research Council, Bulletin 51, 1943; Luis Jimenez de Asua, *Psicoanalisis criminal*, Buenos Aires: Losada, 1947, Fourth Edition. See also, Gerard S. Blum, *Psychoanalytic Theories of Personality*, New York: McGraw-Hill, 1957. For a milder criticism and an attempted integration between psychoanalytic and legal concepts, see Camargo y Marin, 'La definición psicoanalítica del delito', *Rev. jur. Veracruz* (1962) **12**:2:101–128.

164. The need for the introduction of cultural concepts in psychoanalytic theory is widely accepted today. For a recent article on this topic, see E. Becker, 'Anthropological Notes on the Concept of Aggression', *Psychiatry* (1962) **25**:4:328–338.

165. George B. Vold, *Theoretical Criminology*, New York: Oxford University Press, 1958, 125.

166. See F. E. Hartung, 'Observation, A Social Psychological Analysis', Detroit: 1961, mimeographed copy; also, Silvano Arieti, 'Schizophrenia: The Manifest Symptomatology and the Psychodynamic and Formal Mechanisms', in Silvano Arieti (ed.), *American Handbook of Psychiatry*, New York: Basic Books, 1959.

167. Several papers listed *supra*, note 160, are relevant.

168. See Chapter III, notes 124, 125; also, Karl Menninger, Martin Mayman, and Paul Pruyser, *The Vital Balance*, New York: The Viking Press, 1964; see also Melanie Klein, Paula Heimann, and Roger Money-Kyrle (eds.), *New Directions in Psycho-Analysis*, London: Tavistock Publications; New York: Basic Books, 1955.

169. See *supra*, Chapter II, note 126.

170. See *supra*, Chapter II, note 127.

171. See *supra*, Chapter II, note 128.

172. See Don C. Gibbons, *Changing the Law Breaker*, Englewood Cliffs, N.J.: Prentice-Hall, 1965, pp. 97–128. Specifically, two of the types postulated by Gibbons (X: Personal Offender, One Time Loser, and XI: Psychopathic Assaultist) describe violent offenders.

173. See *supra*, note 151 and Chapter V, note 125.
174. The theoretical statements of Lewis Yablonsky, *The Violent Gang*, New York: Macmillan, 1962, of Cloward and Ohlin (*op. cit.*), and of Leonard Berkowitz (*op. cit.*, 1962) have not been followed by extensive clinical application.
175. Arnold H. Buss, *op. cit.*, 1961, Chapters 8 and 9.
176. Arnold H. Buss and Ann Durkee, 'An Inventory for Assessing Different Kinds of Hostility', *Journal of Consulting Psychology* (1959) 23:510–513.
177. Agostino Gemelli, *La personalità del delinquente nei suoi fondamenti biologici e psicologici*, Milano: Giuffrè, 1948, Second Edition.
178. Karl F. Schuessler and Donald R. Cressey, 'Personality Characteristics of Criminals', *American Journal of Sociology* (1950) 55:5:476–483.
179. For a discussion of the Schuessler and Cressey paper, see Franco Ferracuti, 'The Contribution of Psychological Testing to Criminological Theories and to Diagnosis of Mentally Abnormal Criminals', in Gerhard Mueller (ed.), *Essays in Criminal Science*, London: Sweet and Maxwell, 1961, pp. 63–74.
180. Carl Murchison, *Criminal Intelligence*, Worcester: Clark University, 1926, p. 187. For a full bibliography on the relationship of intelligence and crime, see *supra*, note 122.
181. Eleanor T. Glueck, 'Mental Retardation and Juvenile Delinquency', *Mental Hygiene* (1935) 19:549–572.
182. I. A. Berg and Vernon Fox, 'Factors in Homicide Committed by 200 Males', *American Psychologist* (1946) 1:461. For a full text of this paper, see *Journal of Social Psychology* (1947) 26:109–119.
183. Renato Lazzari, Franco Ferracuti, Giovanni B. Rizzo, 'Applicazione della Scala di Intelligenza Wechsler-Bellevue, Forma I, su un gruppo di detenuti italiani', *Rassegna di Studi Penitenziari*, *Atti del I Convegno Int. di Criminologia Clinica* (1958), 449–456.
184. Franco Ferracuti, Renato Lazzari, and Marvin E. Wolfgang, 'The Intelligence of Puerto Rican Inmates', *Archivos de Criminologia, Neuropsiquiatria y Disciplinas Conexas* (1964) 12:47:490–509.
185. Zygmunt A. Piotrowski and David Abrahamsen 'Sexual Crime, Alcohol and the Rorschach Test', *Psychiatric Quarterly Supplement* (1952) 26: Part II:248–260. See also, New York State Department of Mental Hygiene, *Report of the Study of 102 Sex Offenders at Sing Sing Prison*, Albany: State Hospital Press, 1950.
186. We have, at several points, touched briefly on the consistent association found between alcoholic intoxication and violent crimes, and the data available (for example, Wolfgang, *op. cit.*, 1958) would seem to indicate a certain amount of specificity. Yet not all intoxicated subjects become violent. Alcohol appears to be merely a releaser of violent traits and forms of behavior which are ordinarily kept under cortical control. The Piotrowski study seems to indicate a means for predicting the probability of the emergence of violent behavior while under intoxication. The specific level of intoxication

capable of eliciting violent behavior seems to remain, however, an individual variable.

187. E. Ochneider, 'Rorschachversuche mit Mördern', *Z. diagnost. Psychol.* (1955) 3:154–169.

188. A. Paolella, *Résultats au test de Rorschach chez des Homicides*, Proceedings of the XIII Congress of Applied Psychology, Rome, 1958, 668–669.

189. Carlo Romano and A. Paolella, 'Primi risultati dell'indagine sulla personalità di alcuni detenuti per omicidio', *Difesa Sociale* (1958) 37:41–72.

190. Takayuki Tsuboi and Nobuyashi Takemura, 'A Study of Parricides', *Journal of Correctional Medicine* (1960) 9:Special Issue:53–63. Seventy-three cases of the murder of parents were examined, and in 30 'parricide' cases the Rorschach Test was applied.

191. Th. Kohlmann, 'The Possibility of Projection of the Psychopathic in the Rorschach Test', *Rev. Psychol. Appl.* (1961) 11:3:221–231.

192. A. I. Rabin, 'Homicide and Attempted Suicide: A Rorschach Study', *American Journal of Orthopsychiatry* (1946) 16:516–524. On this same issue, Samuel Beck has commented on this case study, emphasizing the difference between the first Rorschach protocol, showing danger signs consisting in dammed-up affect, and the other two Rorschach protocols, which show a broader and relaxed prevalent mode of reaction (or *Erlebnistypus*).

193. William C. Perdue, 'Rorschach Responses of 100 Murderers', *Corrective Psychiatry and Journal of Social Therapy* (1964) 10:6:322–328.

194. Ralph S. Banay, 'Study in Murder', *Annals of the American Academy of Political and Social Science* (1952) 284:26–34.

195. M. Schachter and S. Cotte, 'Nouvelle contribution à l'étude des homicides et tentatives d'homicide chez les mineurs. A propos de deux nouvelles observations', *Aggiornamento Pediatrico* (1963) 14:4:141–156.

196. E. Pakesch, 'The Influence of Imprisonment on the Psyche of the Prisoner', *Mschr. Kriminol. Strafrechtsref.* (1961) 44:3–4; 65–85, reviewed in *Excerpta Criminologica* (1962) 2:2:218:item 560.

197. See particularly the following:

Julio Endara, 'Psicodiagnostico de Rorschach y delincuencia. La representacion de la figura umana', *Archivos de Criminologia, Neuropsiquiatria y Disciplinas Conexas* (1957) 20:547–574.

Julio Endara, 'Psicodiagnostico de Rorschach. Reserches de clinique psychologiques', *Zeitschrift für Diagnostische Psychologie und Personlichkeitsforschung* (1955) 4:311–374.

Julio Endara, 'Degradaciones y desvitalizaciones en los delincuentes a través del test de Rorschach', *Archivos de Criminologia, Neuropsiquiatria y Disciplinas Conexas* (1959) 7:26:167–182 (Also in *Quaderni di Criminologia Clinica* (1960) 1:21–36).

198. Bernard Serebrinsky, *El psicodiagnostico de Rorschach en los homicidas*, Cordoba, Argentina: Imprenta de la Universidad, 1941.

199. For a description of the 'scale', which combines psychoanalytic and perceptual elements, see Myriam Orr, *Le test de Rorschach et l'Imago Maternelle*, Paris: Group Français du Rorschach, 1958.

200. Giovanni B. Rizzo and Franco Ferracuti, 'Impiego del test di Rorschach in Criminologia Clinica', *Rassegna di Studi Penitenziari* (1959) 1:23-50.

201. The ratio between movement and color responses (or *Erlebnistypus*) corresponds to a basic, poorly differentiated typology ranging from, but not exactly corresponding to, extroverts and introverts.

202. Within the color responses, the more the color dominates the less the subject is able to control his emotional expressions. Thus, the ratio between pure color (C) and color-form (CF) responses, versus the form-color (FC) responses is a measure of emotional control.

203. For the importance of the FC (form-color) responses, see *supra*, note 202.

204. In a recent study by Canestrari and Battacchi (Renato Canestrari and M. Walter Battacchi, *Strutture e dinamiche della personalità nella antisocialità minorile*, Bologna: Malipiero, 1963, p. 220) 32 per cent of a group of 193 juvenile delinquents did not give any human-content response on the Rorschach Test. For further analysis of the value of the human-content Rorschach response for the diagnosis of aggressive trends, see the papers by Endara listed in note 197, and also Bruno Klopfer and collaborators, *Developments in the Rorschach Technique*, New York: World Book Co., 1954, Vol. I, p. 379; Zygmunt A. Piotrowski, *Perceptanalysis*, New York: Macmillan, 1957, p. 344; E. Bohn, *Traité du Psychodiagnostic de Rorschach*, Paris: P.U.F., 1955, pp. 95, 280.

205. Leslie Phillips and J. G. Smith, *Rorschach Interpretation: Advanced Technique*, New York: Grune & Stratton, 1953. In the opinion of these authors, anatomical content responses in general are a contraindication of direct bodily assault and acting-out; however, 'bony' anatomical responses are a repression of aggression, while 'visceral' anatomical responses indicate an inclination to open verbal expressions of hostility. Hostility has been found to be associated with 'white space' responses in the Rorschach, but this sign is unreliable and responses of this type are rare. For an analysis of the value of 'white space' responses, see Ephraim Rosen, 'MMPI and Rorschach Correlates of the Rorschach White Space Response', *Journal of Clinical Psychology* (1952) 8:3:283-288.

206. For a detailed and careful analysis of the Rorschach content scales as a measurement of aggression, see Arnold H. Buss, *op. cit.*, 1961, pp. 128-135 and 137-138. The first, and one of the most frequently used, content scales for aggression was designed by Elizur (Abraham Elizur, 'Content Analysis of the Rorschach with Regard to Anxiety and Hostility', *Journal of Projective Techniques* (1949) 12:1:247-284). According to Buss, the content scoring systems measure a personality variable of aggressiveness, but they relate only to long-term trends in aggression and not to transient and experimentally induced

aggressive trends. The hostility that is elicited is consciously present to the subject, and is not subconscious. This would seem to make the Rorschach Test of particular value in subcultural analyses, for the subcultural personality variables should be long-term; moreover, it should be useful in the examination of criminal subjects who may be aware of their hostility but unwilling to express it.

207. Alan P. Towbin, 'Hostility in Rorschach Content and Overt Aggressive Behavior', *The Journal of Abnormal and Social Psychology* (1959) 3:312–316.

208. For an analysis of cross-cultural studies, see the chapter on this topic in B. Klopfer and collaborators, *op. cit.*, Vol. II. For a specific Rorschach study of subcultural variables, see Seymour Fisher and Rhoda Lee Fisher, 'A Projective Test Analysis of Ethnic Subculture Themes in Families', *Journal of Projective Techniques* (1960) 24:4:366–369.

209. Beck (Samuel J. Beck, *The Rorschach Experiment*, New York: Grune & Stratton, 1960) describes a 'symptomatic aggressiveness' (pp. 228–229) characterized by white space responses, a color-dominated *Erlebnistypus*, CF and C responses, poor form responses, and an 'adaptive aggressiveness' (pp. 234–235). The identifying Rorschach signs are the same in both defensive syndromes and they also present aggressive contents. Their positive, adjusted, or negative symptomatic character is a matter of degree of concomitant personality traits.

210. A. Paolella, *Résultats au TAT chez des homicides*, Rome: Proceedings of the XIII Congress of Applied Psychology, 1958, pp. 669–670.

211. H. Stone, 'The TAT Aggressive Content Scale', *Journal of Projective Techniques* (1956) 4:445–452. The scale used by Stone identified murder cases correctly with a t value of 2·98 ($p < 0.01$).

212. Giovanni B. Rizzo, *Studio di un gruppo di 20 omicidi con il metodo MAPS*, Atti dell'XI Convegno degli Psicologi Italiani, Milano: Vita e Pensiero, 1956. This study is based on 20 homicide subjects compared with 20 property offenders. The MAPS stories were examined 'blindly'. A reliability coefficient of +0·89 was obtained between two independent judges for a sample of the stories. The p value for the identification of the homicide offenders was less than 0·01. The scoring system used for the MAPS stories was that proposed by Fine (R. Fine, *Manual for Scoring Scheme for Verbal Projective Techniques, TAT, MAPS, and the Like*, University of Southern California: unpublished manual, 1948) and utilized by Walker (Robert G. Walker, 'A Comparison of Clinical Manifestations of Hostility with Rorschach and MAPS Test Performances', *Journal of Projective Techniques* (1951) 15:1:444–460).

213. Herbert C. Goldenberg, 'A Résumé of Make-A-Picture-Story (MAPS) Test Results', *Journal of Projective Techniques* (1951) 15:1:79–86.

214. Zygmunt A. Piotrowski, 'A New Evaluation of the Thematic Apperception Test', *Psychoanalytic Review* (April, 1950), 101–127.

215. See end of Chapter III. A recent study by Peterson, Pittman, and O'Neal on 19 cases found more aggression in assaultive, violent offenders (R. A. Peterson, D. J. Pittman, and P. O'Neal, 'Stabilities in Deviance: A Study of Assaultive and Non-Assaultive Offenders', *Journal of Criminal Law, Criminology and Police Science* (1962) 53:1:44–48. Another study, by Rizzo, failed to differentiate between 50 homicides and 30 thieves, examined with the Rosenzweig Picture-Frustration Study (Giovanni B. Rizzo, *Il Rosenzweig P-F Study applicato ad un gruppo di omicidi e ad un gruppo di autori di reati contro la proprietà*, V Congresso Internazionale Rorschach, Freiburg, 1961). In an interesting study of the relationship between length of incarceration and direction of aggression, based on two groups of 40 inmates each, Peizer was able to assess the changes in the direction of aggression (in the sense of less extra-aggression and more intra-aggression) after three years of incarceration, with the Rosenzweig P-F Study. (Sheldon B. Peizer, 'Effect of Incarceration on the Direction of Aggressive Behavior', *The Journal of Correctional Psychology* (1956) 1:1–2; 26–31.)

216. For a discussion of this point, of basic importance to all projective-test analysis of offenders' behavior, see Saul Rosenzweig, 'Levels of Behavior in Psychodiagnosis with Special Reference to the Picture-Frustration Study', *American Journal of Orthopsychiatry* (1950) 20:63–72, and also the more recent paper, Saul Rosenzweig, 'Validity of the Rosenzweig Picture-Frustration Study with Felons and Delinquents', *Journal of Consulting Psychology* (1963) 27:6:535–536. This last study reviews all pertinent published researches on offenders with the P-F test. An 'assaultive' convict may well respond to the test situation at an opinion level and give non-extrapunitive responses.

217. P. Coppola, 'Il test di Luescher in criminologia', *Rassegna di Studi Penitenziari* (1953) 539–546.

218. Hans Walder, *Drive Structure and Criminality. Crimino-biologic Investigations*, Springfield, Ill.: C. C. Thomas, 1959. This author assumes a close correspondence between character traits, or drives, and type of offense and even proposes that the Szondi Test be used as a method of *criminal inquiry*, to rule out those subjects whose drive structure does not conform to the criminal behavior under investigation. The validity of the Szondi Test is far from being proved, and the conclusions of Walder appear unwarranted and over-enthusiastic.

219. F. Oliver Brachfeld, 'El fatoanalisis de Szondi y la criminologia', *Archivos de Criminologia, Neuropsiquiatria y Disciplinas Conexas* (1955) 11:457–467.

220. P. Spadaro, 'Contributo allo studio del test di Goodenough in varie categorie di criminali', *Quaderni di Criminologia Clinica* (1960) 4:459–468.

221. M. Schachter, 'Su di una tematica significativa nel test di Goodenough in minori accusati di aggressione criminale', *Quaderni di Criminologia Clinica* (1960) 1:37–46.

222. U. Vaccaro, 'Il reattivo dell'albero degli omicidi', *Bollettino di Psicologia Applicata* (1960) **40–41–42**:29–37.
223. Barry Brieldin, Zygmunt A. Piotrowski, and Edwin E. Wagner, *The Hand Test*, Springfield, Ill.: C. C. Thomas, 1962. This new test, based on the interpretation of actions performed by hands drawn in various ambiguous poses, is short, easy to administer and score, and, at least from the initial results, valid. In two groups of 32 normal adults and 59 inmates, aggressive responses were 7 per cent and 15 per cent respectively. The 'acting-out score' differentiated successfully between 'acting-out' and 'non-acting-out' inmates, and between recidivists and non-recidivists. The test also seems capable of differentiating aggressive from non-aggressive hospitalized schizophrenics. See Edwin E. Wagner and Eugene Medvedeff, 'Differentiation of Aggressive Behavior of Institutionalized Schizophrenics with the Hand Test', *Journal of Projective Techniques* (1963) **27**:1.
224. See Buss, *op. cit.*, Chapter 9.
225. For Buss's questionnaire, see *supra* note 176. For the Collins and Wrightman study, see W. Collins and E. L. S. Wrightman, 'Indicators of the Maladjustment in Preadolescent and Adolescent Boys', *American Psychologist* (1962) **17**:**16**:318. (Abstract of paper presented at the 17th Annual Convention of the American Psychological Association, St Louis, 1962.)
226. Ephraim Rosen, *op. cit.*, 1952. See also *supra*, note 205.
227. Marvin W. Kahn, 'A Comparison of Personality, Intelligence, and Social History of Two Criminal Groups', *Journal of Social Psychology* (1959) **49**:3–40.
228. Marvin W. Kahn, 'A Factor-Analytic Study of Personality, Intelligence and Social History Characteristics of Murderers', paper read at the 73rd annual meeting of the American Psychological Association, Chicago, September 3–7, 1965.
229. See Ernest L. V. Shelley and Hans H. Toch, 'The Perception of Violence as an Indicator of Adjustment in Institutionalized Offenders', *Journal of Criminal Law, Criminology and Police Science* (1962) **53**:4:463–469. Also, Hans H. Toch, 'The Stereoscope. A New Frontier in Psychological Research', *The Research Newsletter* (1961) **3**:18–22; Hans H. Toch and R. Schulte, 'Readiness to Perceive Violence as a Result of Police Training', *British Journal of Psychology* (1961) **52**:389.

V · Social Investigations of Homicide and Treatment and Research Related to Subculture of Violence

Many of the methodologically critical comments we have made about biological, psychiatric, and psychological studies can be applied to what may be called social investigations and sociological researches on aggressive crime, particularly homicide. If endocrinological and electroencephalographic (EEG) examinations have been made on homicide offenders without reference to sociological data, it is equally the case that social categories of homicide offenders have been established by sociologists who have by-passed all or most of the other disciplines that could have contributed to their analyses.

This disciplinary insularity is not only the classic case of the several blind men separately examining the elephant and separately discovering distinctly different parts; more than this, these are scientists with sight but little peripheral vision and inadequate communication among themselves. The domain of ignorance is only slowly and sparsely punctured by isolated probes. Like the child with a picture composed of numbered dots, the worker with an interdisciplinary approach seeks to draw lines between these probes in the hope that from such linkage a general abstraction will emerge. Unless teams of different talents mount the attack of researching the problems, neither the age, race, and sex of a thousand cases, nor the hypoglycemia of six homicide offenders, will add up to anything very meaningful.

As in the earlier chapters of this volume, our major purpose is to present a summary analysis and to draw upon references to determine the interplay of correlative forces that appear to contribute to our notion of a subculture of violence. In previous publications we have examined homicide studies in detail;[1] there is no need to dwell on the abundance of statistical computations from officially published rates or from special sociological studies on limited populations. The present review, therefore, is focused on the subculture of violence and includes: (1) a set of interpretative conclusions generated by relatively systematic research that has analysed data; (2) a display of culture case studies on homicide from different countries; and (3) a brief discussion of the control, prevention, and treatment of violent crime. These sections, as we shall see, appear to contribute substantially to the emphasis we have placed on culture values in conflict and to the delimited, socially circumscribed parameters within which the use of violence occurs.

The level and types of statistics used in sociological research on homicide and other assaultive crimes vary considerably. Some researchers, for instance Harlan[2] and Wolfgang,[3] have predominantly used police statistics, others have used court convictions and still others, for example Gillin,[4] prisoner populations. Rates will vary, of course, according to the official level chosen, but for general theorizing purposes these differences are not serious impediments. Moreover, although the level of police efficiency in apprehending offenders, and the probability of offense reporting, may also vary considerably between and within culture areas, homicide anywhere still remains one of the most highly visible crimes. Consistency of social variables over time and space tends to reduce the impact of valid criticisms which these probability functions may have in a detailed critique of international criminal statistics.

THE MAIN VARIABLES EMPLOYED
IN SOCIOLOGICAL INVESTIGATIONS

AGE AND SEX

If aggression in general is associated with age and sex, homicide, as an explicit behavioral form of aggression, is especially so. Almost universally it can be asserted that the highest incidence of assaultive crimes such as homicide is found among young offenders, most of whom are in their twenties, many of whom are in their late teens or early thirties.[5] Males predominate everywhere.[6] But, as Verkko has pointed out, when the general criminal homicidal rate is low in a given culture, the percentage of female offenders is generally higher than when the homicide rate is high, thus suggesting a greater stability in the amount of female homicide.[7]

It would appear to be incorrect to claim that, as women experience a social status more closely resembling equality with men, female homicide increases. If we can judge by the United States and other Western countries, woman's right to vote, her greater participation in the labor force and in family decision-making episodes, and so on, have not significantly raised her rate of assaultive crime. The anthropological evidence from societies with more than the usual amount of female responsibility and economic activity does not clearly indicate woman's greater criminal aggression.[8] It would, perhaps, be revealing to construct a culture rating scheme on the basis of some kind of masculine-feminine continuum, and then to obtain rates of crimes of violence committed by men and by women in each rated culture. It may be argued that in the United States, where the homicide rate has been steadily declining from the 1920s to the 1960s while the status of the sexes in many social spheres of activity has been approaching equality, there has been an increasing feminization of the culture. Instead of females becoming more like males, males have increasingly taken on some of the roles and attributes formerly assigned mostly to females. Add to this notion the suggestion that, with the continual diminution of earlier frontier mores, which placed a premium on male aggressiveness, other attributes of masculinity have gained currency. The gun and fist have been substantially replaced by financial ability, by capacity to manipulate others in complex economic or political bureaucracies, even, among some groups, by intellectual talents. The thoughtful wit, the easy verbalizer, the computer programmer, even the striving musician or artist, represent, in the dominant culture, equivalents of male assertiveness where the broad shoulders and fighting fists were once the major symbols. The young culture heroes may range from Van Cliburn to the Beatles, but Billy the Kid is a figure from an earlier age or from fantasy.

That the rates of violent crimes are high among certain male groups in a culture suggests that these groups still, and strongly, retain notions of *maschismo*, continue to equate maleness with overt physical aggression.[9] Because the young male is better equipped physically than the very young, the middle-aged, or the very old to manifest this form of masculinity; because the youthful male, once having learned this normative value, needs no special education to employ the agents of physical aggression (fists, feet, lithe agility); and because he seeks reinforcement from others for his ego, as do we all, and for his commitment to these values of violence, he comes to play games of conflict within his own subcultural value groups. So does the artist when he competes for a prize, the young scholar for tenure, the financier for new holding companies, and nations for propaganda advantage. But the prescribed rules for street fighting are more deadly quarrels (excepting wars) with weapons of knives, guns, and knuckles instead of the brush, the treatise, or a moon-shot.

In reviewing the literature from various disciplines on the topic of homicide, we are struck with the fact that very violent crimes are rarely committed by children, even males, under fourteen or by persons over forty years of age. When these cases occur, causal agents most frequently concentrate around individual pathologies such as brain damage and abnormal EEG patterns, or clear-cut and marked psychic disturbance, often without the usual accompanying social pathologies or immersion in a cultural milieu where violence is a more common mode of interpersonal action.[10] The child who kills his playmate or sibling and the middle-aged and middle-class woman who kills her husband are regularly perceived by officialdom as having engaged in behavior alien to their past personality performances and are often excused by reason of insanity or some similar social sinecure of exoneration. The slum delinquent gang member who slays in a fight, and the bar-room brawler who ends a drunken drama with death are officially indicted for homicides that appear to culminate lives dethroned of propriety and dignity, devoted to destruction of property and person. (We are not here arguing on behalf of the persons from our latter example as also being subjects for social protection, although we would strongly maintain that social determinism needs as much judicial recognition as does psychic determinism relative to the 'not-guilty-by-reason-of' plea.)

In general, a review of the statistical and clinical literature from many societies indicates that the age–sex category of youthful males exhibits the highest association with violent crime and that physically aggressive behavior for this group converges with notions about the masculine ideal.

SOCIAL CLASS

Social class, whatever the position of a society on a closed–open class continuum, looms large in all studies of violent crime. Although some exceptions may be noted, the finding of higher-class suicide and lower-class homicide has been so widely and firmly documented that Morselli[11] long ago posited a kind of social organic law about it, Verkko[12] and others have speculated about it as two streams of violence stemming from the same river of aggression, and Henry and Short[13] have elaborately discussed social-psychological variables of the strength of internal and external restraints in relation to self- and other-directed aggression. Henry and Short review relevant studies and, with minor exceptions, conclude that the higher the class status, the higher the incidence of suicide, and the lower the class status, the higher the incidence of homicide. In 1958 Wolfgang,[14] reporting on his own Philadelphia study of homicide and reviewing previous sociological studies with rates according to social-class indicators, noted that in the five-year Philadelphia study all homicides had been committed by representatives of the blue-collar, lower social and economic class, especially the laboring, unskilled working group.

Studies reported since 1958 and in many other languages consistently report the same observation: namely, that the overwhelming majority of homicides and other assaultive crimes are committed by persons from the lowest stratum of a social organization. Of course, it must be noted that most crimes in general, except the white-collar variety, are attributed to this same social class. Still, the rate difference between the social classes is significantly greater for physically aggressive than for purely acquisitive crimes. It is highly doubtful whether the increasing number of self-reporting studies,[15] even the recent and expertly executed ones by Christie, Andenaes, and Skirbekk[16] in Norway and by Elmhorn[17] in Sweden, will alter this conclusion based upon officially recorded crimes. Homicide has rarely – perhaps because it is not a frequent crime – been included in these studies, the serious transgressions of aggression are not usually listed, and there is considerable doubt whether people will report, even anonymously, that they have ever committed homicide.

From Ferri[18] in Italy to Brearley[19] in the United States, and, more recently, to Bensing and Schroeder[20] in Cleveland, Svalastoga[21] in Denmark, Morris and Blom-Cooper[22] in England, Verkko[23] in Finland, Jayewardene[24] and Wood[25] in Ceylon, Bustamante and Bravo[26] in Mexico, Lamont[27] in South Africa, Franchini and Introna[28] in modern Italy – these and many other authors in these and other places report the same general relationship between economic class and homicide.

This is not to say that upper- and middle-class homicides do not occur, nor that in some societies or subsocieties the rates for these groups may not be singularly higher than in other societies. Whites in Southern United States have homicide rates four to five times higher than whites in New England. Moreover, the percentage participation of the middle and upper classes in homicide, relative to the total volume of homicide in a society, may be developed into a valid generalization akin to Verkko's statement about sex and the volume of homicide. We cannot be sure, because cross-cultural studies have not examined this topic, but material from England, for example, which has a relatively low rate, suggests that there is a higher proportion of middle- and upper-class offenders than in countries such as the United States, which has a moderately high rate, or Mexico and Colombia, which have very high rates.[29]

As we have earlier indicated, when homicide is committed by members of the middle and upper social classes, there appears to be a high likelihood of major psychopathology or of planned, more 'rational' (or rationalized) behavior. Thus for them to commit an act of willful murder, which is in diametrical opposition to the set of values embraced by the dominant social-class establishment of which they are a part, often means that these persons are suffering severely from an emotional crisis of profound proportions. Or they have been able, like Cressey's[30] embezzler, to meditate and mediate with their own internalized value system until they can conceive of the murder act without the consequence of an overburdening guilt, and thereby justify their performing the deed. This self-justificatory behavior undoubtedly requires of the actor considerable time and much introspective wrestling in order to remain within, yet contradict, his supportive value system. The infrequency of middle- and upper-class homicide, even in societies such as Colombia, Mexico, and, on a lower level, Sardinia or the Southern part of the United States, must attest to the fact that this kind of rationalization of killing is not only extremely unlikely to occur but also very difficult to promote.

In preparing for the rational, premeditated murder, the middle- or upper-class actor also reasons that he has a considerable portion of his ego-involvement and investment in social life to lose should his blatant, legally antithetic act become detected. In a ponderous assessment of the probabilities of apprehension, this 'prudent' and 'rational' man is surely more likely than the explosive knife-carrier, prepared for battle, to be inhibited even by the highest of statistical odds against apprehension. We are not suggesting that the 'average' middle-class man is primarily deterred from committing homicide by reason of the threat of severe penalty, but neither can we deny such threats some power to restrict and to prevent the commission of these criminal acts. However, our thesis contains principally the notion that the man from a culture system that denounces the use of interpersonal violence will be restrained from using violence because of his positive perspective that conforms to his value system, not because of a negation of it. The absence of that kind of value system is hardly likely to be a vacuous neutrality regarding violence. Instead, it is replaced by a value system that views violence as tolerable, expected, or required. As we approach that part of the cultural continuum where violence is a requisite response, we also enter a subculture where physically aggressive action can quickly and readily bleed into aggressive crime. The man from this culture area is more likely to use violence, similarly because of a positive perspective that requires conformity to his value system. Restraint from using violence may be a frustrating, ego-deflating, even a guilt-ridden experience. Questions of the risks of being apprehended, and the distant, abstract notion of the threat of punishment are almost irrelevant to one who acts with quick, yet socially ingrained aggressivity. Neither reasoning nor time for it are at his disposal.[31]

The rarity and complexity of middle- and upper-class criminal homicide are eloquent reasons for its prominence as a literary theme and for the criminologists' primary concern with the frequent type of homicide that is more 'normal', i.e. statistically more common and reflective of the learned, habituated aggressive reaction to sets of stimuli perceived as noxious.

RACE

Whenever a culture is racially heterogeneous, with a minority that is subservient, suppressed, or in some other manner superordinated by a ruling majority, the minority group is likely to be viewed as socially inferior and to have a high proportion of its members in the lower social and economic class. The Negro protest that burst into the history of the United States is still so recent that for a long time validity will be retained in economic statistics that indicate the prevalence of Negroes in the lower-class structure of that country. Restricted and isolated from the institutionalized means to achieve the goals of the dominant culture, many more Negroes than whites are caught in what Merton,[32] Cloward and Ohlin,[33] and others refer to as the differential opportunity structure, and are more likely to commit crime. The massive mobilization of federal and other public monies to provide new economic opportunities is in part an official testimony to this thesis. And as one of us recently remarked in a review of the literature on crime and race: '. . . if a careful, detached scholar knew nothing about crime rates but was aware of the social, economic and political disparities between whites and Negroes in the United States, and if this diligent researcher had prior knowledge of the historical status of the American Negro, what would be the most plausible hypothesis our scholar could make about the crime rate of Negroes? Even this small amount of relevant knowledge would justify the expectation that Negroes would be found to have a higher crime rate than whites.'[34]

Statistics on homicide and other assaultive crimes in the United States consistently show that Negroes have rates between four and ten times higher than whites. Aside from a critique of official arrest statistics that raises serious questions about the amount of Negro crime,[35] there is no real evidence to deny the greater involvement that Negroes have in assaultive crimes. What *is* forcefully denied is any genetic specificity for committing crime and any biological proclivity peculiar to Negroes or any other racial group for engaging in criminal behavior. There is reason to agree, however, that whatever may be the learned responses and social conditions contributing to criminality, persons visibly identified and socially labeled as Negroes in the United States appear to possess them in considerably higher proportions than do persons labeled white. Our subculture-of-violence thesis would, therefore, expect to find a large spread to the learning of, resort to, and criminal display of the violence value among minority groups such as Negroes.

OTHER VARIABLES

As we have said earlier, we are not prepared to account for the genesis of the subculture, but a thesis that points to the descriptive parameters of a phenomenon (the subculture of violence) theoretically presumed to be causally linked to another phenomenon (homicide and other crimes of violence) can provide a useful basis for social intervention, prevention, and treatment.

There is a bundle of other variables commonly collected in homicide studies. These include references to marital status, broken homes, level of intelligence, police-recorded motives, methods and weapons used, the presence of alcohol, previous criminal record, census-tract, or other ecological data, patterns of social disorganization, and anomie.[36] When these types of information have been available to the researchers, they have generally been included as part of the internal analysis of the data on homicide offenders, and sometimes, but rarely, on homicide victims. Although these items make for interesting descriptive analysis in a comparison of homicide offenders and victims with other types of offender, or even with other cultures, they have contributed little to a higher order of abstraction and general theory construction.[37] Perhaps the item of IQ is a mild exception, for as we stated in an earlier section, most assaultive offenders have been shown to have mean IQs significantly lower than those of property offenders, and certainly lower than those of the general population.

But this last point – i.e. comparison with the population at large – is an important one generally overlooked or unavailable to the investigators. Groups of non-homicide subjects matched with homicide offenders are almost never obtained, except in the case of very specialized studies such as that carried out by Rizzo in Italy with five plates from the MAPS test.[38] The control group in this study, however, consisted of inmates who had committed property crimes, and the homicide offenders were found to be significantly more aggressive than the matched group.

Random representatives from the general noncriminal population are not compared with assaultive offenders, and base-line statistics from the population at large are commonly not mentioned. For example, the presence of alcohol in two-thirds of the homicide situations, where alcohol had been ingested just prior to the homicide by the offender, the victim, or both, is a statistic that has not been (and perhaps cannot be) stated in relation to the abundance of many other occasions of social intercourse in which alcohol was an ingredient.[39] Almost trite questions arise: Although alcohol may be an inhibition-reducing agent, on how many other occasions did the homicide offenders imbibe? If we knew the incidence of alcohol-related homicide among all alcohol-related social interactions, would we be at all impressed by the coefficient? Among persons from broken homes, or with working mothers, inadequate fathers, low educational levels, and an ecological residence characterized by poverty, general physical deterioration, transiency, and density, very few persons commit homicide or other aggressive crimes. Neither the *length of exposure* to many of these conditions (how long was the father absent or 'inadequate'? when was the home broken? when did

K

the mother start working? have poverty and density always been present?) nor the *quality* of them (how was the home broken? would it have been better unbroken? did the mother provide supervision, even though she worked? was it a poor but wholesome family? just what does 'density' mean?) is generally accounted for in the references.

Motives for homicide, as described by the police or court records, do not differ widely between the many studies, although frequency distributions sometimes vary, as might be expected, from tribes in Africa to cities in Western countries.[40] 'Jealousy', 'domestic quarrels', 'altercations', and so forth, are terms that are commonly used by researchers because they rely upon officially recorded items. Obviously, these are 'motives' only in the sense used in the vernacular; they are not finely differentiated, and they convey little of the dynamics of personal interaction that lead to homicide. Still, the terms used almost universally express the recognized generalization that most homicides represent a form of behavior from a wider pool of aggression that is in a ready state for use. Again we would ask, if the data were available, how many domestic quarrels end in homicide. Why do *some* domestic quarrels, why do *some* jealousies, why do *some* arguments over dice in a back-alley game in New York, over property boundaries in Ceylon, or over family honor in Sicily, end in criminal slayings? Neither the information on incidence nor the explanation for these events seems to be readily available without reference to cultural and subcultural variations on the theme of violence; or without resort to a psychopathological condition, which in the ultimate analysis begs the question and succeeds only in removing the case from the field of criminology to that of forensic psychiatry. The need remains for a 'differential social psychology' which must be theoretically constructed within an integrated frame of reference. As we have mentioned, the concept of a subculture of violence may provide these requisites.

There is another pattern of homicide that is almost universal: namely, its intragroup character and the small proportion of cases in which there is a stranger relationship between victims and offenders. Relatives, close friends of both sexes, acquaintances with residential proximity, members of the same ethnic, tribal, or other similarly denoted social group, constitute the main targets of aggression. The enormous number of *vis-à-vis* relationships experienced by all members of society makes the number of intragroup homicide appear high, although if it were possible to count the number of fleeting, impersonal, secondary types of contact an individual has in a lifetime, a year, or a day, this number would also be enormous and would increase with the complexity and population of the society. Clearly, it is more than the number of exposures to primary or secondary relationships that results in high rates of intragroup targets and agents of assault. And it is more than the fact that primary, *vis-à-vis* relationships are charged with high emotional content, for there is no reason to believe that intensity of personal interaction is greater in number or degree among specific social groups, among lower classes, minority groups, the unskilled, or the young adult or the male population. The sentiments of attraction and hostility are widely and probably randomly distributed. Professional and managerial occupational groups, the better-educated and higher-income families also have arguments, domestic quarrels, and love triangles. But within a portion of the lower class, especially, there is a 'life style', a culturally transmitted and shared willingness to express disdain, disgruntlement, and other hostile feelings in personal interaction by using physical force. The repertoire of response to unpleasant stimuli is delimited for them; it is not simply that more stimuli are displeasing. And in this limited repertoire of alternatives, the ultimate weapon in efforts to control others, violence, not only is available but also has been incorporated into the personality structure through childhood discipline, reinforced in juvenile peer groups, confirmed in the strategies of the street. The aggressive male is socially 'castrated' only for short periods of time in school, at work, and in other encounters with external controls. But the fighting routine in his personal milieu is continued, for his subcultural group is prepared to use the same violence as he, to respond in similar fashion to his attack, to be governed by the same norms containing the same values. Within this value set, the external expectations of aggression more readily activate the internal physiological responses of excitation, and the circle of violence circumscribes a situation containing the essential ingredients for assaultive crime. It should also be noted that, as we have seen in the previous chapter, a number of physiological and pathological conditions, often of a subclinical kind, may influence the ease of violent response to aggressive or stressful factors. Because of their generally inferior circumstances at birth and their less healthy environment, the lower classes are more vulnerable and more predisposed than are the middle and upper classes to physiological conditions that increase the risk of a situation that is psychologically and sociologically criminogenic.

ANOMIE

We have mentioned anomie in several places throughout the book, and we draw attention to it again only in order to indicate reasons for our not dwelling on the concept as part of our theoretical formulation.[41] While some authors employ the concept of 'normlessness' as a synonym for anomie, it is difficult to conjure up a situation in which a completely new set of stimuli appears to which existing norms for the individual could in no way be applied. Even if new and different circumstances might occur in which no prevailing and known norms were specifically applicable, other known and related norms would be called into play to operate as governing rules for the new congeries of events. The response of doubt about how or what to do in a new situation is born from individual ignorance or confusion of norms, not from the total social absence of some group's conception of normative behavior. And even if a collective normlessness existed, it is not a concept that could be applied specifically to violence, nor especially to homicide.

Reference to anomie as a confusion of norms, or as an encounter of conflicting norms, begins to approach the general notion of subcultures. If, in this sense, anomie is viewed from a broad, macroscopic frame of reference, the culture–contraculture social mass may be said to contain anomic features. But the conception does not itself delineate distinctive features of the culture conflict and provides little more than convenient parsimony of nomenclature for a set of variables equally well or poorly understood under other labels. The term is widely used by social scientists and some psychologists, and it will continue to be used by us because it conveys much meaning.[42] But its conceptual breadth is somewhat self-defeating so far as its capacity for being operationalized and differentiated is concerned. The emergence of a sociology and a social psychology of subcultures seems to have diminished the utility of the concept of anomie both in theory and in empirical research. What may be said by using anomie may be said in broader scope and with better parameters through a subcultural analysis, for anomie may or may not be present in a given subculture. Moreover, sociological theories of subcultures, we believe, are more adaptable to principles of psychology and psychiatry. The psychological studies of anomie have been few and of limited impact. None has been conducted in criminology.[43]

In short, our thesis of a subculture of violence may be perceived as anomie only from the broad overview of the entire social organization that contains some dysfunctional qualities. To express this notion we have used culture conflict. From within the culture, there is neither normlessness, nor confusion, nor conflict.

THE CORRELATION OF THESE VARIABLES WITH ASSAULTIVE CRIME

From the foregoing, it is obvious even to the casual observer that only a few males in their twenties commit homicide or other crimes of violence. Only a few of those who are in the lower social and economic class, who have below average IQs, whose families are disrupted, who live in poor neighborhoods, etc., kill others or even act aggressively. We should add, of course, that not all persons suffering from hyper-thyroidism, other hormonal imbalances, hypoglycemia, or psycho-pathology, commit assaultive crimes.

By reversing the coin of initiating inquiry, as is frequently done in clinical studies, and asking how many aggressive offenders possess these attributes in total or in large measure, we note that the resulting per-centages appear relatively high compared with those for non-assaultive offenders or for non-offenders. Still, no factorial analysis designed to weigh the loading of these variables would produce a coefficient of very high predictability.

If in the criminological study of violent crime we exclude the few psychopathological and premeditated murders and add to the known correlated ingredients of most assaultive crimes the socially inspired, and habit-reinforced experience of physical aggression – in short, the social value of violence – the theory posits that there will be a statistically highly significant and etiologically meaningful association with assaultive crime.

DEVELOPING COUNTRIES

There appears to be increasing concern with an apparent rise of crime in developing countries throughout Asia, the Middle East, Africa, and much of Latin America.[44] Where valid data are available, these areas of the world are experiencing crime increases, mostly in property offenses and particularly in juvenile delinquency. These forms of criminality, along with crimes of violence, have often been interpreted in terms of culture conflict resulting from social change.[45]

The thesis appears to be most easily adapted to the kinds of situations that arise when a country is involved in new and rapid urbanization and industrialization. We would slightly amend the culture conflict formulation by suggesting that the very process of developing creates heterogeneity and subcultural pockets, either of newly developed value systems or of isolated retainers of older value systems more adapted to primitive and underdeveloped conditions. The larger, dominant culture is often diffused and not yet clearly formulated. The thrust of its new values related to city dwelling, increasing complexity of social life, and an industrial labor force is still weak and amorphous. The political elite and the cadre controlling economic forces are often attacked by the subcultures around them, which are composed of large numbers of people who do not hold the same values as the established fraternity. It probably makes little difference in the long run whether the Establishment engaged in the development process is the representative of a metropolitan culture, or whether it is indigenous and has the cultural consanguinity of a parent to the rebellious subcultural offshoots.

Social change in most developing countries means increasing Westernization, the adoption of many functional items of Western culture. In this process, the indigenous culture itself often becomes a subculture to the emerging culture. To retain their original identity, their self-respect, and their historical continuity, the culture-retainers seek to wrest control, and, over time, they become a smaller but more firmly committed group, thereby forming a subculture in opposition to the dominant developing culture.

In a developing country, it is not disturbance of the social equilibrium alone that may make violence a viable way of life for many people. It is a culture, or contraculture, that makes physical aggression a virtue, often with political or religious justifications. Both the Indians and the whites on the western plains of the United States in the nineteenth century placed a premium on the need for and use of violence against one another. Both the Mau Mau and the British colonists in Kenya employed violence as a solution.[46] When the dethroned cannot accept the invading system and play the game of accommodation within the rules of the conquistadores, the ultimate weapon is violence. Nonviolent disobedience is employable only when and if the dominant system tolerates it and, while viewing it as a disruptive force, will not sacrifice its own functional harmony by resorting to totalitarian tactics to destroy the adherents of the movement. Gandhi's measures were successful in large part because the British administration in India respected the rights of others; the Negro nonviolent protest in the United States has been successful for this same reason.

In an emerging nation, newly urbanized and industrialized groups are confronted not only with new types of social contact, role, and function but also with great increases in their number. This sheer increase in social complexities may contribute to an increase in the volume of criminal and other deviant acts. To this notion, however, must be added the kind of analysis Thomas and Znaniecki[47] provided for the Polish peasant in Europe and America. From that point, then, it is only a slight change in terminology that moves analysis to culture conflict and subcultural considerations.

SELECTED CULTURE CASE STUDIES

To have generalizability, the subculture-of-violence theory should be expected to explain the appearance of explosive, aggressive crime in a variety of places, times, and cultures. Thus, time and space confirmations not only increase the number of instances embraced by a theory; they also validate its level of abstraction and explanatory power. The subculture-of-violence thesis was generated principally by recent observations in the United States and Europe. Heterogeneity through ethnic clustering, urbanization, industrialization, open social-class systems, residential juxtaposition of rich and poor, and so forth, which are part of these cultures and these times, may be key factors in causing subcultures and contracultures to emerge. Hence there is the possibility that the theory may be unduly limited, provincial, and specific in scope. Moreover, we have relied heavily upon social-class differences, drawing special attention to the concomitants of class, identifying the middle class with the dominant numbers and power in society as well as with the law and values of nonviolence. However, a strong middle social class should be viewed only as a sufficient, but not as a necessary, element of the theory. Wherever the modulus of morality exists, and whatever the political framework, so long as nonviolence is the governing principle within the social and political life of the group, a subculture of violence could exist. The principal culture may sometimes be violent or have elements of violence; but it cannot be a culture of violence, not unless it is attacking a group outside itself. If a dominant cultural group uses heavy force to suppress a rising opposition to its authority, if it maintains itself in power through violence, it is still fighting a group outside itself. Even dictators who gain control of nations prefer sub-servience through genuine willingness to submit to the necessity of using force.

We do not know whether history and anthropology would find in other times and other cultures concurrence with the modalities of homicide consistently reported in this century for many countries. Whatever the case, the subculture-of-violence thesis is assumed to be operative for this modal form, the passionate killing. The theory is certainly not meant to apply to all aggression, to all crime, nor even to all homicide. Where rates of homicides and other assaults are high, there would seem to be a reasonable likelihood of a subculture of violence. However, low rates for a nation-state do not rule out the possibility of a subcultural pocket containing sufficient commitment to the use of violence to qualify as a subculture of violence. Research simply is not available to permit us to designate where in the world all of these subcultures may be. Survey studies would first be needed to indicate areas of high probability; and then research on values, as proposed in Chapter III, might provide some social meaning to statistical variations, average scores on a value scale, significant differences, and other standard tests. Until such measurements are made across, among, and between cultures and subcultures, we can do little more than rely upon the isolated, often parochial, methodologically uneven studies that appear in existing literature.

We have scanned the criminological literature and have located some culture case studies that seem to indicate the presence of subcultures of violence in different parts of the world. These studies are mentioned here only as illustrative examples, for we cannot claim to be exhaustive in any way. Historical and anthropological researches would probably be most rewarding in adding temporal and spatial dimensions to the concepts and perhaps thereby could embellish the theory. The Thugs[48] of India, the Ismalian[49] community of 'assassins' begun in the eleventh century, which spread to various parts of the Middle East, the Haitian 'Sect Rouge'[50] based on certain aspects of Voodoo religion, the earlier vendettas or blood feuds of Macedonia,[51] Albania,[52] Cyprus,[53] and the early stages of secret societies such as the Camorra of Naples and the Mafia of Sicily are but a few examples requiring detailed examination to determine whether they fit the theory of a subculture of violence and whether they contribute to our understanding of such a subculture.

Perhaps a further brief note is needed about the current phase of the Sicilian Mafia.[54] In the course of its now long evolution it has lost its original character of reactive violence and has become a network of organized crime. As such, it does not resort systematically, or even by preference, to violence. When violence occurs, it is planned, and is engaged in in accordance with the norms rather than for its own sake; it is exercised by young members, who are frequently dropped from the association or kept in a lower rank. Violence for the Mafia is an ultimate weapon of social and economic control, not unlike the death penalty in organized society, and not a set of values. It is interesting to note that the 'long arm' of the police on Mafia activities has caused an increase in violence. Perhaps the point needs to be stressed here that, although the *mafiosa* began as a vendetta system over a century ago, it was transformed into a social form of political and economic control not dissimilar to organized crime in the United States. As such, the Mafia in Sicily today exists for economic reasons. In general it may be stated that when an organized group uses violence merely as a tool to obtain economic rewards, the group probably does not fall within the meaning of the concept, subculture of violence.

INTERNATIONAL CRIMINAL STATISTICS

International criminal statistics are woefully inadequate for well-known reasons. The table of homicide death rates below is presented with a cautious reminder of the abundant qualifications necessary regarding the validity of these statistics for comparative purposes. A country's omission is due to its failure to report appropriate data to the United Nations. It cannot accurately be said that subcultures of violence are more frequent in countries with rates above rather than below the average. An hypothesis of this kind could be entertained, for present evidence seems to point in this direction, but the picture is unclear, mostly from lack of adequate research. The emergence of new nations and the poverty of their criminal statistics compound the problems of international analysis. Another factor of potential importance must be kept in mind: the reduction of homicide rates does not mean *per se* the reduction of violent crime. Better communication and transportation systems and improvement in medical technology and facilities may be significant factors in reducing the number of homicides and increasing the number of aggravated and other legally denoted forms of criminal assaults while the total number of assaultive crimes may remain constant or even rise.[55] We cannot at present be certain of the functional interplay of these factors.

TABLE I HOMICIDE DEATH RATES BY COUNTRY AND
YEAR OF REPORT*

Rate per 100,000	Country	Year
34·0	Colombia	1960
31·1	Mexico	1958
22·8	Nicaragua	1959
21·2	South Africa	1959
10·8	Burma	1959
9·9	Aden Colony	1956
9·8	Guatemala	1960
6·1	Turkey	1959
5·9	Panama	1960
5·3	Puerto Rico	1959
5·3	St Vincent	1955
4·9	Chile	1957
4·6	Uruguay	1955
4·6	Trinidad/Tobago	1960
4·5	United States	1960
4·4	Nigeria	1960
4·3	Ceylon	1959
3·9	Dominican Republic	1955
3·2	Costa Rica	1960
3·0	Channel Islands	1959
3·0	Reunion	1956
2·9	Finland	1960
2·7	Bulgaria	1960
2·6	North Borneo	1960
2·5	Barbados	1960
2·3	United Arab Republic	1958
2·2	Peru	1959
2·1	Poland	1959
1·9	Japan	1960
1·8	Fed. Rep. of Germany – West Berlin	1959
1·8	Singapore	1960
1·7	France	1960
1·6	Hungary	1960
1·5	Australia	1960
1·5	Greece	1960
1·4	Canada	1960
1·4	Italy	1959
1·2	Australasia	1960

* Item BE50 (E964, E965, E980–E999) from *Demographic Yearbook*, Thirteenth Issue, New York: United Nations Publications, 1961, pp. 398–471.

TABLE I—*Contd.:*

Rate per 100,000	Country	Year
1·2	Jordan	1960
1·1	New Zealand	1960
1·0	Hong Kong	1960
0·9	Mauritius ex. dep.	1960
0·9	Northern Ireland	1960
0·9	Portugal	1960
0·9	Switzerland	1959
0·8	Spain	1959
0·7	Belgium	1959
0·7	Ryukyu Islands	1960
0·7	Scotland	1960
0·7	Sweden	1959
0·6	England/Wales	1960
0·6	Iceland	1959
0·6	Luxembourg	1960
0·6	Sarawak	1958
0·5	Cape Verde Islands	1959
0·5	Denmark	1959
0·5	Norway	1959
0·4	British Guiana	1958
0·3	Malta/Gozo	1960
0·3	Netherlands	1960
0·2	Ireland (Eire)	1960

COLOMBIA – VIOLENCIA

One of the most striking examples of large-scale violence is the case of Colombia. The phenomenon of the so-called *violencia colombiana* is well known and we shall therefore not attempt here a detailed description and reconstruction of its history.[56] A few notes, however, seem necessary to reveal its main characteristics.

Colombia has exhibited for the past eighteen years a fantastic increase in homicides owing to a combination of political causes which gave rise to the outbreak of a kind of undeclared civil war, or, as Caplow[57] calls it, an 'epidemic of disorder', between the two main parties (the Liberals and Conservatives), which had almost equal political strength. After a few episodes of political bloodshed in the thirties, a very popular political leader, Dr Jorge Eliezer Gaitan, was assassinated in 1948 by a person who was immediately lynched and whose political affiliations were never identified. From 1946 the political fights had assumed a particularly violent character, but, after the assassination of Gaitan, a wave of violence swept the country. With alternate outcomes, Liberals and Conservatives fought bitterly, and entire sections of the country fell under the control of armed groups, the *guerrilleros* or *anti-sociales*.

A temporary peace at one time occurred between the two parties, but the fighting continued. New political forces, occasionally external to the country, became involved in the national scene, but meanwhile many of the guerrilla groups became devoid of political meaning and assumed a purely antisocial character.

The army slowly regained control of the situation and today the fighting is much less acute. Still, bloodshed continues and Colombia remains with the highest homicide rate in the world. The *violencia* was primarily a rural phenomenon, but now, with large numbers of people migrating to cities to escape the violence in the countryside, a new problem of urban violence has been created.

The total number of deaths due to the *violencia* is unknown, but some estimates place it as high as 200,000. The table opposite from official death statistics shows how rates rose after the Gaitan assassination and have remained extraordinarily high since 1949.

In several districts, the rate of homicide has been nearly twice as high as the national rate. For example, in Tolima the rate in 1960 was 63 per 100,000.[58] In the age group 15 to 44 years, homicide has been the leading cause of death in the years covered by the official statistics since 1957. An analysis of criminal statistics and of other information media shows a very high concentration of crime in those departments associated with the action of the *violencia* groups.

It should be pointed out that homicide which is directly attributable to guerrilla action takes place almost exclusively in rural areas. The traditional pattern of attack is against cars or buses in transit and against small *veredas*; there are also sporadic open fights with government forces. Homicide in the guerrilla operations generally takes an extremely sadistic form. Several most brutal and painful ways of killing have become popular and have acquired special names: *Picar para tamal* (to cut up the body in little pieces), *Bocachiquiar* (to make transversal and longitudinal cuts in the body in a way similar to that of preparing fresh-water fish, *bocachica*, for cooking), *corte de corbata* (in which the throat is split longitudinally and the tongue is pulled down to hang like a tie). Almost all the brutal and senseless paraphernalia of slaying known to history have been exhibited in Colombia. Cases of cannibalism are recorded, bodies are uncared for and exposed to the public, and violent death has become a commonplace. The battle names of the guerrilla leaders echo this violent pattern (*Sangre Negra, Diablo, Neron*, etc.), and

TABLE 2   NUMBER AND RATE OF DEATHS FROM HOMICIDE WITH AN INDEX OF 100 FOR 1938

Colombia 1938–1960*

Year	Number	Rate per 100,000	Base Year 1938 = 100
1938	1,280	14·6	100
1943	765	8·1	55·5
1944	1,111	11·2	76·5
1945	1,290	12·7	87
1946	1,184	11·5	79
1947	1,214	11·4	78
1948	1,715	15·9	109
1949	3,285	31·03	212
1950	3,227	28·4	195
1951	3,608	32·8	225
1952	4,670	39·2	269
1953	3,772	31·05	216
1954	3,121	25·18	174
1955	4,156	33·0	230
1956	5,187	39·9	273
1957	5,471	41·3	281
1958	6,966	51·4	351
1959	5,513	39·8	272
1960	4,799	33·8	232

* Data for this table have been collected directly from the office in charge of death statistics in the Colombian Ministry of Health.

many new expressions concerning killing have been introduced into the language. Frequently, homicide is carried out against whole families and, especially in the past, it has followed a pattern of extermination and genocide. Another practice of the guerrilla operation is *no dejar la semilla* (not to leave the seed), which involves emasculation of males and extermination of women and children.[59]

The population in the affected areas occasionally supports the guerrilla groups. Leaders often become idealized figures in the daily games of children in these districts. Entire farm districts have been abandoned, and migration to the cities has swollen the urban population to the point of creating seemingly unmanageable problems. Recently, the army and the police have abandoned the tactic of acute armed repression and have enlisted the help of the local population, but the *violencia* has not yet ended. Only in 1964 was the area of Marquetalia (which the guerrilla bands had taken over and organized as an 'independent' republic) restored to some semblance of order.

Several explanations have been offered for the *violencia colombiana*, but a valid and objective study of the phenomenon is not yet available. Although political and economic factors are at the base, many elements contributed to its genesis and to its perpetuation. Anomie,[60] a structural–functional interpretation,[61] frustration of aspirations for upward mobility,[62] have been hypothesized by some authors as possible explanations, but these same notions have also been rejected by other observers. Some of the guerrilla groups established autonomous legislatures which have been analyzed from a legal standpoint.[63]

Among the different causes of the *violencia* phenomenon, the hypothesis of a subcultural transmission, as a problem-solving mechanism, can easily be formulated. Apart from the geographical, age, and social-class concentration, and the development of folklore and language, other elements can be isolated to uphold a subcultural approach. In addition to the broader political and economic factors, the transmission of violence is sustained by the constant presentation of violent stimuli and values to the children. The ever-present feeling of menace, fear, and death, the actual visual presentation of mangled bodies and of other sadistic manifestations, together with the desire for revenge in those children whose parents or relatives have been victims of the violence, all tend to perpetuate a situation which possibly has no equal in contemporary Western civilization. Similar violent political clashes have occurred elsewhere; Mexico has provided tragic examples of political extermination. But nowhere in the Western world in recent times since the Second World War has senseless brutality, a genocidal pattern, and a non-war pattern of violence been so nearly total as in the Colombian tragedy. The average age of present guerrilla members is estimated to be about twenty-four. This identifies them as having been six or seven years of age when the *violencia* began. Moreover, most guerrilla leaders today appear to be sons of parents killed in the *violencia*. Thus, the general appearance and expectation of brutality reinforce the acceptance of violence as a chief value, and indoctrination of children about methods of killing is a widely practiced addition to the almost daily experience provided by the guerrilla forces.

SARDINIA – THE BARBARICINO CODE

The island of Sardinia, and particularly its internal mountainous regions referred to as 'Barbagia', provides another interesting example of a violent culture. The label of subculture can be attached only when Sardinia is viewed in relation to the larger Italian political culture; otherwise, the *barbaricino* culture is autonomous and almost self-contained, with its own characteristic economic, social, historical, linguistic, and folklore features. The use of violence, particularly of vendetta homicides, is regulated by a set of norms which Pigliaru[64] has studied from the viewpoint of the philosophy of law. In his careful and detailed analysis, which constitutes an excellent example of a normative approach to the study of subcultures, Pigliaru traces the value-norm sets in their intricate actualization. The 'habituality' (*consuetudine*) of the norms, apart from proving their validity as a 'code', expresses their subcultural character. The indoctrination process is almost total, for the Italian criminal code is accepted passively as a political, externally imposed necessity, but is discarded whenever it conflicts with the *barbaricino* code. The long history of this code is expressed in Sardinian folklore, and daily behavior is carefully regulated by its norms. For the Sardinian who breaks the code, violent death or escape are the only alternatives. Similar patterns exist in other regions of Southern Italy, but nowhere have they reached the open normative level of Barbagia.

MEXICO – FATALISTIC ACCEPTANCE OF DEATH

Mexico has experienced high rates of homicide for years. From 1931 to 1954 there were 257,000 cases of homicide in that country, although rates per 100,000 have been decreasing from a high point of 60·1 in 1937–1938 to 38·0 in 1954 and in 1960 to 31·1.[65] The mean five-year rate from 1950 to 1954 ranged from 82·9 in the Morelos area to 5·4 in the Baja California Territory. While homicide rates are high throughout the whole country, those for the coastal and rural areas are considerably higher than those for the peninsulas and urban areas. Citing data from the Laboratory of Biostatistics, Jorge M. Velasco Alzaga notes that in the Federal District 'the risk of dying in this zone [from homicide], in accordance with the information in the study, is greater than the risk that existed in London from bombardment during World War Two'.[66]

This author, along with other Mexican social analysts, asserts that in the areas of high homicide rate, physically aggressive forms of behavior 'constitute positive values of the particular ethics of some social groups'.[67] Although references are made in the Mexican criminological literature to 'impersonal tension', 'resentment against society', 'anxiety', 'hunger, lack of adequate clothes, inadequate dwelling, lack of affection and tense relations between parents', there is an emphasis on a kind of fatalistic expectation of violence and death, with many 'folklore expressions that show an admiration toward destructive symbols and toward death itself'.[68] We are told that common folklore expressions include: 'We were born to die.' 'If I should be killed tomorrow, I might as well be killed now.' 'They'll kill me, but I have killed more than four.' Clinicians and social observers report that among laborers and much of the lower classes there is a rationalized attitude of becoming used to the idea of death, and that, by perceiving death through homicide as something quite concrete, the magical part of the fear of death disappears.

The high rates of criminal homicide in Mexico, the convergence of such social factors as male sex, membership of the working class, and a tradition of employing physical aggression, suggest that there exist in that country subcultural areas of violence. Where the use of violence is taken for granted and homicide is a common form of death, subcultural values encouraging the use of violence can surely be assumed to be present.

ALBANIA – THE BESA TRADITION OF VENDETTA

Crisafulli and Di Tullio[69] reported in 1942 the results of an unusual study conducted in Albania among Italian and Albanian soldiers, of whom the latter were incorporated into the Italian army and subjected to the Italian military code. Using the records of criminal offenses brought before the military courts in Albania, supplemented with clinical examinations and interviews, the two authors described the differential incidence of various criminal acts. Only the Albanian soldiers had records of committing homicide. It is interesting to note that, although the detailed clinical analysis was based primarily on a biological perspective, the authors none the less emphasize the importance of the cultural factor of the so-called *besa* (pacification of blood) as a determinant of violent behavior. The *besa* was a cultural tradition of the vendetta which was transmitted from generation to generation and constituted a moral code from which most Albanians from the mountain regions could not readily escape. It is a rule of life and a code of honor, say Crisafulli and Di Tullio. Ferri had already presented the hypothesis that the colonies of Albanians in southern and eastern Italy and in some parts of Switzerland accounted for the high rates of homicide in these areas, although he attributed them to an ethnobiological causality. No socio-cultural studies of Albania are available since the Crisafulli and Di Tullio study, but the character and extent of the Albanian violence as outlined by these authors conforms to the definition and meaning of the subculture of violence.

ALBANOVA, ITALY – THE VENDETTA IN AN ISOLATED COMMUNITY

Another example of a violent subculture may be found in the small community of Albanova, Italy. This is an aggregate of three villages, Casal di Principe, San Cipriano d'Aversa, and Casapesenna, located in the district of Caserta near Naples. The total population is about 30,000, characterized by an agricultural economy. It has had the highest rate of violent crimes in Europe. For example, in 1954 this community experienced 6 homicides, 68 attempted homicides, and 3 armed robberies; 418 persons were indicted for different crimes and 254 were arrested. There are no criminological studies of this community, but recently two articles vividly described its characteristics.[70] A combination of ruthless vendetta practices, a proclivity for violence, a high number of available weapons, and a largely shared and totally accepted code of honor, make violence an almost inevitable pattern of behavior which several repressive attempts by the police have failed to control. In the perception of the Albanovesi, weapons have an almost ritualistic value. A gun is a common gift of the godfather to the child at the time he is baptized.[71] The community has lived in almost total isolation for centuries and even today is almost separate from the relatively peaceful surrounding area.

Although no study has ever been made, several hypotheses have been advanced[72] to explain the extraordinary phenomenon of violence in this community. Outbreaks of violence appear to be spontaneous, caused by offenses that in nearby areas would be solved peacefully or go unnoticed. The Albanovese *must* kill to redeem an offense. The common saying goes: 'If you are slapped, you must wash the slap from your face.' This means, as in Sardinia, that one should react to an offense with a more serious, more damaging offense, even to the point of causing a violent death.

The person who does not exact revenge is considered inadequate and is ostracized. Violent juvenile crime is frequent, and in one year three juvenile homicides occurred. The geographical isolation of the village has certainly contributed to the perpetuation of the violent behavior pattern. Alternative 'explanations' sometimes offered include reference to inherited characteristics (in Roman times, apparently, the area was a penal colony) and even to specific violence-causing characteristics of the local wine, the Asprinio, not dissimilar from Hungarian Tokay. In 1890 a famed religious image of the Virgin Mary was accidentally burned in Albanova, and because of the resentment of the surrounding populations, the community became even more isolated. Cultural transmission of violent values appears to be the only explanation that fits the known facts about this puzzling area of unleashed violence in Southern Italy.

ACAN, MEXICO – THE VENDETTA AND POLITICAL VIOLENCE

Another interesting example of isolated cultural transmission of violent values has been described by Friedrich[73] in a village called Acan, in the Tarascan area of Mexico. In a population of 1,500 persons, 77 homicides, 100 woundings, and hundreds of exchanges of fire took place over 35 years. The homicide rate reached the unparalleled figure of 200 per 100,000 in one year. Homicide in Acan is limited to males and is due to vendetta or to political reasons. Political controversies include violence as a normal means of struggle. Homicide is not sadistic and is carried out by the quickest possible means. It goes almost uncensured by local mores, provided it conforms to the social vendetta and political expectations. Men must demonstrate their 'valor' or face loss of prestige and estrangement from political and social life. Homicide is justified and even prescribed. Violence erupted at the beginning of the century during the agrarian revolution and has never been abandoned as an accepted means of achieving political success.

INDIA – CRIMINAL TRIBES

Another interesting example, although not primarily a violent one, is that posed by the Indian criminal tribes. These are several groups of persons, mostly of a nomadic, gypsy-like character, which devote most of their activities to criminal acts, particularly consisting of crimes against property. Special legislation, consisting of a 'notification', or legal identification as criminals, has been in force for many years and has only recently been repealed. These tribes are many, and several have recently been well described by Panakal and Punekar.[74] No clear-cut racial differentiation is present in these highly specific groups (the Banjaras, the Bawarias, the Berads, the Bhamptas-Takari, the Bhamptas-Rajput, the Bhils, the Daffers, the Hingoras, the Iranis, the Kaikadis, the Katkaris, the Kolis-Gujarat, the Kolis-Mahades, the Mangs, the Mang-Garudis, the Myanas, the Pardhis, the Ramoshis, the Sansis, the Thakars, the Vachers, the Vaghris, the Waddars). Transmission of criminal patterns and of the sometimes highly specific *modus operandi* follow clear cultural lines, with early training, indoctrination, and ostracism and punishment for non-acceptance of the criminal behavior. Efforts by the central government have been moderately successful in eliminating the problem posed by these tribes, whose wandering nature aggravates the difficulty of every large-scale treatment program. The earlier legal process of 'notification', though of dubious value, has perhaps contributed to the identification and isolation of these cultural groups. The genesis of these tribes is unknown or mainly conjectural. One interesting aspect is the global participation of the community, with different roles, in criminal behavior. The original 'notification' (Criminal Tribes Act XXVII of 1871) was modified in 1911, 1924, 1931, and repealed first in Bombay State in 1949 and by the Government of India in 1953.

There are a few culture areas that have been reported with considerable clarity regarding what appear to be values common to a subculture of violence, and of theft in the case of the Indian tribes. The researches by Bohannan[75] on African homicide and suicide, by Straus[76] and Wood[77] on homicide and suicide in Ceylon, and by Jayewardene[78] on Ceylon, and reports by other scholars on homicides in other cultures,[79] do not indicate the presence of subcultures of violence among the peoples studied. The African study includes descriptions of seven tribes relatively unaffected by social change. None of them could be said to have formed a subculture of violence. In Ceylon, culture conflict derived from social change is claimed by Wood and by Jayewardene to be the explanation for many of the homicides. Jayewardene[80] explicitly denies that a subculture of violence as yet exists in Ceylon, but the increasing number of land disputes in rural areas owing to over-population and land shortage, the shift from a caste system and traditional values to secular beliefs and achieved status, and other indices of change could promote conditions associated with the development of a subculture of violence.

CONTROL, PREVENTION, AND TREATMENT

ACTS, ACTORS, AND POLICY DECISIONS

Society does not appear to denounce all violence, nor is there scientific support for the notion that all violence is bad for a society. 'Bad' is, after all, a value-laden term, and the social functions of violence have been described both by intellectuals and activists.

Yet, the social machinery of political institutions, police organizations, and policy-making bodies is geared to control and prevent crimes of violence as these forms of conduct are codified in penal law. Although property rights sometimes may seem to supersede human rights in legislative action concerned with minority groups, there is little doubt that crimes of personal violence are viewed by the public in general as more serious than crimes against property or any other type of offense.

There may be many ways by which society could reduce the number of violent crimes, but research is needed to determine which is the most effective, efficient, rapid, and enduring method. Even more fundamental questions need answers:

1. How much cost are we willing to tolerate for an X amount of reduction in violent crime?
2. What do we consider a 'significant' reduction of violent crime, whatever the cost?
3. To what extent are we willing to change the traditional democratic constraints that normally function to restrict society's manipulative control over behavior, even the conduct of criminals, in order to reduce crimes of violence?

Cost analyses and operations research studies are tools for providing alternative answers to some of these questions. With finite resources of money, men, talent, and power, priority allocations and decisions will be made. Whether these assignments are made in unplanned, non-rational, haphazard ways or with conscious design and rational selection is also a decision placed upon a society that is made aware of the difference.

The public appears to be unwilling to tolerate the current rate, amount, and increase of crimes of violence. A program that would reduce these crimes by 10 per cent during a given year would probably be viewed as important and effective. But other variables must be included in the equation of change in order to interpret that 10 per cent and to evaluate society's willingness to have it. If the cost of the reduction drains resources from other social projects that are deemed more worthy of attention, the 10-per-cent reduction in violent crime may be viewed as intolerable. Executing all three-time recidivists could conceivably yield the 10-per-cent reduction, but at an unacceptable price. Moreover, building a new superhighway to satisfy demands for a rapid mode of vehicular movement may become the choice for expenditure and replace programs known to reduce crime.

Another kind of decision involves the population to be prevented from committing crimes of violence. On the basis of past criminological research experience, there appear to be three major groups:

I   the set of all persons who have never been known officially to have committed a crime;

II the set of persons who have been known to have committed only one crime;

III the set of persons who are known to have committed more than one crime.

There are several ways of approaching these three categories. One is to establish a single group as the target population; e.g. to have as the goal prevention of crime before it occurs (group I), and to concentrate new and creative efforts on this goal while maintaining a traditional containment policy with respect to the other two groups. A second way is to distribute equally whatever resources are available among all three groups and prevention goals. This approach assumes either a lack of information for making rational choices or information that suggests equal efficacy among the three goals. A third way is to discover relative weights for the effectiveness of crime-control action applied to each group; then, to allocate resources according to the weighting system.

Group I is an obvious designation. The whole process of socialization is meant to transmit culture values, attitudes, desires, wishes to each new generation. Prescriptions of conduct are presented not only to assist the child to adjust to the demands placed upon him, but also to prevent his committing socially unacceptable (including criminal) acts. The larger social organizations outside the family assume some responsibility in this socialization process when they seek to prevent persons from ever becoming delinquent or criminal. Efforts to predict delinquency when children enter first grade focus on this group as the goal of prevention. Community welfare programs, slum clearance, improvement in police efficiency, etc., are part of this type of prevention.

Group II is treated as an important target population because various studies indicate that only about half of the juveniles taken into custody by the police for the first time recidivate. This means that if we were able to predict successfully which first-time delinquents continued and which did not, we could concentrate prevention efforts on the predicted recidivists in order to reduce their continued criminality. It could be that the sheer reduction in the size of this target group over the first one would improve our efficiency and reduce the costs instead of engaging in massive efforts to prevent any crime before it occurs.

Group III is the regular recidivistic, 'hard-core' delinquent or criminal population. They constitute a group most often found at some time within walls of confinement and subject to manipulative efforts of extended and intensive therapy.

It is this last group which most vividly dramatizes another question, other issues, and another major area for social decision. We know that offenders who have already committed two offenses have a statistically significantly higher probability of committing the third offense than do first-time offenders for committing a second offense. The three-time offender has a higher probability of becoming a four-time offender than has the two-time offender of becoming a three-time offender; and so on.[81] The issue here is whether we are more interested in (a) preventing *individuals* from ever becoming criminal, or more criminal, or (b) preventing criminal *acts*. A hypothetical question, using extremes, makes the issue quite clear. Which is worse? – 1,000 boys committing 1,000 criminal acts, each boy for the first and only time; or 100 boys committing the same 1,000 criminal acts, each boy committing 10 such acts. If the former is considered worse, it is because we view the more extended distribution of delinquent behavior, albeit short-run, throughout the community as worse than a more restricted and confined distribution among a smaller group with a stronger and longer delinquent orientation. The number of criminal acts can, of course, be altered in either direction so that, for instance, the 1,000 boys commit only 500 criminal offenses (two boys in each offense), and the 100 boys still commit 1,000 offenses; or, vice versa, the 1,000 boys commit 1,000 offenses and the 100 boys only 500 offenses.

When variations in the severity of the crimes are introduced into the question, a new dimension is involved and attention is more likely to shift from actors to acts. If the 500 acts committed by only 100 boys are of a much more serious character than the 1,000 acts by the 1,000 boys, the former set of circumstances may be viewed as much worse. Thus, 500 robberies are worse than 1,000 bicycle thefts. Moreover, it should be evident that each of the original target groups contains a subset of violent offenders and each of the additional issues raised about criminal acts can also involve violent offenses.

In the real world of much greater complexity, where acts and actors are varied in multiple ways, methods are needed for clarifying all these issues so that equations of choice in prevention techniques can be computed and compared.

In another context, Daniel Glaser has succinctly pointed to some of the difficulties of predicting future behavior of one of the target groups; namely, those persons who have been imprisoned and are to be released on parole. 'Even if a board were given all the psychiatrists, sociologists, statisticians, and other experts it desired to make a thorough investigation and analysis of each case, it is doubtful,' he asserts, 'if it could achieve 80 percent accuracy in identifying the less-than-5 percent of parolees who commit clearly violent offenses after release. Eighty percent accuracy is about the greatest precision that has been demonstrated by any man or any prediction system, applied to a cross-section of prisoners, for predicting parole violation in general, rather than the more difficult task of predicting violence on parole.'[82] Pursuing this point further in terms of statistical probabilities and decision theory, Glaser remarks:

'If a board were 80 percent accurate in identifying the most violent parolees, they would still make more than 2 erroneous predictions in 10 as long as the violence they sought to predict occurred in less than 20 percent of the cases. This is simply a matter of mathematics. For example, if violence were committed by 5 percent of prison releases in every 1,000 releasees, a parole board would have to identify 50 men who would commit violence among 950 who would not. With 80 percent predictive accuracy, we could expect the board to predict violence for 20 per cent of the 950, or 190 cases, and for 80 percent of the 50, or 40 cases. However, in this total of 230 designations as probably violent, one could not know in advance which actually would be the 40 who would be violent. They would make a total of 200 erroneous predictions, the 190 nonviolent designated as violent and the 10 violent not designated as violent, in identifying correctly the 230 cases in 1,000 which include 40 of the 50 violence cases. These errors are apart from others they might make in predicting more common types of parole infraction, such as nonviolent theft, burglary or return to narcotics.'[83]

Predicting rare events, such as homicides or rapes from among the universe of all major crimes, is extremely difficult and forms part of statistical decision theory known as the problem of antecedent probability.[84] Even with the smallest target group (III, referred to previously) of criminal repeaters, predicting with high degrees of accuracy their probabilities of committing crimes of violence is not a facile operation. And as has been noted, the number of false positives (predicted violence in cases with no violence) is usually large, whether predicting delinquency before it occurs or violent offenses for men on parole. The high number of false positives therefore means that a considerable amount of resources will be used to control, prevent, or deter many individuals who do not need such attention and for whom restraints may amount to an unwarranted imposition of authority.

Efforts to determine the most propitious point for intervention in the life cycle of the individual in order to prevent the onset or the repetition of violence are still in an exploratory stage of scientific analysis. Both the complexity of human behavior and the use of relatively unsophisticated methods have been responsible for the lack of effective decisions for action. No treatment strategy, no social action program of prevention or deterrence has yet reached a level of significant and repetitive demonstration of success. Negative, segmental findings which indicate that a new form of treatment does not produce a greater increase of recidivism than the older form have been the most common results of research, and tend to converge with changing notions of humanitarianism. With adequately designed experimental and control groups it has been noted that probation can be used instead of imprisonment, men can be released on parole six months earlier than ordinarily, that short-run group therapy can be used instead of the more expensive individual therapy, that a treatment milieu can replace a punitive prison culture – all without significant increases (or decreases) in the amount of future crime or criminality. Thus, historically, society's reaction to the criminal and the approach to treatment have changed without significantly affecting offenders or their amount of criminal deviance.

Psychotherapy in almost any form – group counseling, psychoanalysis, guided group interaction, conditioning, etc. – has not demonstrated its power of success significantly above the normal course of change that occurs without it.[85] Medical models of illness applied to criminal deviance may be analytically useful, but offer little of value in treatment or prognosis. Speaking about the mass murderer in general, and particularly about Charles Whitman in Houston, Robert Coles correctly described the current condition: 'For every quiet, apparently harmless individual who becomes a criminal are there not dozens of manifestly angry and even crazy people who not only commit no crimes, but live extremely useful lives? Do not many so-called "ordinary" people share whatever pattern we find in a gifted person's personality? These are riddles, not ones to shame any profession, but not ones to go unacknowledged, or be buried in a display of wordy and dogmatic psychiatric interpretations.'[86]

Inability to predict outcome in individual cases should not, however, cause undue pessimism about the control or prevention of violence. Science is concerned with clusters, groups, categories as units of analysis, and is not bound by the uniqueness of individual personalities. Moreover, understanding causation or etiology is not always essential for purposes of prediction and prevention. One set of independent factors correlated with a dependent factor or another set of factors, even in inexplicable ways, may still produce predictive and preventive power.[87]

Society's desire to control crimes of violence is furnished with interesting clues that form the *a priori* material of experimental research. It is not that society is without suggestions from the public, public officials, and scholars. Rather, it is the difficulty of deciding which of the host of ideas would be the most operationally efficacious. The history of the processes that translate ideas into action, and of the politics of appropriation would surely indicate that the interaction of research with policy and action has been minimal with respect to efforts to control crimes of violence.

A variety of action research designs, attractive to both the intellectual community of scholars and the agents of public decision, could be piloted throughout the country in such a way that all of them would be integrated into a macroscopic schema of testing, evaluating, and weighting of the results. Each attack on a specific area could be catalogued and calculated in terms of its relative contribution to control and reduction of violence. Within the master plan there would be no isolated or uncoordinated research. (This is not to say that all supported research should fall within the plan; but that the plan contain only coordinated, centrally controlled, and integrated research.) The insularity of scientific disciplines and the parochialism of some community findings would yield to the integrative function of coordinated research and outcome.

TECHNOLOGICAL CONTROL

This section is concerned not directly with criminal attitudes or values but more with technical innovations that are aimed at physical devices or accoutrements in the physical space around us, and that, when employed, may aid the police and other agencies of community protection in producing more effective crime-control measures.

Alarm Systems and Gun Control

In Florence, Venice, and other Italian communes of the late Middle Ages and early Renaissance there were *tamburi*, or accusation boxes, available to all citizens.[88] These were small boxes in strategic public places where one could write citizen complaints (*tamburazioni*), anonymously or otherwise, accusing persons of having committed various crimes. The note-writer was often a witness to crime, did not want to get involved personally, and yet could act as additional eyes of public protection by alerting the proper authorities. Opportunities for false accusations were obvious, as were other untoward consequences of such accusation boxes when viewed from a contemporary perspective.

Still, the notion of direct communication between citizen and police is a tantalizing suggestion for crime-reporting. Especially is some kind of alarm system like a wristband or otherwise small portable instrument relevant to danger of violence from strangers in the street. In fantasies about the future, based on increasing miniaturization of materials, one can easily conceive of almost everyone's possessing two-way Dick-Tracy-type wrist-radios tuned into household or police headquarters. The corner police telephone box of today would probably have been a more fantastic suggestion over a century ago. Without neglecting the problems about the law of evidence, uncorroborated witnesses, false accusations, etc., a citizen seeing a woman attacked, or perhaps the woman herself, could instantly call for assistance. While the stealth of offenders might overcome much of the advantage which the possessor of such an instrument might have, the ubiquitous and instant alarm system would most probably function as a considerable deterrent to many potential offenders.

Most serious crimes are discovered by citizens and not by the police,[89] and most appear to be reported to the police. There is also good reason to believe that there is an inverse relationship between the amount of time that elapses from commission of crime and the proportion of offenses cleared by arrest. It could be argued, therefore, that the more rapidly a crime is reported to the police, the higher the probability of apprehending the offender. From this hypothesis, we could accept (or test) the orthodox assumption that the higher the probability of detection and arrest, the greater will be the deterrent effect. The greater the deterrent effect, the more effective is the crime-control system and the lower will be the rate of crime.

Behavioral scientists may sometimes dismiss better lighting of streets and property as superficial means of reducing night crime, arguing that motives, values, attitudes of criminal orientation are the crucial causative forces. Yet improved lights or even television block-scanners relaying street scenes to the police, and stationed strategically throughout a city, are suggestions that also may deserve evaluative research. Notwithstanding the technological feasibility of wrist-radios and television cameras (protected, of course, from stones tossed by playful juveniles), highly placed on corner lamp-posts, the costs of such a network of communication and serious questions of having a population subject to constant surveillance except in controlled privacy indoors, might be intolerably oppressive to many people. The parameters of these problems need to be explored.

The ready access to guns, not just rifles for hunting, but pistols and automatic guns used for human killing, is viewed by many observers as a major factor contributing to acts of violence. We shall not here pursue this topic in documentary detail nor debate with the U.S. National Rifle Association. The dramatic and ugly consequences of an Oswald or a Whitman alerted and alarmed the nation to the fact that there are millions of guns easily available to almost anyone who would have one. Restricting access to guns has again been vigorously debated since Oswald. Although it may be true that anyone determined to kill will find a weapon, including a gun, even under the most restrictive legislation, most slayings involving guns are not committed by determined murderers. The handy gun has usually become the method of impulse, the vehicle of violence. Coles is most clear and succinct on this point:

'Every psychiatrist has treated patients who were thankful that guns were not around at one or another time in their lives. Temper tantrums, fits, seizures, hysterical episodes all make the presence of guns an additional and possibly mortal danger. In this country today children can obtain guns by mail-order. I have treated delinquents who have grown up with them, not toy guns but real ones. We cannot prevent insanity in adults or violent and delinquent urges in many children by curbing guns, but we can certainly make the translation of crazy or vicious impulses into pulled triggers less likely and less possible.'[90]

Systems Analysis

Major urban police departments have been using computers for some years, mainly or merely to tabulate criminal complaints, police services, and arrests for annual reporting purposes. But today there can be computerized analyses of police activity and models for predicting crime and determining the most effective methods for allocating police resources. Quantitative, operational research techniques are capable of being applied to the normal police functions of prevention, deterrence, protection, and apprehension. Police departments do not use formal techniques to analyze their own data in such a way as to provide the basis of a valid, repeatable, and practical tool for the prediction of crime. Usually, intuitive judgement and experience have been employed to provide the police with reasonable estimates of crime location and occurrence. But these latter tools are severely limited by the complexity, extent, and interaction of the many elements that must be considered in determining the probability of crime occurrence.

Without reference to underlying 'cause', a crime-predictive model can be constructed on the basis of variables associated with the incidence of crime.[91] Through statistical multiple-regression techniques, multidimensional analysis, or predictive attribute analysis, or a series of simultaneous linear equations, etc., it is now feasible to produce a model that optimizes deployment of special forces within limits of time, space, and cost. After the parameters of the problem have been described, the accuracy and completeness of police record-keeping assured, and data collected for programming, independent variables can be tested for significance and their coefficients (weights) computed. A prediction equation model giving the incidences of a particular class or subclass of crime over time–space dimensions would be the goal of such a systems analysis. Up-dating, modification, and recalibration routines would be integral parts of the prediction model and deployment strategy. Evaluating the accuracy of the model would also become part of the process, and the extent to which operations of the model itself cause perturbations in the rates of crime would have to be carefully monitored and included in the feedback loops of the system.

Only in quite recent years has some attention been given to the ways in which systems analysis can be applied to crime control. Greenhalgh,[92] of the Home Office in London, engaged in multiple-correlation analysis as a starter in this direction. He attempted to determine specific rates of crime in different sectors of a city at varying time-periods, relative to the migratory flow of people, as an aid to police deployment. Roy[93] proposed an 'expected total cost' model for crime including the costs to the victim (material loss, physical and psychological trauma, etc.), the costs to the state (police efforts, court procedure, incarceration, and rehabilitation), and the costs to the criminal and his family. His proposed measure of 'undesirability' is expressed in monetary units. The weighted scale of crime researched by Sellin and Wolfgang[94] suggests methods for measuring the effectiveness of crime-control activities in terms of subjective public reaction to the resulting crime situation. The report of the Space-General Corporation in California[95] used the rudimentary techniques of systems engineering in an examination of a broad spectrum of criminal justice, including law enforcement, courts, probation, institutions, and parole. Shumate and Crowther[96] have applied quantitative methods to the problem of optimizing the allocation of police resources by calculating probabilities of the number of events requiring service relative to time intervals of delay, essentially a queueing problem. Wolfgang and Smith[97] addressed themselves to the ways in which an inter-disciplinary team of operation analysts, working with mathematical techniques, including mathematical modeling, mathematical programming, game theory, Markov-process theory, queueing theory, etc., may help to improve the operations of various crime control activities. The extent to which any type of systems analysis is capable of promoting measures to reduce crimes of violence is still not clear. Most success is presumed to relate to the risk-reward system connected with acquisitive crime. However, it is conceivable that socio-psychological variables can be included in a model in such a way as to effect rates of rape, aggravated assaults, and even homicide. For example, in one study it was noted that two-thirds of homicide offenders had prior police arrest records, and of these, three-fourths had prior records of aggravated assaults.[98] An intervention model could include this kind of variable as a parameter that, when acted upon at the propitious moment in the biographies of potential killers, could alter their progression of aggressivity from assault to murder. Moreover, patterns of statistical regularity of many crimes of violence suggest the feasibility of social control. There are diurnal, weekly, and monthly bulges of frequency to homicides, rapes, and aggravated assaults. The movement of assaultive offenders from residence to target areas is not a 'random walk', nor are the methods employed or victims assaulted merely chance selections. As we have noted in earlier chapters, there are clusters of variables that have been traditionally noted to be associated with homicide and other assaultive crimes. No formal, systematic effort known to the present writer has yet been made to develop a predictive model designed to prevent these crimes. The fact that many homicides are the outcome of domestic quarrels between husbands and wives should not automatically preclude an effort to predict, and hence prevent, them. Nor should consideration of these types of homicide divert concern from other less privately displayed acts of violence. In a subsequent section we shall briefly discuss family factors related to crimes of violence and the features of community action that might reduce their occurrence.

Communication, Transportation, and Medical Technology

In a previous work[99] it has been noted that over several decades the rates of homicide have steadily decreased while rates of aggravated assault have steadily increased. In addition, examination of the time span between commission of a homicidal assault and death of the victim raised several interesting questions. The data combined to suggest that something other than a greater repugnance against committing crimes of personal violence may have entered our mores. Of course, many variables are involved in examining changing rates of homicide, such as the age composition, business cycles, etc. But because crimes of violence against the person, excluding homicide, appear to have increased during the past several decades, it is logical to assume that if these gross social variables affect homicide, they should affect other crimes of violence in the same way. Perhaps the following explanation, which remains on the level of an *a priori*, untested assumption, provides a partial explanation of the lower homicide rate in recent years.

It was noted that the time between assault of a victim and pronouncement of death varies according to the method by which death was inflicted. It would be interesting to have this same type of information for a period twenty or twenty-five years ago. It would also be valuable to know the recovery rate for those who are today grievously assaulted but who would have probably died under medical and other conditions of a generation ago.

It may be that three major factors present in our culture today, and absent a generation ago, make it possible for many victims of aggravated assault and other serious offenses against the person to recover from their wounds, to continue living and thereby swell the police statistics of major assaults, while simultaneously reducing the number of criminal homicides. These three factors are:

1. quick communication with the police by telephone and radio shortly after a homicidal attack;
2. rapid transportation to a hospital after a serious stabbing, shooting, beating, etc.; and,
3. advanced medical technology, such as the development of the many 'wonder drugs' since the late nineteen-thirties.

A complete analysis of these three factors has not been made, but the importance of them today can hardly be denied. In most cases of assault crimes, either the police are notified almost immediately, or someone is available to transport the victim to a nearby hospital. The motorized police in most urban communities are capable of transporting an assault victim to the hospital within a very short period of time. Upon notification, the police in several major cities arrive at the scene of a crime within an average of two minutes. Such speed of communication and transportation was undoubtedly less possible twenty-five or thirty-five years ago.

Once in a hospital, a victim of an assault probably has a much better chance of recovery and survival today than earlier. Development during the middle thirties and the more extensive years since the Second World War of sulfonamids and antibiotics is partially responsible for the differential recovery rate. Since the early nineteen-fifties cortisone has been used as a standard shock treatment in many acute stages of stress, in cases of severe body damage, and as a means of providing a general supportive effect to the organism. Within the past twenty years there has been a virtual revolution in preventing loss of blood and other fluid. Fluid-replacement therapy today means that probably many lives are saved that would have been lost before because of our ability to maintain fluid and electrolyte balance in proper chemical relationships. Today, there are better emergency teams in our hospitals capable of preventing and controlling infection and shock after a stabbing or shooting or other kind of assault. Techniques in surgical repair, whereby whole sections of blood vessels and nerve sheaths are replaced, are amazing developments which have matured within the past ten years. Heart manipulation and chemical or electrical stimulation after cardiac arrest are now almost common practice in our major hospitals. The alcoholically debilitated victim can now be supported with vitamins, hormones, and other means so that life is often sustained when such would not have been possible previously. Studies of the changes in mortality rates resulting from combat wounds during the First World War, the Second World War, and the Korean War,[100] add convincing evidence to the assumed importance that these medical advances have had in reducing homicide rates in the civilian population.

Thus, quick communication, rapid transportation, and such medical-technological advances as those mentioned above, as well as many others, may mean that many cases of physical assault are kept in the column of aggravated assault statistics and are thereby prevented from being listed as criminal homicides. Empirical research testing the hypothesis suggested by these factors might be useful in explaining some of the decrease in homicide.

If there is any validity to the thesis, then it would appear obvious that accelerating the flow of information about an assault to the police and the transportation of a victim to a medical center would further reduce the rate of homicide. Perhaps an improvement in any one of the three items (communication, transportation, medicine) would show an effect in reduced rates. Altering all three would have a multiple probability function. Our previous references to alarm systems and computerized police operations are clearly related to this thesis of technological control of violent crime.

COMMUNITY CONTROL

Criminogenic Forces of the City [101]

We have earlier inferred that crime statistics to some extent reflect the efficiency and intensity of police action, from patrols to paperwork. But there are probably mightier forces within an urban community than in rural areas that generate conditions conducive to criminality. Urban living is more anonymous living. It releases the individual from community restraints more common in tradition-oriented societies. But more freedom from constraints and controls also provides greater freedom to deviate. And living in the more impersonalized, formally controlled urban society means that regulatory orders of conduct are often directed by distant bureaucrats. The police are strangers executing these prescriptions on, at worst, an alien subcommunity and, at best, an anonymous set of subjects. Minor offenses in a small town or village are often handled without resort to official police action, and as eufunctional as such action may seem to be, it none the less results in fewer recorded violations of the law, compared to the city. Although it may perhaps cause some difficult decision for the police in small towns, the villagers are unwilling to tolerate formal, objective law enforcement.

Urban areas, with mass populations, greater wealth, more commercial establishments, and more products of technology, also provide more frequent opportunities for theft. Victims are impersonalized, property is insured, consumer goods in greater abundance are vividly displayed and are more portable.

Urban life is commonly characterized by population density, spatial mobility, ethnic and class heterogeneity, reduced family functions, and, as we have said, greater anonymity. All of these traits are expressed in comparison to non-urban life, or varying degrees of urbanism and urbanization. When, on a scale, these traits are found in high degree, and when they are combined with poverty, physical deterioration, low education, residence in industrial and commercial centers, unemployment or unskilled labor, economic dependency, marital instability or breaks, poor or absent male models for young boys, overcrowding, lack of legitimate opportunities to make a better life, the absence of positive, anticriminal behavior patterns, higher frequency of organic diseases, a cultural minority status of inferiority, it is generally assumed that social-psychological mechanisms leading to deviance are more likely to emerge. These include frustration, lack of motivation to obey external demands, internalized cultural strains of inconsistency between means available and ends desired, conflicting norms, anomie, and so forth. The link between these two conditions – physical features of subparts of a city and the social-psychological aspects – has not been fully researched to the point where the latter can safely be said to be invariable or highly probable consequences of the former. Thus, to move onto a third level, namely a tradition of lawlessness, of delinquent or criminal behavior, as a further consequence of the physical and social-psychological conditions of much urban life, is an even more tenuous scientific position. None the less, these are the assumptions under which the community of scholars and public administrators operate today. The assumptions are the most justified and logically adequate we can make unless or until they are successfully refuted.

It has often been suggested that high-crime areas of a city (meaning both residence of offenders and places of crime occurrence) contain, in high numbers, new migrants, the residue of earlier residential groups that have mostly moved out, and competitive failures from better districts who were forced to move back to the cheaper rent areas. This 'selective migration' thesis may have some validity, as Taft[102]

L

discovered in a study of Danville, Illinois, many years ago. But he also noted that most of the criminals in the high-crime areas had been reared in delinquency areas of other cities.

It is abundantly clear even to the most casual observer that Negroes in American society are the current carriers of a ghetto tradition, that they, more than any other socially defined group, are the recipients of urban deterioration and the social-psychological forces leading to deviance from the law. And for this reason, crime in the urban community is commonly a matter of Negro crime. Although there are good reasons for raising serious questions about criminal statistics that report race of the offender and the fact that Negro crime rates are in general three or four times higher than white rates,[103] and although Negroes probably suffer more injustices than whites in the law-enforcement process from arrest to imprisonment, it is no surprise that the most valid efforts to measure crime still find Negro crime rates high. When the untoward aspects of urban life are found among Italians, Germans, Poles, or almost any other group, their crime rates are similarly high. Relative deprivation and social disqualification are thus dramatically chained to despair and delinquency.

All of this is not meant to obscure the fact that poverty also exists in small towns and rural areas. But when multiplied by thousands, congested, and transmitted over generations, poverty becomes a culture. The expectations of social intercourse change, and irritable, frustrated parents often become neglectful and aggressive. Their children inherit a *subculture of violence* where physically aggressive responses are either expected or required by all members sharing not only the tenement's plumbing but also its system of values. Ready access and resort to weapons in this milieu may be essential to protection against others who respond in similarly violent ways in certain situations. The carrying of knives or other protective devices becomes a common symbol of willingness to participate in violence, to expect violence, and to be ready to retaliate against it.

A subculture of violence is not the product of cities alone. The Thugs of India, the *vendetta barbaricina* in Sardinia, the *mafioso* in Sicily have existed for a long time. But the contemporary American city has the accoutrements not only for the genesis but also for the highly accelerated development of this subculture. From this subculture, we have suggested, come most violent crimes like homicide, rape, robbery, and aggravated assaults.

Dispersion of the Subculture of Violence

To intervene socially means taking some kind of action designed to break into the information loop that links the subcultural representatives in a constant chain of reinforcement of the use of violence. Political, economic, and other forms of social action sometimes buttress the subculture by forcing it to seek strength and solace within itself as a defense against the larger culture and thereby more strongly establishes the subcultural value system. Social inaction probably does the same in lesser degree, for inaction is not generally indifference, and thereby does not produce zero response.

The residential propinquity of the actors in a subculture of violence has been noted. Breaking up this propinquity, dispersing the members who share intense commitment to the violence value, could also cause a break in the intergenerational and intragenerational communication of this value system. Dispersion can be done in many ways and does not necessarily imply massive population shifts, although urban renewal, slum clearance, and housing projects suggest feasible methods. Renewal programs that simply shift the location of the subculture from one part of a city to another do not destroy the subculture. In order to distribute the subculture so that it dissipates, the scattered units should be small. Housing projects and neighborhood areas should be small microcosms of the social hierarchy and value system of the central dominant culture. It is in homogeneity that the subculture has strength and durability. (Some of these same notions have been presented by Cloward and Ohlin[104] in their brief discussion of controlling the conflict subculture, and by Peter McHugh[105] in his paper on breaking up the inmate culture in prison before resocialization can begin.)

For all their apparent, but still questionable, virtues and victories, the detached-worker programs of handling juvenile and delinquent gangs must still be viewed as a kind of holding action, or containment policy, until a more or less 'spontaneous remission' of gang members occurs through aging, marrying, or moving away. The occasionally reported solidifying[106] of formerly diffused or 'near-group' activities is an untoward turn of events in the detached-worker programs. The point is, however, that detached-worker action, like any program from outside a subculture that moves into it, even with the language and dress associated with it, is designed to introduce values from the dominant culture by subtly and slowly bending the subculture values to parallel the former. (Where deviant values are not delinquent, it is probably more propitious for the dominant culture to become more flexible and permit the deviancy to function freely.) But such purposeful action by the larger society has been only piecemeal, outnumbered and outmaneuvered by the subculture, which, to the invading team, itself becomes the dominant culture within this setting.

In a sense, then, the larger culture sets up its own outposts within a subculture and seeks by subversive action to undermine the subcultural values. The police in these neighborhoods are like enemy troops in alien territory; they are the most blatant bearers of the wider culture. The detached workers, while still not undercover agents, are the more subtle subversives. With neither form of control, however, has society been able to record much success; and certainly no, or at best few, claims can be made for destroying the subculture of violence by these means.

While operating within a subculture that uses non-legal methods, the legal nonviolence methods of the invaders often appear to have little or no utility. In many cases, the invaders from the larger culture who seek to control the subculture of violence ultimately resort to violence themselves and hence use the very methods of the subculture to subdue it. This usage reinforces and provides new subcultural justification for violence.

Before one set of values can replace another, before the subculture of violence can be substituted by the establishment of nonviolence, the former must be disrupted, dispersed, disorganized. The resocialization, relearning process best takes place when the old socialization and old learning are forgotten or denied their validity. Once the subculture is disintegrated by dispersion of its members, aggressive attitudes are not supported by like-minded companions, and violent behavior is not regularly on display to encourage imitation and repetition.

To be most immediately effective beyond this point, however, the normative system of the larger culture must be presented as a reasonably clear, if not codified, statement. But neither national goals nor the middle-class value system in a democratic society constitutes a dogma. One virtue of a more doctrinaire system lies in its clarification of principles. To remain fluid and flexible is another kind, and perhaps a more enduring quality, of strength. To reconvert, retrain, reform may require some exaggeration of the elements of the value system, i.e. a presentation of an ideal and idealized type. With respect to violence, and especially to criminal homicide, most cultures can be more explicit and have stronger consensus against it than with respect to any other item. Except for a somewhat schizoid attitude toward war, the values of the larger culture contain strong prescriptions for nonviolence. Thus, if the dominant middle-class ethic is clearly opposed to the use of violence in interpersonal relationships, the clarity of its opposition should be a useful element in its efforts to resocialize the dispersed members of a former subculture of violence.

We shall return to this suggestion of wider dispersion of the subculture of violence in a subsequent section on 'territory'.

Community Service Centers

Community service centers are expanding in number and function. Mental health programs, marriage and school counseling, medical care, job opportunities, legal aid, home economics, child care for working mothers, rent and shopping advice, and so forth, are some of the services provided today in the heartland and on the periphery of poverty quarters in major cities.

Relative to our principal concern with crimes and criminals of violence, observers have suggested that all of these services and the structures of the centers that provide them be further elaborated and more fully integrated with the subcommunities they serve. If there is value in their existence, it is logical to promote their extension, staff improvement, and increase in functions. It has been suggested that the interservice referral system be improved; that a central registry be established; that all, not merely 'multiple-problem', families be treated as 'total' families in terms of the growing field of social psychiatry; that gang-control units of police departments become intimately acquainted with community service centers, refer individual juveniles and gangs to these centers for non-police attention; that all accumulated information on troubled families in poor neighborhoods be shared with, sifted by, and acted upon by community organization staffs of city welfare boards who are presumed to be in the best position for overviewing and coordinating the complex machinery of social service.

A particularly intriguing innovation suggested as a special function of community centers is the 'emergency domestic quarrel team' of specialists.[107] With a staff of sufficient size and training to provide twenty-four-hour service on call, the team is viewed as capable of offering rapid social intervention, quick decisions and accelerated resolutions to families caught in a conflict crisis. Traditionally, the police are called into service when domestic quarrels erupt into public complaints. The police are trained principally to interrupt fights in verbal or physical form. Their chief function is to prevent assault and battery at the moment of arrival, to arrest assaulters on complaint, and then to go about their business of patrolling their sector. It is well known that some of the most potentially dangerous calls police officers act upon are reports of domestic quarrels. About one-fifth of all policemen killed on duty are those who responded to 'disturbance' calls which include family quarrels.[108]

The suggestion of an emergency domestic quarrel team is meant to include the police as part of the group, primarily to protect the team itself from violent attack. After the initial danger has subsided, the police could withdraw, leaving the team of psychological and social work specialists to talk with the family, to suggest the best solution to the immediate problem, and work out a program for a more enduring resolution.

It should be kept in mind that a relatively high proportion of criminal homicides are classified as emerging from domestic quarrels. These are acts usually committed indoors, not normally subject to observation by patrolmen on the street, and therefore considered virtually unpredictable and unpreventable. An emergency domestic quarrel team might, therefore, function from a community center as an effective homicide-prevention measure. Intervening in earlier stages of physically aggressive strife in the family, the team could conceivably thwart the progression of family violence to the point of homicidal attack. The strategies for resolving domestic conflict are details too specific to pursue further here, but, clearly, experience would accumulate to provide increasing sophistication. In addition to information shared in an adequate referral system, these teams would soon develop expertise in handling many difficult family situations. It should be further noted that twice as many homicides among Negroes as among whites are known to develop from quarrels within the family, usually between husbands and wives.[109] These are almost invariably lower-class, poor Negro families. The emergency teams to which we refer would operate out of centers often located in areas with high concentrations of the Negro poor.

Various indices to measure the success of these teams can easily be imagined. Keeping in mind our focus on crimes of violence, one index of the value of emergency intervention could be changing rates of domestic homicides and aggravated assaults. Perhaps even rate changes in general throughout an ecological area would be influenced. After all, an unresolved family conflict may cause some family members to displace their cumulative aggressivity on close friends, neighborhood acquaintances, or even strangers. For we do not know the number of homicides and aggravated assaults recorded by the police as due to 'altercations' which may have had their genesis in a hostile exchange in the family.

Territory

Building upon many anthropological findings and socio-psychological studies of aggression and the meaning of life-space, Robert Ardrey has recently written an able and provocative book entitled *The Territorial Imperative*.[110] Briefly stated, his main thesis is that from fiddler crabs to gibbons to *Homo sapiens*, there is from genetic structure an instinctive attachment to territories, to a familiar living-space. This inward compulsion to possess and defend such a space makes man, as well as lower creatures in the evolutionary scale, a territorial animal. Possession of a territory is, he asserts, a mysterious source of extra energy to the proprietor. Referring to Konrad Lorenz (*On Aggression*), as we have done in a prior section, Ardrey argues that intraspecific aggression is not only ritualized and inevitable, but also serves an integrative function. Amity is expressed by members for their own group, but is equal to the sum of the forces of enmity and hazard which are arrayed against it ($A = E + h$). By enmity he refers to forces of antagonism and hostility originating in members of one's own species. Hazard means threats that do not originate in one's own group.

Both from statements by Ardrey and by projections from his thesis of the territorial imperative, gigantic theoretical leaps can too readily be made to gang delinquency and international conflict. The 'turf' of delinquent gangs, the opposition to slum clearance by slum-dwellers, the skid-row resident who fights removal, the white protest against Negro property invasions, the burglarizing intrusion on the territory of others, the frequency of intragroup crimes of violence, etc., are facile translations of Ardrey's propositions. But as Loren Eiseley remarks in his review of Ardrey's book, 'He makes a strong case, but in spite of a few hasty qualifications it is, to the social anthropologist, simplistic. . . . Life is easily convicted of being "biological" simply by being life.'[111]

Even without acceptance of the validity of a genetic proclivity to have attachment to a living-space, there appear to be at least social and psychological propensities manifested behaviorally toward territory. Pride in possession and the congealed labor which property represents are probably not unique to the middle-class ethic of contemporary man, although they may be more highly placed in the middle-class than in the lower-class value system.

There is a relationship between this territorial notion and what we have previously said about community service centers and the dispersion of the subculture of violence. Regardless of the apparent value as an immediate ameliorative, the establishment of service centers within the communities or neighborhoods of need does endorse the territory. In one sense, an area of deprivation becomes officially labeled, the territory is known as troubled, and the residents are, by the services, unintentionally encouraged, if not required, to remain. It could even be argued that the ecological parameters of poverty become more solidified. When there is added the ingredient of self-help and developing indigenous leadership,[112] there is further coalescence of forces to retain group and territorial identification.

These remarks should not be interpreted as opposition to the kinds of community action programs currently in progress. Viewed in terms of a long perspective of time, they may substantially reduce poverty, increase opportunities, and change allegiance to violence to commitment to nonviolence. But the territory will remain. Ghettos may change to ethnic guilds; but group identity and unintended residential separation may remain.

On the other hand, our earlier remarks about more massive efforts to disperse, dissipate, and relocate the members of a subculture of violence suggest that the community-center-action programs are stop-gap measures of temporary containment of conflict. The pressures toward crimes of violence and riots of protest can be arrested by direct and immediate action within the recognizable communities of need. But if the terrain of deprivation is to be changed, its inhabitants should be spread and made an integral part of a more mosaic, heterogeneous pattern of an urban structure. The original territory of poverty would, of course, be replaced by another heterogeneous cluster of groups. Supporting this notion of socially planned heterogeneity is a recent paper by Paul Eberts and Kent Schwirian,[113] who examined the crime rates of 212 communities identified as Standard Metropolitan Statistical Areas in 1960, within the theoretical framework of relative deprivation. These authors found, among other things, that rates for major crimes in general as well as for crimes involving violent personal attack are lowest in those cities where the class structure is balanced instead of being characterized by a high proportion of upper-class or a high proportion of lower-class members. The use of the term 'balanced' by Eberts and

Schwirian is not synonymous with our reference to heterogeneity of community structure. Their term refers to a relatively even spread of the population by social and economic classes. Our reference has been to a relatively even ecological spread of these same classes throughout the community. But if efforts to provide economic security and other services of community action continued simultaneously with the dispersion of the population of the poor, there is reason to believe that the class structure would also have a high probability of becoming balanced.

The Masculine Protest and Its Transformation

Social scientists have long stressed the importance of the theme of masculinity in American culture and the effect that this image of the strong masculine role has had on child-rearing and the general socialization process. The inability of the middle-class male child to match himself to this masculine model and the neuroticism that is the consequence of this increasingly futile struggle was vividly brought to our attention years ago by Arnold Green.[114] The continuity of this masculine role in the lower classes has often been asserted and was made one of the 'focal concerns' in Walter B. Miller's[115] profile of the lower-class milieu. There is reason to believe, however, that this once-dominating culture theme is dissipating, especially in the central or middle-class culture, and that this dissipation is diffusing downwards through the lower classes via the youth subculture.

It may well be true that in many lower-class communities violence is associated with masculinity and may be not only acceptable but admired behavior. That the rates of violent crimes are high among lower-class males suggests that this group still and strongly retains notions of *machismo*, continues to equate maleness with overt physical aggression. In the Italian slum of the Boston West End, Herbert Gans[116] describes families dominated by the men in which mothers encourage male dominance. On the other hand, lower-class boys who lack father or other strong male figures, as in the case of many Negro families, have a problem of finding models to imitate. But rejecting female dominance at home and at school and their association of morality may be a means of their asserting their masculinity, and such assertion must be performed with a strong antithesis of femininity, namely by being physically aggressive. Being a bad boy, Parsons[117] has said, can become a positive goal if goodness is too closely identified with feminity.

Jackson Toby[118] has recently suggested that, if the compulsive masculinity hypothesis has merit, it ought to generate testable predictions about the occurrence of violence, and lists the following: '(1) Boys who grow up in households headed by women are more likely to behave violently than boys who grow up in households headed by a man. . . . (2) Boys who grow up in households where it is relatively easy to identify with the father figure are less likely to behave violently than in households where identification with the father figure is difficult. . . . (3) Boys whose development toward adult masculinity is slower than their peers are more likely to behave violently than boys who find it easy to think of themselves as "men". . . . (4) Masculine ideals emphasize physical roughness and toughness in those populations where *symbolic* masculine power is difficult to understand. Thus, middle-class boys ought to be less likely than working-class youngsters to idealize strength and its expression in action and to be more likely to appreciate the authority over other people exercised by a physician or a business executive.'[(119)] As Toby indicates, it is unfortunate that evidence at present is so fragmentary that these predictions are not subject to rigorous evaluation.

Should the lower classes become more like the middle class in value orientation, family structure, and stability, there is reason to believe the emphasis on masculine identification through physical prowess and aggression would decline. The need to prove male identity may not disappear, especially if Parsons is correct about the importance of this problem for the middle-class male child. But even being 'bad' in order to sever the linkage of morality and femininity may become increasingly difficult to achieve in a purely masculine way. And if there are available, as some writers believe, new and alternative models for demonstrating masculinity, ways that may be neither 'bad' nor physically aggressive, then we should expect masculine identity to be manifested differently, that is, symbolically, even by lower-class boys. Symbolic expressions have always been available, and some contemporary vulgar types are closer than others to the use of physical force. Cars, motorcycles, boots and helmets; football and other sports with body contact; debating societies, musical virtuosity, and literary talent – in gross terms these represent gradations of distance from the more earthy, mesomorphic masculinity. As the larger culture becomes more cerebral, the refined symbolic forms of masculinity should be more fully adopted. And as the disparity in life style, values, and norms between the lower and middle classes is diminished, so too will be reduced the subculture of violence that views ready resort to violence as an expected form of masculine response to many situations.

SOCIALIZATION FOR NONVIOLENCE

In the Community

In our previous section on community control of violence, with reference to dispersion of the supportive subculture and expansion of community service centers, there is set by inference a corresponding preparatory stage for transmission of the dominant-culture value of nonviolence. By new patterns of residential propinquity to families, schools, and peer groups that contain very few and muted expressions of violence in child-rearing, marital life, playground activities, and other episodes in the dramas of personal interaction, the former members from the subcultural territory would be expected to introject a new set of norms and values. In the subtleties of daily social life, without the vast network of a previous subcultural communication system that reported events of violence as commonplace, the resocialization process can take place. To buttress the otherwise slow shift in attitudes and values are the community service centers, now less locked in the zones of poverty and deviance and widely distributed throughout the city.

Recreational facilities, child guidance clinics, boy and girl scout clubs hobby clubs, Police Athletic League Centers, Little League baseball, neighborhood associations, and the like could now function as demonstrably effective vehicles for conversion to nonviolent activities. There is no solid empirical evidence that the catalogue of clubs and playgrounds in American cities has been effective in preventing delinquency or reducing violent crime. A common criticism is that these positive community agencies do not reach the delinquent, or highly potential delinquent, population. If these centers are placed in congested neighborhoods with high crime rates, the clubs are many times viewed as unwanted invaders of the territory and are consequently often unattended, except by 'good boys' in the bad areas.

When the families from the subculture of violence had been distributed and increasingly absorbed by the surrounding middle-class milieu, they would become conditioned to the behavioral expectations around them. Instead of the old and consistent role models from generations before them and peers beside them, the territorially transplanted families could see, not inadequate images of middle-class conformity and life style from mass-media projections, but nearby neighbors with whom they could interact. The nearly compulsive adoption of middle-class roles by Negro families in integrated communities is already well known. We are drawing attention here to the general social-psychological processes of norm-learning, empathy, projection, identification, internalization, and the influence of ego-ideals, primary reference groups, and differential association.

There may be some concern that the middle-class value system too often requires over-conformity, is 'bourgeois' in a pejorative sense, produces neurotics, and is too strongly permeated with mediocrity and banality in esthetic matters and in life itself. It may also be regretted by some observers that certain features of the life style of the Negro poor and of criminal subcultures might disappear if the middle-class value system destroyed them in a kind of cultural homogenization. The concern in the former statement is overdrawn; the regret in the latter may be a form of romanticism or of vicarious titillation in observing the forbidden games of deviants. As Melvin Tumin has eloquently said, some social analysts do not view some social problems as problems 'because we see them as indirect expressions of laudable human spirit and verve and honesty or straightforwardness breaking through the hypocritical bounds of our ordinary norms . . . [and] the actors in delinquency, crime, adultery and divorce often tend to command our positive sympathies because, I suggest, they are doing things many of us would like to be able to do'.[120]

One might well ask what the alternatives to the middle-class ethic are to which our policy decision-makers would have criminal deviants rehabilitated or resocialized. The diversity of human expression, the range of alternative forms of behavior and attitude within the broad spectrum of the middle class, appear to be sufficiently great to avoid the stultifying and stagnant homogenization that may be feared by some observers.

Finally, under the suggestions of dispersion and newly found attachments to the middle-class milieu, community treatment of delinquents and placement of offenders on probation or return to the community on parole should facilitate the retraining process. Instead of a return to the old criminal subculture or subculture of violence, the offender would be placed in an environment predominantly nonviolent.

In Prison

In a correctional setting, the problem of treatment must be viewed from the perspective of (a) the population involved, i.e. juveniles versus adults, and (b) the kind of institutional orientation, i.e. traditional institutional treatment versus more active group or individual psychotherapeutic efforts. The conception of the subculture of violence implies that two areas will be involved in a treatment approach. One is primarily concerned with values, the other with the specific technique to be employed. These areas may be referred to as intent and technique. The context of a treatment is restricted to values in the sense that this is a useful psychological construct to indicate the most visible element in the general personality structure involved in a subcultural affiliation, which must be established before a new cultural allegiance can be built. The personality must undergo a process of weakening of the subcultural ties by means of one of a variety of techniques until allegiance is decreased and a new value system can be introduced. Implicit in this process is the emergence of an anomic state of confusion which should reflect the moment in which different value sets coexist within an individual and exercise an ambivalent pull over his conscious and unconscious motives. This process may express itself in anxiety states, it may cause regression, it may channel itself through psychosomatic symptomatology. It must be kept within tolerable limits, but it does constitute a healthy sign of modifiability. The process may be totally negative and the subject may consistently resist any effort to change his allegiance; still the presence or absence of anxiety is probably the best indicator of this resistance.

In the process of trying to change values, the therapist faces the difficult step of having to learn the subcultural group orientation of the subject. This is an obvious prerequisite of the therapeutic efforts and is made necessary by the fact that the subculture, or even more broadly the social class, from which the criminal comes, is in many instances radically different from the subculture and class from which the therapist comes. It is also obvious that the therapist must be clear about his own values and commitments because, in a multitude of subtle as well as overt ways, these are constantly being probed by the criminal patient. In fighting off treatment the subcultural delinquent can do this all the more successfully if he repudiates the values which he expects the therapist, as an agent of the community, to represent. Obviously, this objective of the delinquent is more easily obtained if he can find the therapist's values weak and inconsistent.[121]

The need for the therapist to participate in the patient's value system or at least to be aware of it, is certainly not a new notion in psychotherapy. It has very often been stated that the therapist's personality and background should be congruent with the patient's personality and needs relative to such factors as sex, age, race, nationality, religion, and socio-economic background.[122] As Ellis[123] puts it, when the therapist works with clients whose cultural background is radically different from his own, he should understand as fully as possible both the general importance of culture in normal and abnormal behaviour and the influence of the specific cultural background in which the patient was reared. It has even been suggested by Kennedy[124] that when the patient belongs to a minority group it might be advisable to have two therapists working with him, one of whom is also of this minority group. All of these suggestions are especially essential to keep in mind when working with criminal subcultures.

The specific methods and techniques, the procedural guidance to be exercised in the process of subculturally oriented therapy, can be commented upon only very briefly, for no direct experimentation using the notions of a subculture of violence, and obviously no evaluative results, are available. Some practical suggestions include trying to break and disperse the subcultural groups that establish themselves together in the prison community. Some of these groups establish themselves by age or regional affiliation and come to assert so much influence in the prison environment as to controvert efforts of a prison administration to provide a correctional climate favorable to a positive value change.[125] Efforts should be made to avoid reinforcement of negative subcultural values by the prison personnel. Not infrequently, the social class and region of origin of the prison personnel closely match those of the inmate population. The close daily contact and the high number of associations, particularly in isolated penitentiary settings, may cause an absorption of the prison staff into the inmate subculture, with the result that the guards retain values only nominally oriented to the larger society. Moreover, the present institutional mode of classification procedures is generally vague and crude, and tends to throw together inmates who are alike, particularly with respect to their use of violence, and may thereby provide a systematic, unanticipated reinforcement of the subculture of violence. A much more individualized approach to classification than currently exists seems desirable, and greater awareness is needed of the socio-cultural and psychological implications of the criminal behavior and anamnestic patterns present in the developmental and life history of the individual. Subcultural factors, if any, should always be assessed as part of the routine diagnostic process in a correctional classification system.

The treatment aspects we have briefly discussed above are concerned with general institutional care and can be classified under the 'milieu therapy' techniques.[126] Perhaps more important and more provocative are the approaches which constitute a *direct* intervention through individualized or group manipulations on the personality of the violent offender.

We cannot discuss here in detail either the different therapeutic techniques that impinge upon the subcultural hypothesis, or many of the common analytic methods of therapy and day-to-day institutional devices (as outlined in the Redl and Wineman volumes)[127] that may have relevance to a subcultural orientation. The psychoanalytic approach tended to ignore the social factors in the personality make-up of the patient, but the more modern emphasis on ego psychology has modified this attitude. However, the validity of the classical psychotherapeutic techniques has been seriously questioned in many fields, including that of delinquent groups, and the introduction of subcultural factors might help to make these techniques more amenable to scientific validation. The subcultural approach is not in conflict with an hypothesis of dynamic personality structure, but it is more akin to learning theory or perceptual conceptualization. From cognitive theory, Festinger's dissonance theory offers some models that may help in initiating attitude change. A similar approach has been proposed by Stagner[128] for the reduction of international tension, and conceivably it could be transferred to the individual or small-group level. It could be postulated that at least part of what goes on in a group psychotherapy session is a striving toward consonance with norms accepted by the therapist.

The links existing between the subcultural hypothesis and the theory of social learning would tend to direct therapeutic efforts toward the utilization of conditioning therapies. These techniques are today enjoying a new currency in the field of clinical psychiatry, and many different kinds of experimental studies on their validity are in progress. They have been strongly advocated for a variety of reasons, and under the name of behavior therapy have been proposed by Eysenck for criminal subjects. Extrovert criminals (the less 'subcultural' in Eysenck's formulation) require discipline and firmness. The introverts obviously should be approached with reconditioning techniques. The therapeutic effect of benzedrine-like substances could temporarily help to shift the balance of extroverts toward the introverted end of the axis, thus enhancing the possibility of favorable conditioning.[129]

The different possibilities for modification of behavior according to a social-learning approach have been analyzed in detail by Bandura and Walters.[130] Extinction, counter-conditioning, positive reinforcement, social imitation, and discrimination learning have all been postulated as attempts to modify undesirable or deviant behavior. The varied application of operant conditioning in institutional settings, if conducted with a view to changing the subcultural allegiance of the subjects, might improve the chances of success. Punishment *per se* is certainly a confirmed failure as a treatment technique.[131] 'Brainwashing' and repression can be, at the price of dignity, only temporarily successful.[132] Probably systematic conditioning within a subcultural frame of reference can be a happy medium. It certainly warrants further study of its therapeutic possibilities.

RESEARCH ON THE SUBCULTURE OF VIOLENCE

The amount of material which has been presented in the preceding pages could be examined in detail to provide clues to existing research gaps. We shall limit our comments to brief indications of areas of investigation which, in our experience in research and in clinical practice, appear to be of primary importance. This priority listing is admittedly subjective and reflects our joint interdisciplinary interests.

Basic evidence for the existence of a subculture of violence is still missing or tautological. It may be found either in theoretical formulations or in phenomenological studies of particular kinds of crime which are presumed to be committed mostly by persons whose normal patterns of conduct are based upon values shared by groups that support assaultive reactions. While a criminal assault is an obvious indicator of resort to violence, the act *per se* does not prove the existence of supportive groups, for it may be an idiopathic, not a normatively prescribed, response, i.e. it may belong to the idioverse and not to the universe of the criminal.

We have tried to define and describe the meaning of subculture in general, with a view to establishing some tangible theoretical parameters to this, at present, elusive term. At the same time, it is important to state clearly the necessity of moving interchangeably from sociological to psychological theory and concepts, as well as from empirical data in the one discipline to empirical data in the other, in the study and analysis of a subculture of violence. But, perhaps most important of all, attempts should be made to establish a disciplinary duality in binding theory to scientific data; to move smoothly and in both directions from the gross to the refined, from the macroscopic to the individual perspective without distortion or loss of either sociological theory or psychological data. Of the area specialties in sociology, criminology especially has suffered from disciplinary isolation while having more abundant opportunities than most other areas for integration. Perhaps it has been the breadth and scope of criminological investigation in etiology and treatment that have encouraged scholars from many disciplines to study in this field and at the same time have permitted insularity to develop.

That (1) a subculture of violence exists and that (2) it exists in representative, identifiable individuals, are assumptions that underlie research in this area. The first statement requires further development of the theory with a subset of propositions and hypotheses that can be tested. The second statement requires application of validated psychological instruments for determining differences between individual subjects whom the theory identifies as belonging to the subculture. The types of research needed could not provide complete conclusions on these issues but would be attempts to produce some findings that could perhaps firmly establish a subculture of violence and provide meaningful suggestions for further research.[133] In addition, the case-history approach could be utilized extensively in order to collect anamnestic evidence of subcultural allegiance. This could be done in groups where other known parameters help to postulate the existence of a violent subculture.

The differential diagnostic 'power' of different projective and questionnaire types of psychological instrument for the identification of subcultural values related to violence should be carefully examined in order to provide the researcher (and the clinician) with an assessment test for a construct which may prove to be of relevant significance in understanding the personality of the offender.

A study of the effect on conditioning and behavior therapy, perhaps using a stochastic reference model for long-term changes,[134] might help to validate in clinical practice some of the theoretical implications of the subcultural hypotheses.

A cross-cultural search for violent subcultures, through an analysis of their histories, developments and, when applicable, their termination, would provide useful reference data.

SUMMARY

In brief, the theory of a subculture of violence does not include all aggression, socialized or not; it does not include all crime or even all criminal homicide. It does include most aggression manifested in physical assaults that are prohibited in criminal codes under such designations as homicide and assaults.

The notions of a subculture of violence are built upon existing (a) sociological theory on culture, social and personality systems, culture conflict, differential association, and value systems; (b) psychological theory on learning, conditioning, developmental socialization, differential identification; and (c) criminological research on criminal homicide and other assaultive crimes.

The principal propositions of the theory, we have said in Chapter III, include the following, some of which apply in part to the meaning of all subcultures:

1. No subculture can be totally different from or totally in conflict with the society of which it is a part.

2. To establish the existence of a subculture of violence does not require that the actors sharing in this basic value element express violence in all situations.

3. The potential resort or willingness to resort to violence in a variety of situations emphasizes the penetrating and diffusive nature of this culture theme.

4. The subcultural ethos of violence may be shared by all ages in a subsociety, but this ethos is most prominent in a limited age group ranging from late adolescence to middle age.

5. The counter-norm is nonviolence.

6. The development of favorable attitudes toward, and the use of, violence in this subculture involve learned behavior and a process of differential learning, association, or identification.

7. The use of violence in a subculture is not necessarily viewed as illicit conduct, and the users therefore do not have to deal with feelings of guilt about their aggression.

Hypotheses included in these propositions and that constitute suggestions for further research are the following:

1. The parameters of a subculture of violence can be partly established by measurement of social values using a ratio scale (as in

psychophysics) focused on items concerned with the behavioral displays of violence.

2. Psychometric and projective techniques show high correlations between their assessment of aggression and the psychophysical scale scores.

3. Social correlates of criminal assaultive behavior have high correlations with the psychometric and projective techniques and with the psychophysical scale scores.

4. By means of these scale scores and techniques, it is possible to designate the personality and social attributes of the representatives of a subculture of violence, which in turn makes possible the identification of ecological areas and boundaries of the subculture that interact with the dominant culture.

5. Such designated actors and identified regions allow for significantly accurate predictions to be made about future violent criminal behavior among (a) persons who have not yet engaged in such behavior, or (b) persons who have previously committed at least one assaultive crime that has come to the attention of the public authorities.

6. Persons not members of a subculture of violence who none the less commit crimes of violence have psychological and social attributes significantly different from violent criminals from the subculture of violence; i.e. violent criminal offenders from a culture of nonviolence have more psychopathological traits, more guilt, and more anxiety about their violent behavior.

7. Predictable and positive prevention of additional crimes of violence is possible by social action that is designed (a) to disperse, disrupt, and disorganize the representatives of the subculture of violence, and at the same time (b) to effect changes in the value system.

8. Therapy in correctional institutions is most effective with assaultive offenders from a subculture of violence if (a) the offenders are not permitted to retain their collective and supportive homogeneity in prison; (b) values contrary to the subculture of violence are infused into their personality structure and into the prison social system with clarity and commitment by the therapists; (c) these inmates are brought to the point of anomic anxiety; and (d) they are not returned to their subculture of origin.

* * *

At the end of this interdisciplinary excursion, we close the search and hope that forthcoming research will help to firm up some of the assumptions we have derived from our analysis. We hope that our work might be considered useful as a bibliographical guide, as a review of the current stage of criminology and of criminological research and theory, as a clear statement of our thesis of a subculture of violence, as a comprehensive summary of criminological knowledge about homicidal and other assaultive behavior, and as an encouragement to the development of integrated scientific theory and research.

NOTES AND REFERENCES

1. Marvin E. Wolfgang, *Patterns in Criminal Homicide*, Philadelphia, Penna.: University of Pennsylvania Press, 1958; Franco Ferracuti, 'La personalità dell'omicida', *Quaderni di Criminologia Clinica* (October–December, 1961) 4:419–456.
2. Howard Harlan, 'Five Hundred Homicides', *Journal of Criminal Law and Criminology* (1950) 40:736–752.
3. Wolfgang, *Patterns in Criminal Homicide*.
4. J. L. Gillin, *The Wisconsin Prisoner*, Madison, Wisconsin: University of Wisconsin Press, 1946.
5. This generalization about age and homicide appears in almost every sociological study. For example, see the following:

   Ralph S. Banay, 'A Study of 22 Men Convicted of Murder in the First Degree', *Journal of Criminal Law and Criminology* (July, 1943) 34:106–111, p. 110.
   R. C. Bensing and O. J. Schroeder, *Homicide in an Urban Community*, Springfield, Ill.: C. C. Thomas, 1960.
   H. C. Brearley, *Homicide in the United States*, Chapel Hill, N.C.: University of North Carolina Press, 1932, pp. 78–79.
   J. H. Cassidy, 'Personality Study of 200 Murderers', *Journal of Criminal Psychopathology* (1941) 2:296–304, p. 297.
   J. V. De Porte and E. Parkhurst, 'Homicide in New York State. A Statistical Study of the Victims and Criminals in 37 Counties in 1921–30', *Human Biology* (1935) 7:47–73, p. 57.
   L. I. Dublin and Bessie Bunzel, 'Thou Shalt Not Kill: A Study of Homicide in the United States', *Survey Graphic* (March, 1935) 24:127–131, p. 128.
   Evelyn Gibson and S. Klein, *Murder*, London: H.M. Stationery Office, 1961, pp. 24–27.
   Andrew F. Henry and James F. Short, Jr., *Suicide and Homicide*, Glencoe, Ill.: The Free Press, 1954, pp. 88–89.
   Frederick L. Hoffman, *The Homicide Problem*, Newark, N. J.: The Prudential Press, 1925, p. 23.
   J. J. Kilpatrick, 'Murder in the Deep South', *Survey Graphic* (October, 1943) 32:395–397, p. 396.
   Terence Morris and Louis Blom-Cooper, 'Murder in Microcosm', London: *The Observer*, 1961, pp. 3–26.
   Stuart Palmer, *A Study of Murder*, New York: Thomas Y. Crowell, 1960.
   Otto Pollak, *The Criminality of Women*, Philadelphia, Penna.: University of Pennsylvania Press, 1950, p. 156.
   Royal Commission on Capital Punishment, 1949–1953 Report, London: H.M. Stationery Office, 1953, pp. 308–309.

Saverio Siciliano, 'Risultati preliminari di un'indagine sull'omicidio in Danimarca', *La Scuola Positiva* (1961) 4:718–729, p. 723.
Hans von Hentig, *Crime; Causes and Conditions*, New York: McGraw-Hill, 1947, p. 115.

6. There is no need to document this generalization about sex and homicide. Every study known to the authors reports this fact.
7. Veli Verkko, *Homicides and Suicides in Finland and their Dependence on National Character*, Copenhagen: G.E.C. Gads Forlag, 1951, pp. 51–57.
For further comments on Verkko's 'static and dynamic laws' relative to sex and homicide, see Wolfgang, *Patterns in Criminal Homicide*, pp. 61–64.
8. See, for example, the tables of data and findings that supplement Margaret K. Bacon, Irwin L. Child, and Herbert Barry III, 'A Cross-Cultural Study of Correlates of Crime', *Journal of Abnormal and Social Psychology* (1963) 4:291–300. This study included 48 societies in Africa, Asia, North America, South America, Oceania. All information was obtained from ethnographic studies available in the literature or in the Human Relations Area Files. Comparisons can be made of the division of labor by sex and the frequency of theft and of personal crime.
9. There are many discussions of this notion in sociological and psychological literature. Walter Miller, especially, has drawn attention to the concept of 'toughness' and the lower-class male. See, for example, Walter B. Miller, Hildred Geertz, and Henry S. G. Cutter, 'Aggression in a Boys' Street-Corner Group', *Psychiatry* (1961) 24:283–298. See also the analytic comment and reinterpretation of this article by J. D. Douglas in *Psychiatry* (1962) 25:281–284.
Relative to our reiteration concerning the use of violence as normal conduct in a subculture, these authors conclude: '. . . the Junior Outlaws could scarcely be characterized as abnormal. On the contrary, they appear as an organized, efficient, and dynamically balanced system, performing stabilizing and integrative functions for both the group and its members. From this perspective, this type of adolescent group appears not as a defective or pathological organism, but as a highly effective device for accommodating a universal human problem in a manner particularly well geared to the conditions of its cultural milieu' (*Ibid.*, p. 298).
10. There are some exceptions, of course, to this generalization, but the fact that children under 14 who kill constitute a statistical deviancy from the mean, median, and mode renders them more vulnerable to the social machinery that requires their being examined for biopsychological and psychiatric abnormalities. References to child offenders appear in Chapter IV.
11. Enrico Morselli, *Il suicidio*, Milano: Dumolard, 1879.
12. Verkko, *Homicides and Suicides in Finland and Their Dependence on National Character*, Chapter XV, pp. 145–162.

13. Henry and Short, *Suicide and Homicide*. For further discussions of these twin phenomena, major sources include Emile Durkheim, *Suicide*, Glencoe, Ill.; The Free Press, 1951; Enrico Ferri, *L'omicidio*, Torino: Fratelli Bocca, 1895; and Enrico Altavilla, *Il suicidio*, Napoli: Alberto Morano, 1932.
14. Wolfgang, *Patterns in Criminal Homicide*, pp. 36–39.
15. A bibliographical compilation and discussion of these self-reporting studies appears in Robert H. Hardt and George E. Bodine, *Development of Self-Report Instruments in Delinquency Research*, Syracuse, N.Y: Youth Development Center, Syracuse University, 1965.
    Another recent listing with additional data appears in James F. Short, Jr. and Fred L. Strodtbeck, *Group Process and Gang Delinquency*, Chicago, Ill.: University of Chicago Press, 1965.
16. Nils Christie, Johs. Andenaes, and Sigurd Skirbekk, 'A Study of Self-Reported Crime', in *Scandinavian Studies in Criminology*, Vol. I, London: Tavistock, 1965, pp. 86–116.
17. Kerstin Elmhorn, 'Study in Self-Reported Delinquency among School Children in Stockholm', *Scandinavian Studies in Criminology*, Vol. I, London: Tavistock, 1965, pp. 117–146.
18. Enrico Ferri, *L'omicidio*, pp. 710–712.
19. Brearley, *Homicide in the United States*, pp. 43–45, relative to education.
20. Bensing and Schroeder, *Homicide in an Urban Community*, pp. 119–157.
21. Kaare Svalastoga, 'Homicide and Social Contact in Denmark', *American Journal of Sociology* (1956) **62**:37–41.
22. Terence Morris and Louis Blom-Cooper, *A Calendar of Murder*, London: Michael Joseph, 1963.
23. Verkko, *Homicide and Suicide in Finland and Their Dependence on National Character*.
24. C. H. S. Jayewardene, 'Criminal Homicide. A Study in Culture Conflict', Ph.D. Thesis, University of Pennsylvania, 1960; 'Criminal Cultures and Subcultures', *Probation and Child Care Journal* (June, 1963) **2**:1–5; 'Criminal Homicide in Ceylon', *Probation and Child Care Journal* (January, 1964) **3**:15–30. Cf. Herbert Bloch, 'Research Report on Homicide, Attempted Homicide and Crimes of Violence', *Colombo, Ceylon Police Report*, 1960; Edwin D. Driver, 'Interaction and Criminal Homicide in India', *Social Forces* (1961) **40**:153–158.
25. Arthur Wood, 'A Socio-Structural Analysis of Murder, Suicide, and Economic Crime in Ceylon', *American Sociological Review* (1961) **26**:744–753; *Crime and Aggression in Changing Ceylon*, Transactions of the American Philosophical Society, New Series, Vol. 51, Part 8, December, 1961. For an earlier study in Ceylon, see J. H. Strauss and M. A. Strauss, 'Suicide, Homicide and Social Structure in Ceylon', *American Journal of Sociology* (1953) **58**:461–469.
26. Miguel E. Bustamante and Miguel Angel Bravo B., 'Epidemiologia del homicido en Mexico', *Higiene* (1957) **9**:21–33. Also, Paul

Friedrich, 'Assumptions Underlying Tarascan Political Homicide', *Psychiatry* (1962) **25**:315–327.

27. A. M. Lamont, 'Forensic Psychiatric Practice in South African Mental Hospital', *South Africa Medical Journal* (1961) **35**:40:833–837.
28. Aldo Franchini and Francesco Introna, *Delinquenza minorile*, Padova: Cedam, 1961, pp. 611–618.
29. See *infra*, *Table* 1 for homicide rates for these countries.
30. Donald R. Cressey, *Other People's Money*, Glencoe, Ill.: The Free Press, 1953.
31. It might further be pointed out, relative to our discussion of physiological forces in the preceding chapter, that adrenalin discharges are most likely to occur in this latter type of actor but not in the more reasoning middle- and upper-class offender. This does not mean that middle- and upper-class offenders do not possess adrenal reactivity, but it means that their aggressiveness will not, frequently, be mediated by uncontrolled neurovegetative 'storms'.
32. Robert K. Merton, *Social Theory and Social Structure*, Rev. Ed., Glencoe, Ill.: The Free Press, 1957, esp. Chapters 4 and 5.
33. Richard Cloward and Lloyd Ohlin, *Delinquency and Opportunity*, Glencoe, Ill.: The Free Press, 1960.
34. Marvin E. Wolfgang, *Crime and Race: Conceptions and Misconceptions*, New York: Institute of Human Relations Press, 1964, p. 31.
35. See *ibid.* both for a critique of general crime statistics by race and for a selected bibliography on criminal homicide by race.
36. Most of the studies previously cited in this chapter have references to one or more of these items. Some additional studies that may be consulted, containing similar findings for specific variables, are set out below, in chronological order:

Albert W. Stearns, 'Homicide in Massachusetts', *American Journal of Psychiatry* (1925) **4**:725–749.
Calvin F. Schmid, 'Study of Homicides in Seattle', *Social Forces* (1926) **4**:745–756.
A. Raven, 'A Theory of Murder', *American Sociological Review* (1930) **22**:108–118.
K. E. Barnhart, 'A Study of Homicide in the United States', *Social Science* (1932) **7**:141–159.
L. I. Dublin and Bessie Bunzel, 'Thou Shalt Not Kill: A Study of Homicide in the United States', *Survey Graphic* (1935) **24**:127–131.
Emil Frankel, 'One Thousand Murderers', *Journal of Criminal Law and Criminology* (1939) **29**:672–688.
Lewis Lawes, *Meet the Murderer*, New York: Harper and Brothers, 1940.
I. A. Bery and Vernon Fox, 'Factors in Homicides Committed by 200 Males', *Journal of Social Psychology* (1947) **26**:109–119.
Hans von Hentig, *The Criminal and His Victim*, New Haven, Conn.: Yale University Press, 1948.

Harold Garfinkel, 'Research Note on Inter- and Intra-Racial Homicides', *Social Forces* (1949) 27:369–381.

Howard Harlan, 'Five Hundred Homicides', *Journal of Criminal Law and Criminology* (1950) 40:736–752.

Viscount Templewood, *The Shadow of the Gallows*, London: Victor Gollancz, 1951.

Austin L. Porterfield, 'Indices of Suicide and Homicide by States and Cities: Some Southern-Non-Southern Contrasts with Implications for Research', *American Sociological Review* (1952) 57:331–338

Henry Allen Bullock, 'Urban Homicide in Theory and Fact', *Journal of Criminal Law, Criminology and Police Science* (1955) 45:565–575.

Albert Morris, *Homicide: An Approach to the Problem of Crime*, Boston: University Press, 1955.

John Macdonald, *The Murderer and His Victim*, Springfield, Ill.: Charles C. Thomas, 1961.

John M. Macdonald, 'The Threat to Kill', *American Journal of Psychiatry* (1963) 120:125–130.

37. For an especially keen and concise analysis of some theories abou homicides, see Frank E. Hartung, *Crime, Law and Society*, Detroit: Wayne State University Press, 1965; see especially pp. 136–153 and the footnote references to this section. It should be noted that Hartung accepts the validity of the concept of a subculture of violence (*ibid.*, p. 147).

That many of the social variables found to be associated with homicide are also characteristic of the offense, offenders, and victims of other assaultive crimes may be confirmed in Richard A. Peterson, David J. Pittman, Patricia O'Neal, 'Stabilities in Deviance: A Study of Assaultive and Non-Assaultive Offenders', *Journal of Criminal Law, Criminology and Police Science* (1962) 53:44–48; and in David Pittman and William Handy, 'Patterns in Aggravated Assault', *Journal of Criminal Law, Criminology and Police Science* (1964) 55:462–470.

Pittman and Handy conclude: 'This comparison of findings concerning acts of homicide and aggravated assault indicates that the pattern for the two crimes is quite similar. Both acts, of course, are reflections of population subgroupings which tend to externalize their aggression when confronted with conflict situations' (*ibid.*, p. 470).

38. See *supra*, Chapter IV, note 212.

39. An effort was made to deal with this problem analytically in Marvin E. Wolfgang and Rolf Strohm, 'The Relationship between Alcohol and Criminal Homicide', *Quarterly Journal of Studies on Alcohol* (1956) 17:411–425.

40. For interesting comparisons between homicide in Western studies and homicide in several African tribes, see Paul Bohannan (ed.),

African Homicide and Suicide, Princeton, New Jersey: Princeton University Press, 1960.

41. The literature on anomie is vast and it would serve little purpose to cite many references other than those already noted in earlier chapters. The most comprehensive review of the concept has recently appeared in Marshall Clinard (ed.), *Anomie and Deviant Behavior: A Discussion and Critique*, New York: The Free Press of Glencoe, 1964. Particularly useful is the Appendix, which provides an inventory of empirical and theoretical studies of anomie (*ibid.*, pp. 243–311). It is interesting to note that in a recent article, Jaffe suggested that 'both feelings of powerlessness and ambivalent parental identification result from a lack of *value consensus* among family members, and that these three variables taken together define family anomie' (Lester D. Jaffe, 'Delinquency Proneness and Family Anomie', *Journal of Criminal Law, Criminology and Police Science* (1963) 54:146–154, p. 154 cited and emphasis added).

42. But the meaning anomie conveys is at about the same level as 'existential vacuum', 'maladjustment', 'sick', and, unfortunately, 'juvenile delinquency'. Note, in this context, the similarity between the concept of anomie and the Adlerian concept of 'lack of social interest' (Heinz L. Ansbacher: 'Anomie, The Sociologist's Conception of Lack of Social Interest', *Journal of Individual Psychology* (1959) 15:2:212–214).

43. For an analysis of psychological studies of anomie, see Davol and Reimanis's article, cited above, p. 181.

44. The most comprehensive bibliography (259 items) with references to support this statement is still to be found in the 1960 General Report to the Second United Nations Congress on the Prevention of Crime and the Treatment of Offenders, by Wolf Middendorf, entitled *New Forms of Juvenile Delinquency: Their Origin, Prevention and Treatment*, New York: United Nations, Department of Economic and Social Affairs, A/CONF 17/6, 1960. See also the Secretariat document on the same subject: 'New Forms of Juvenile Delinquency: Their Origin, Prevention and Treatment', A/CONF. 17/7.

Other references of use for examining the problems of crime and delinquency in developing countries include the following:

Charles Abrams, 'City Planning and Housing Policy in Relation to Crime and Delinquency', *International Review of Criminal Policy* (1960) 16:23–28.

R. G. Andry, 'Juvenile Delinquency in Developing Countries', *International Annals of Criminology* (1964) Part 1:87–92.

Karl O. Christiansen, 'Industrialization and Urbanization in Relation to Crime and Delinquency', *International Review of Criminal Policy* (1960) 16:3–8.

Marshall Clinard, 'The Organization of Urban Community Development Services in the Prevention of Crime and Juvenile Delinquency, with Particular Reference to Less-Developed

Countries', *International Review of Criminal Policy* (1962)
19:3–12.
Abdellatif El Bacha, 'Quelques aspects particuliers de la délinquance
juvénile dans certaines villes du royaume du Maroc', *International Review of Criminal Policy* (1962) 20:11–26.
Manuel Lopez-Rey, 'Economic Conditions and Crime with Special
Reference to Less-Developed Countries', *International Annals of Criminology* (1964) Part 1:33–40.
Manuel Lopez-Rey, 'Preliminary Considerations on Formulation of
Policy for the Prevention of Juvenile Delinquency in Developing Countries', *International Annals of Criminology* (1964) Part 1:73–86.
A. K. Nazmul, 'Crime in East Pakistan Since 1947', *International Review of Criminal Policy* (1960) 16:47–53.
J. J. Panakal and A. Khalifa, *Prevention of Types of Criminality Resulting from Social Changes and Accompanying Economic Development in Less-Developed Countries*, New York: United Nations, Department of Economic and Social Affairs, A/CONF. 17/3, May, 1960. Also, the corresponding Secretariat paper with the same title: A/CONF. 17/4.
Evelyne Pierre, J.-P. Flamand, and H. Collomb, 'La délinquance
juvénile à Dakar', *International Review of Criminal Policy* (1962) 20:27–34.
Paul Raymaekers, 'Prédélinquance et délinquance juvénile à Léo-
poldville', *International Review of Criminal Policy* (1962) 20:49–57.
S. P. Tschoungui and Pierre Zumbach, 'Diagnostic de la délinquance
juvénile au Cameroun', *International Review of Criminal Policy* (1962) 20:35–47.
United Nations Secretariat, 'Quelques considérations sur la pré-
vention de la délinquance juvénile dans les pays africains subissant des changements sociaux rapides', *International Review of Criminal Policy* (1960) 16:43–44.
Herman J. Venter, 'Urbanization and Industrialization as Crimino-
genic Factors in the Republic of South Africa', *International Review of Criminal Policy* (1962) 20:59–71.
Kirson S. Weinberg, 'Juvenile Delinquency in Ghana: A Compara-
tive Analysis of Delinquents and Non-Delinquents', *Journal of Criminal Law, Criminology and Police Science* (1964) 55:471–481.
This topic has again been discussed particularly in relation to
social change, at the Third United Nations Congress on the Prevention of Crime and Treatment of Offenders, held in Stockholm in 1965. Only the Secretariat paper is, however, available so far: 'Social Change and Criminality', A/CONF. 26/1.

45. Especially:

Shlomo Shoham, 'The Application of the "Culture-Conflict" Hypothesis to the Criminality of Immigrants to Israel', *Journal of*

Criminal Law, Criminology and Police Science (1962) **53**:207–214.

C. H. S. Jayewardene, 'Criminal Homicide. A Study in Culture Conflict', Ph.D. Thesis, University of Pennsylvania, 1960.

C. H. S. Jayewardene, 'Criminal Culture and Subcultures', *Probation and Child Care Journal* (1963) **2**:1–5.

C. H. S. Jayewardene, 'New Forms of Crime and Delinquency', *Probation and Child Care Journal* (1963) **2**:9–16.

Amilijoes Sa'danoer, 'Crime and Delinquency in Developing Countries', (April 1965), mineographed report.

46. For an excellent and comprehensive discussion of this problem as it existed for several years in Kenya, see F. D. Corfield, *Historical Survey of the Origins and Growth of Mau Mau*, London: H.M. Stationery Office, 1960.

47. W. I. Thomas and Florian Znaniecki, *The Polish Peasant in Europe and America*, 2 Volumes, 2nd Revised Edition, New York: Dover Publications, 1958.

48. James L. Sleeman, *Thug, or a Million Murders*, London: Sampson Low, Marston, 1933.

   We acknowledge reliance upon material cited by R. H. Ahrenfeldt and T. C. N. Gibbens in the working paper 'Cultural Aspects of Delinquency, Preliminary Report' for a conference on 'Cultural Factors in Delinquency', held by the World Federation for Mental Health at the Menninger Clinic, Topeka, Kansas, September 8–17, 1964. The proceedings and the reports of the conference have been published in the volume *Cultural Factors in Delinquency*, edited by T. C. N. Gibbens and R. H. Ahrenfeldt, London: Tavistock Publications; Philadelphia: Lippincott, 1966.

49. D. S. Margoliouth, 'Assassins', *Encyclopedia of Religion and Ethics*, 1909, **11**:138–141.

50. Z. Hurston, *Voodoo Gods: An Inquiry into Native Myths and Magic in Jamaica and Haiti*, London: 1939.

51. V. Bujan, 'Decrease of Vendetta in the Macedonia People's Republic', Paper presented at the 5th Congress of the International Academy of Legal and Social Medicine, Vienna, May, 1961. (Cited by *Excerpta Criminologica*, 1961, Volume 1, No. 3, abstract 553.)

52. J. D. Bourchier, 'Albania', *Encyclopaedia Britannica*, 11th edition, 1910, **1**:484. 'In all parts of Albania,' Bourchier wrote, 'the vendetta . . . is an established usage; the duty of revenge is a sacred tradition handed down to successive generations in the family, the village and the tribe. . . . It is estimated that in consequence of these feuds scarcely 75% of the population in certain mountainous districts die a natural death' (*ibid.*).

53. W. Clifford, 'Delinquency in Cyprus', *British Journal of Delinquency* (1954) **5**:146–150. 'Throughout the years,' says Clifford, 'crimes of honour and those connected with family vendettas have been a

feature of Cyprus life. There is some improvement today, but up to recent times there have been so-called "criminal" villages not only steeped in personal feuds and the concomitant violence, but also places where assassins could be hired. These murders were almost always connected with family disputes and dishonour by seduction. In such villages the inhabitants do not go out alone at night and they take elaborate precautions against attack through open doors or windows' (*ibid.*).

54. There are many books, articles, and official government reports on the Mafia in Sicily. We believe the following are recent, dependable, and valid summary descriptions of the development and present stage of the Mafia: G. G. Loschiavo, 'La Mafia Siciliana', *Notiziario per l'Arma dei CC.*, 1955; Giovanni Schiavo, *The Truth About the Mafia and Organized Crime in America*, New York: Vigo Press, 1962; Norman Lewis, 'The Honored Society', *The New Yorker* (February 8, 15, 22, 1964); *The Honored Society*, New York: Putnam, 1964.

55. This hypothesis was suggested by Wolfgang in *Patterns in Criminal Homicide*, pp. 116–119, 321, 332–333. In a study using data on homicide and health services in Ceylon, England, and Finland, Jayewardene questioned that improvement in the medical standards of a country is a valid factor in the reduction of homicides. (C. H. S. Jayewardene, 'L'influenza del progresso medico sull'andamento statistico degli omicidi', *Quaderni di Criminologia Clinica* (1961) 2:165–180.)

More research is obviously needed, for no study has thus far gone to primary sources of data for examination of direct connections between police reports of assaults and the techniques of medical practice or therapy in treating the wounds.

56. The literature on the Colombian violence is extensive but not easy to locate outside the country. The data presented in these pages have been collected by one of the authors during a UNICEF mission to Colombia concerned with the planning of institutional care for children orphaned by the *violencia*. Only the main sources of information are listed below, in order of importance and completeness. Two major volumes on the *violencia* have been published only recently: German Guzman Campos, Orlando Fals Borda, and Eduardo Umaña Luna, *La Violencia en Colombia, Estudio de un Proceso Social, Tomo Primo*, 2nd Edition, Bogotá: Ediciones Tercer Mundo, 1962; German Guzman Campos, Orlando Fals Borda, and Eduardo Umaña Luna, *La Violencia en Colombia. Estudio de un Proceso Social, Segundo Tomo*, Bogotá: Ediciones Tercer Mundo, 1964. The first volume caused a major public opinion reaction both inside and outside of Colombia. The volume was acclaimed as a major exposé but was also sharply criticized. One detailed critical analysis was published by Miguel Angel Gonzalez, S. J.: 'La Violencia en Colombia. Analisis de un libro', *Revista Javeriana* (September, 1962) Volume 288.

Other sources include the following:

Eduardo Franco Isaga, *Las guerrillas del llano*, Bogotá: Libreria Mundial, 1959.
Jorge Enrique Gutierrez Anzola, *Violencia y Justicia*, Bogotá: Ediciones Tercer Mundo, 1962.
Primer Seminario sobre la Educacion en las Zonas de Violencia, Ministerio de Educacion Nacional, Gobernacion del Depto de Tolima, Universidad de Tolima, April 26–27–28 de 1963.
Segundo Seminario sobre la Educacion en las Zonas de Violencia, Ministerio de Educacion Nacional, Gobernacion del Valle del Cauca, Universidad del Valle, Universidad Santiago de Cali, Santiago de Cali, June 26–27–28, 1963.
Belisario Betancur, *Colombia cara a cara* (Chapter IV, 'Las caras de la Violencia'), Bogotá: Ediciones Tercer Mundo, 1961.
Camilo Torres Restrepo, *La violencia y los cambios socio-culturales en las areas rurales colombianas*, in Associacion Colombiana de Sociologia, Memoria del Primer Congreso Nacional de Sociologia, Bogotá: Ediciones Iqueiura, 1963, pp. 95–152.
Enrique Benalcazar Saavedra and Gilberto Martinez Rave, *Violencia Politica en Colombia*, Proceedings of the 12th International Course in Criminology, *The Causation and Prevention of Crime in Developing Countries*, 1963, 2:Part 2, Jerusalem, 358–370.

57. Theodore Caplow, 'La violencia', *Columbia University Forum* (1963) Winter, 45–46.
58. These and the following data have been collected from official Colombian sources.
59. Guzman Campos, Fals Borda, and Umaña Luna, Volume I, discusses in detail the phenomenology of homicide and the folklore and language correlates of the *violencia*. A relatively large novelistic literature has emerged and has been analyzed by the three authors. The most effective and powerful novel, now a collector's item, is probably Daniel Caicedo, *Viento Seco*, Buenos Aires: Editorial Nuestra America, 1954, 3rd Edition. In the opinion of informed observers, this last book contains a dramatic and realistic description of the early phases of the *violencia* in the Cali area.
60. Aaron Lipman and A. Eugene Havens, *Effects of the Colombian Violence on Personality: An Ex Post Facto Experiment*, unpublished manuscript.
61. Orlando Fals Borda, in the two volumes quoted above, co-authored with German Guzman Campos and Eduardo Umaña Luna, offers a tentative structural-functional interpretation of the *violencia* phenomenon.
62. Camilo Torres Restrepo, *op. cit.*
63. Eduardo Umaña Luna has analyzed the legal structure of the violencia legislation in the second volume of Guzman Campos, Fals Borda, Umaña Luna, *La Violencia en Colombia*.
64. Antonio Pigliaru, *La vendetta barbaricina come ordinamento giuridico*,

Milano: Giuffrè, 1959. Pigliaru has 'codified' the norms of the *vendetta barbaricina* and has analyzed in detail their meaning and their procedural application. Two 'articles' from his codified norms are presented here to illustrate their subcultural value (pp. 107–108): Art. 1: 'The offense *must* be avenged. The man who does not perform the duty of the vendetta has no honor, unless throughout his life he has proved his virility and gives up the vendetta for a superior moral reason' (*L'offesa deve* essere vendicata. Non è uomo d'onore chi si sottrae al dovere della vendetta, salvo nel caso che, avendo dato, con il complesso della sua vita, prova della propria virilità, vi rinunci per un superiore motivo morale).

Art. 2: 'The law of the vendetta binds all those who for any reason live and operate within the community' (La legge della vendetta obbliga tutti coloro che, ad un qualsivoglia titolo, vivano ed operino nell'ambito della comunitá).

These two 'laws' express the binding, inescapable, social expectation to exact violent revenge, and the power of the dominating values to impose their own fulfillment. The code is very detailed, although remaining structurally simple. As another example, the theft of a goat is not an 'offense', unless the goat's milk is used by the family or there is a clear intent to 'offend' or spite the victim (pp. 116–117). In this case the revenge is progressively more serious, up to death. Death, in any case, as an offense or as a revenge, constitutes a new offense, punishable by death, and has no 'statute of limitations' (p. 120).

65. Jorge M. Velasco Alzaga, 'Epidemiology of Homicide in Mexico, D.F.' (English translation by M. H. C. Manjarrez), Photocopy Report, n.d.
66. *Ibid.*, p. 5.
67. *Ibid.*, p. 6.
68. *Ibid.*
69. Anselmo Crisafulli and Benigno Di Tullio, *Aspetti della criminalità militare nel settore albanese*, Tirana: Tipografia Militare, 1942.
70. Giulio Frisoli, 'La pistola regalo di battesimo', *Epoca* (February 21, 1965), pp. 102–105; Giulio Frisoli and Pietro Zullino, 'Il segreto di Albanova', *Epoca* (March 7, 1965) pp. 34–38.
71. Giulio Frisoli, *op. cit.*
72. Giulio Frisoli and Pietro Zullino, *op. cit.*
73. Paul Friedrich, 'El homicidio politico en Acan', *Revista de Ciencias Sociales* (1964) 8:1:27–51.
74. See J. J. Panakal and V. B. Punekar, 'Challenge to Society. A Study of the De-Notified Communities, Ex-Criminal Tribes', in press, 1965.
75. Paul Bohannan (ed.), *African Homicide and Suicide*, Princeton, New Jersey: Princeton University Press, 1960.
76. J. H. Straus and M. A. Straus, 'Suicide, Homicide and Social Structure in Ceylon', *American Journal of Sociology* (1953) 58:461–469.

77. Arthur L. Wood, *Crime and Aggression in Changing Ceylon*, Transactions of the American Philosophical Society, New Series, Vol. 51, Part 8, December 1961, 'A Socio Structural Analysis of Murder, Suicide, and Economic Crime in Ceylon', *American Sociological Review* (1961) 26:744–753.

78. C. H. S. Jayewardene, 'Criminal Homicide. A Study in Culture Conflict', Ph.D. Thesis, University of Pennsylvania, 1960.

C. H. S. Jayewardene, 'Criminal Culture and Subcultures', *Probation and Child Care Journal* (1963) 2:1–15.

C. H. S. Jayewardene, 'Criminal Homicide in Ceylon', *Ibid.* (1964) 3:15–30.

C. H. S. Jayewardene and H. Ranasinghe, *Criminal Homicide in the Southern Province*, Colombo: The Colombo Apothecaries Co., 1963.

C. H. S. Jayewardene, 'Murder and Sexual Assault of an Old Woman', *Zacchia* (1963) 26:1–8.

79. There are many anthropological references to murder and homicide generally, but without detailed study it is difficult to determine whether any preliterate or even literate group can be said to contain a subculture of violence. For a useful anthropological bibliography, see E. Adamson Hoebel, *The Law of Primitive Man*, Cambridge, Mass.: Harvard University Press, 1954.

Some other relevant homicide references available to the authors and which suggested but did not clearly indicate subcultures of violence include:

M. Pamir, 'Psicopatici nelle Indie Neederlandesi. Loro importanza forense (l'assassinio Atjese e l'amok)', *Archivio di Antropologia Criminale* (1936) 56:571–579.

A. B. Saran, 'Murder among the Munda: A Case Study', *Indian Journal of Social Work*, n.d.

Verrier Elwin, *Maria Murder and Suicide*, London: Oxford University Press, 1943.

H. Lieberz-Wygodzinski, 'Zur Soziopsychologie des Mordes in Chile', *Monatsschrift fur Kriminologie und Strafrechtsreform* (1957) 40:163–175.

M. Mala, 'Problems of Women Offenders of Nari Bandi Niketan, Lucknow', *Journal of Correctional Work* (1960) 7:85–91.

Klaus Lithner, 'Garofalo and Violent Crimes on the Island of Aspo', *Nord. T. Kriminalvidensk* (1961) 49:172–173.

Robert J. Smith, 'The Japanese Rural Community: Norms, Sanctions and Ostracism', *American Anthropologist* (1961) 63:522–533.

D. F. Henderson, 'Settlement of Homicide Disputes in Sakya (Tibet)', *American Anthropologist* (1964) 66:1099–1105.

80. C. H. S. Jayewardene, 'Criminal Cultures and Subcultures', *op. cit.*, p. 30.

81. Alan Little, 'The Increase in Crime 1952–62: An Empirical Analysis of Adolescent Offenders', *British Journal of Criminology* (1965) 5:77–82.
82. Daniel Glaser, Donald Kenefick, and Vincent O'Leary, *The Violent Offender*, Washington, D.C.: U.S. Department of Health, Education and Welfare, 1966, p. 35.
83. *Ibid.*, p. 36.
84. See Paul E. Meehl and Albert Rosen, 'Antecedent Probability and the Efficiency of Psychometric Signs, Patterns or Cutting Scores', *Psychological Bulletin* (May, 1955) 52:3:194–216.
85. See, for example, Hans Eysenck, 'The Effects of Psychotherapy', *International Journal of Psychiatry* (January, 1965) 1:97–144.
86. Robert Coles, 'American Amok', *The New Republic* (August 27, 1966) 155:8:12–15, p. 14 cited.
87. See especially Leslie T. Wilkins on this point, in *Social Deviance*, London: Tavistock Publications, 1964; Englewood Cliffs, N.J.: Prentice-Hall.
88. Gene A. Brucker, *Florentine Politics and Society, 1343–1378*, Princeton, N.J.: Princeton University Press, 1962.
89. See, for example, Sellin and Wolfgang, *The Measurement of Delinquency*, Chapters 11 and 12.
90. Coles, *op. cit.*, p. 14.
91. The Philadelphia Police Department embarked on such a predictions model in July, 1966, under support from the Law Enforcement Assistance Act.
92. W. F. Greenhalgh, 'A Town's Rate of Serious Crime Against Property and Its Association with Some Broad Social Factors', *Home Office Report*, London, England, February, 1964; W. F. Greenhalgh, 'Police Correlation Analysis: An Interim Report', *Home Office Report*, London, England, August, 1964.
93. Robert H. Roy, 'An Outline for Research in Penology', *Operations Research* (January–February, 1964) 12:1–15.
94. Sellin and Wolfgang, *The Measurement of Delinquency*, 1964.
95. *A Study of Prevention and Control of Crime and Delinquency*, Final Report PCCD-7, prepared by the Space-General Corporation, El Monte, California, for the Youth and Adult Corrections Agency of California, July 29, 1965.
96. Robert P. Shumate and Richard F. Crowther, 'Quantitative Methods for Optimizing the Allocation of Police Resources', *Journal of Criminal Law, Criminology and Police Science* (1966) 57:197–206.
97. Marvin E. Wolfgang and Harvey A. Smith, 'Mathematical Methods in Criminology', *International Social Science Journal*, forthcoming.
98. Wolfgang, *Patterns in Criminal Homicide*, 1958.
99. *Ibid.*, pp. 116–119. In a slightly revised and abstracted version, the remainder of the present section is taken from *ibid.*
100. See, for example, Warner F. Bowers, Frederick T. Marchant, and Kenneth H. Judy, 'The Present Story on Battle Casualties from

M

Korea', *Surgery, Gynecology, and Obstetrics* (November, 1951) 93:529–542.

Jayewardeno has added an interesting note on medical technology relative to homicide statistics in Ceylon. See C. H. S. Jayewardene, 'L'influenza del progresso medico nell'andamento statistico degli omicidi', *Quaderni di Criminologia Clinica* (1961) 2:162–180.

101. Abstracted in part from M. E. Wolfgang's paper on 'Urban Crime', for the U.S. Chamber of Commerce, September, 1966.

102. Donald R. Taft, 'Testing the Selective Influence of Areas of Delinquency', *American Journal of Sociology* (1933) 38:699–712.

103. See *supra* for more detailed discussion, and the monograph, *Crime and Race*, 1964, by M. E. Wolfgang.

104. Richard Cloward and Lloyd Ohlin, *Delinquency and Opportunity*, Chapter 8.

105. Peter McHugh, 'Social Requisites of Radical Individual Change', Paper presented at the Annual Meeting of the American Sociological Association, Montreal, Canada, August, 1964.

106. Lewis Yablonsky, *The Violent Gang*, New York: Macmillan, 1962.

107. Suggested to the authors by Victor Gioscia and Martin Timin.

108. *Uniform Crime Reports*, 1965, pp. 33–38.

109. See Wolfgang, *Patterns in Criminal Homicide*, p. 192.

110. Robert Ardrey, *The Territorial Imperative*, New York: Atheneum, 1966.

111. Loren Eiseley, in a review of *The Territorial Imperative*, *The New York Times Book Review*, September 11, 1966, pp. 6, 40.

112. The authors regret that they have not had the benefit of what appears to be an excellent volume by Marshall Clinard on development of indigenous leadership and community self-help programs, viewed cross-culturally. See the forthcoming publication of Marshall Clinard, *Slums and Community Development: Experiments in Self-Help*, New York: The Free Press, 1966.

113. Paul Eberts and Kent Schwirian, 'Crime Rates and Relative Deprivation', Paper presented at the Annual Meeting of the American Sociological Association, Miami, Florida, August 31, 1966.

114. Arnold W. Green, 'The Middle-Class Male Child and Neurosis', *American Sociological Review* (February, 1946) 11:31–41.

115. Walter B. Miller, 'Lower-Class Culture as a Generating Milieu of Gang Delinquency', *Journal of Social Issues* (1958) 14:5–19.

116. Herbert J. Gans, *The Urban Villagers*, New York: The Free Press of Glencoe, 1962.

117. Talcott Parsons, 'Certain Primary Sources and Patterns of Aggression in the Social Structure of the Western World', *Psychiatry* (May, 1947) 10:167–181.

118. Jackson Toby, 'Violence and the Masculine Ideal: Some Qualitative Data', in Marvin E. Wolfgang (ed.), *Patterns of Violence, The Annals of the American Academy of Political and Social Science* (March, 1966) 364:19–27.

119. *Ibid.*, pp. 21–22.

120. Melvin Tumin, 'The Functionalist Approach to Social Problems', *Social Problems* (1965) 12:379–388, pp. 386–387 cited.

121. For a brief discussion of these points regarding value-change during psychotherapy, see:

Ruth Ochroch, 'The Social Reality of the Delinquent', *Journal of Offender Therapy* (1963) 7:2:41–44.

Benjamin I. Coleman, 'Value Construction in the Treatment of the Offender', *Journal of Offender Therapy* (1964) 7:2:45–47.

Franco Ferracuti, 'Values in Criminal Psychotherapy', *Journal of Offender Therapy* (1963) 7:2:48–51, 56.

122. G. Devereaux, 'Cultural Factors in Psychoanalytic Therapy', *Journal of American Psychoanalytic Association* (1953) 1:624–655.

J. A. Kennedy, 'Problems Posed in the Analysis of Negro Patients', *Psychiatry* (1952) 15:313–327.

J. Ruesch, 'Social Factors in Therapy', *Research Publications, Association for Research in Nervous and Mental Diseases* (1951) 31:59–93.

H. A. Savitz, 'The Cultural Background of the Patient as Part of the Physician's Armamentarium', *Journal of Abnormal and Social Psychology* (1952) 47:245–254.

123. Albert Ellis, 'New Approaches to Psychotherapy Techniques', *Journal of Clinical Psychology*, Monographs Supplement (1965) 11.

124. J. A. Kennedy, *op. cit.*

125. California Department of Corrections, 'Final Report of the Task Force to Define Violence Potential in Inmates and Parolees', (mimeographed), June 17, 1963; John Conrad, 'The Nature and Treatment of the Violent Offender', Address delivered at the Youth Trainers Institute, December 6, 1963; Franklin H. Ernst and William C. Keating, 'Psychiatric Treatment of the California Felon', *American Journal of Psychiatry* (1964) 120:974–979.

126. Don Gibbons has recently classified and discussed these different types of treatment settings, although he presents no statistical assessment of treatment strategies. See Don C. Gibbons, *Changing the Lawbreaker*, Englewood Cliffs, New Jersey: Prentice-Hall, 1965.

127. Fritz Redl and David Wineman, *The Aggressive Child*, Glencoe, Ill.: The Free Press, 1963 (a one-volume edition of *Children Who Hate* and *Controls from Within*).

128. For a discussion of this point see: Ross Stagner, *The Psychology of Human Conflict*, Chapter 3 in Elton B. McNeil (ed.), *The Nature of Human Conflict*, Englewood Cliffs, N.J.: Prentice-Hall, 1965, pp. 60–61. A similar approach has been proposed by Charles E. Osgood (cited by Stagner, *op. cit.*, p. 61).

129. Conditioning therapies have been proposed for a variety of conditions and are enjoying a relatively wide popularity. From the vast list of sources on these techniques (which can broadly be divided into two groups, the Skinnerian instrumental conditioning approach and the

Wolpe-Eysenck classical conditioning approach based on Hull's learning theory) we have selected those that appear to be most relevant to the treatment of offenders·

H. J. Eysenck (ed.), *Behavior Therapy and the Neuroses*, New York: Pergamon Press, 1960.

Albert Bandura, 'Psychotherapy as a Learning Process', *Psychological Bulletin* (1961) **58**:143–159.

W. K. Boardman, 'Rusty: A Brief Behavior Disorder', *Journal of Consulting Psychology* (1962) **26**:4:293–297.

H. J. Eysenck, 'Behavior Therapy, Extinction and Relapse in Neurosis', *British Journal of Psychiatry* (1963) **109**:12–18.

Joseph Wolpe, Andrew Salter, and Leo J. Reyna, *The Conditioning Therapies: The Challenge in Psychotherapy*, New York: Holt, Rinehart & Winston, 1964.

J. M. Grassberg, 'Behavior Therapy: A Review', *Psychological Bulletin* (1964) **62**:2:73–88.

John D. Burchard and Vernon O. Tyler, *The Modification of Delinquent Behavior through Operant Conditioning*, American Psychological Association Meeting, Los Angeles, California, September, 1964, mimeographed copy.

H. J. Eysenck, 'The Effects of Psychotherapy', *International Journal of Psychiatry* (1965) **1**:97–144.

This last article, critical of most psychotherapy, is followed by discussions from fourteen scholars, pp. 144–178. It should be stated that conditioning therapies are still in an experimental stage and that it would be inadvisable to foster excessive expectations concerning their validity and their future development and acceptance. L. Breger has recently published (*Journal of Projective Techniques and Personality Assessment* (1965) **29**:2:252–255) a detailed and careful critique of this therapeutic approach as a review of the Wolpe, Salter, and Reyna book quoted above.

For a detailed discussion of the social-learning approach to treatment and prevention see: Albert Bandura and Richard H. Walters, *Social Learning and Personality Development*, New York: Holt, Rinehart, and Winston, 1964. Also A. Bandura and A. C. Huston, 'Identification as a Process of Incidental Learning', *Journal of Abnormal and Social Psychology* (1961) **63**:311–318; A. Bandura, *Social Learning through Imitation*, Symposium on Motivation, 1962, Lincoln, Nebraska: University of Nebraska Press, 1962.

130. Albert Bandura and Richard H. Walters, *Social Learning and Personality Development*, New York: Holt, Rinehart and Winston, 1964.

131. A recent analysis, based on experimental data of the ineffectiveness of punishment in achieving any permanent change of undesirable behavior has been presented by James B. Appel: 'The Control of Behavior by Punishment', mimeographed copy, American Association for the Advancement of Science, American Society of Criminology

meeting, Cleveland, 1963. On the other hand, unusual and punitive correctional practices are at times proposed again. For an extreme example, see Peter McK. Middleton: 'Motor Deprivation or Paralysed Awareness in the Treatment of Delinquency', mimeographed copy, paper presented at the First International Congress of Social Psychiatry, London, August, 1964.

132. Robert Jay Lifton, *Thought Reform and the Psychology of Totalism*, New York: W. W. Norton, 1961; Albert D. Biderman and Herbert Zimmer (eds.), *The Manipulation of Human Behavior*, New York: 1961.

133. Franco Ferracuti and Marvin E. Wolfgang, 'Design for a Proposed Study of Violence: A Socio-Psychological Study of a Subculture of Violence', *British Journal of Criminology* (1963) 3:377–388.

134. Marvin E. Wolfgang, 'Statistical Evaluation of Treatment Programs', Section 3, General Report presented at the Fifth Congress of the International Society of Criminology, Montreal, Canada, August 29–September 3, 1965. For another paper stressing the value of setting up mathematical models in correctional research, see Robert H. Roy, 'An Outline for Research in Penology', *Operations Research* (January–February, 1964) 12:1:1–12.

Index of Names
Analytical Index

Index of Names

Analytical Index

acceptance of leadership regardless of discipline origin, 11
common language or terminology, 11
free information communication and exchange, 11
individual methods subordinated to project aims, 12
members selected for ability in project area, 11
minimum influence from outside the research team, 12
problem-centered activity, 11
reciprocal teaching and learning, 11
results published by group rather than individual members, 12
role flexibility, 11
sharing of suggestions, ideas, data, 11
total participation of members in joint planning, 11
Group homicide (*massen Mord*), 202, 238, 289
Groups
study of
conformity, commitment, and deviance in, 25, 112–113, 120–121
delinquent, 27, 28, 33, 43, 52, 97–98, 115
group culture concept, 102–104
individual's interaction with, 52–53, 97–98, 101–102, 120–121
norms and counter-norms, 101–102, 106–107
small, 52, 120–121
social class, 97–98
subcultural, 97–98, 101–102, 102–104, 106–107, 109, 114–115, 120–121
therapy, 43, 288, 311–312
role theory, 120–121
values and value systems of,

97–98, 101–102, 106–107, 109, 114, 115, 120–121
See also Group functioning, Subcultures, Delinquency, Subculture-of-violence theory
Guilt, 161

Haiti, 'Sect Rouge' subculture of violence, 272
Hand Test, description of and use in homicide studies, 218, 256
Harvard University, 130
'Hierarchy index', 116, 123–124
Hingoras (India), criminal tribe, 283
History, xiv, 19, 20–21, 23–24, 25, 272
criminology and, 19, 20–21, 23–24, 25, 272
criminology compared, 23–24
Holland, *see* Netherlands
Homicide, criminal
anthropology and, 192–193, 195–196
biological study of
alcoholic intoxication and alcoholism, 190, 206, 214, 251–252, 265
frustration–aggression hypothesis, xvii, 98, 140, 143–146, 147–150, 154–155, 208, 209, 218, 226
innate-instinct versus learned-response theory of aggression, 140, 141–142, 192–194, 210–211
somatotypes, 23, 41, 142, 173–174, 195
weather, 191
classification of, 140–141, 187–191, 207–208, 209, 223–224, 262–263, 269, 320
criteria for typologies, 189–191, 203–204
'normal' passionate, 140–141, 189–190, 190–191, 209, 269, 320

For Product Safety Concerns and Information please contact our EU
representative GPSR@taylorandfrancis.com Taylor & Francis Verlag GmbH,
Kaufingerstraße 24, 80331 München, Germany

Printed and bound by CPI Group (UK) Ltd, Croydon, CR0 4YY
01/05/2025
01858543-0001